# AQA

# PE

# for AS

# AQA PE for AS

Graham Thompson
Nesta Wiggins-James
Rob James

DYNAMIC LEARNING
Innovate • Motivate • Personalise
CD-ROM INSIDE

HODDER EDUCATION
A PART OF HACHETTE LIVRE UK

Orders: please contact Bookpoint Ltd, 130 Milton Park, Abingdon, Oxon OX14 4SB.
Telephone: (44) 01235 827720. Fax: (44) 01235 400454. Lines are open from 9.00am – 5.00pm,
Monday to Saturday, with a 24-hour message-answering service. You can also order
through our website www.hoddereducation.co.uk

If you have any comments to make about this, or any of our other titles, please send them
to educationenquiries@hodder.co.uk

*British Library Cataloguing in Publication Data*
A catalogue record for this title is available from the British Library

ISBN: 978 0 340 95905 3

First Edition Published 2008
Impression number 10 9 8 7 6 5 4 3 2 1
Year 2013 2012 2011 2010 2009 2008



Cover photo from Getty Images: (photographer: Scott Thomas)
Typeset by Pantek Arts Ltd, Maidstone, Kent
Printed in Italy for Hodder Education, part of Hachette Livre UK, 338 Euston Road,
London NW1 3BH.

# Contents

# Acknowledgements

**Graham Thompson** would like to thank his friends and family for their support, understanding and patience during the writing of this book.

**Rob James** and **Nesta Wiggins-James** would like to thank Ffion, Ellie, Rees and Cai for putting up with them while they completed the writing of this book.

The publishers would like to thank the following for permission to reproduce their images:

| | |
|---|---|
| 1.1 (a) | Jack Sullivan/Alamy |
| 1.1 (b) | JUPITERIMAGES/PIXLAND/Alamy |
| 1.3 | Neil Tingle/Action Plus |
| 1.5 | Neil Tingle/Action Plus |
| 1.6 | Richard Francis/Action Plus |
| 1.7 | Neil Tingle/Action Plus |
| 1.11 | James Leynse/Corbis |
| 1.12 | Source: The Eatwell Plate, Food Standards Agency © Crown copyright material is reproduced with the permission of the Controller of HMSO and Queen's Printer for Scotland |
| 1.13 | PHOTOTAKE Inc/Alamy |
| 1.14 | Glyn Kirk/Action Plus |
| 2.1 | Helene Rogers/Alamy |
| 2.2 | Richard Wareham Fotografie/Alamy |
| 2.4 | Steve Allen/Brand X/Corbis |
| 2.6 | Neil Tingle/Action Plus |
| 2.8 | Corbis Premium RF/Alamy |
| 2.9 | Neil Tingle/Action Plus |
| 2.13 | Topfoto/Image Works |
| 3.3 | News/DPPI/Action Plus |
| 3.4 | Stefan Matzke/NewSport/Corbis |
| 3.9 | Bob Sacha/Corbis |
| 3.10 | Glyn Kirk/Action Plus |
| 4.8 | Richard Saker/Allsport/Getty Images |
| 4.10 (a) | Neil Tingle/Action Plus |
| 4.10 (b) | Neil Tingle/Action Plus |
| 4.10 (c) | Glyn Kirk/Action Plus |
| 4.14 | Tim de Waele/Corbis |
| 4.16 | Glyn Kirk/Action Plus |
| 4.12 | Photodisc |
| 4.22 (c) | Mark Nolan/Getty Images |
| 4.22 (d) | Glyn Kirk/Action Plus |
| 4.23 | Ahmad Yusni/AFP/Getty Images |
| 4.27 | Steve Bardens/Action Plus |
| 5.8 | Neil Tingle/Action Plus |
| 5.10 | Glyn Kirk/Action Plus |
| 5.11 | Glyn Kirk/Action Plus |
| 5.12 | Chris Barry/Action Plus |
| 5.13 | George Tiedemann/GT Images/Corbis |
| 5.16 | Adam Pretty/Getty Images |
| 5.19 (b) | Glyn Kirk/Action Plus |
| 5.20 | Bradley Kanaris/Getty Images |
| 5.21 (a) & (b) | Neil Tingle/Action Plus |
| 5.22 (a) & (b) | Glyn Kirk/Action Plus |
| 5.23 (a) & (b) | Neil Tingle/Action Plus |
| 5.24 (a) & (b) | David J. Phillip/AP/PA Photos |
| 6.1 | Franck Faugere/DPPI/Action Plus |
| 6.2 | Darren Hauck/epa/Corbis |
| 6.3 | Glyn Kirk/Action Plus |
| 6.4 (a) | Action Plus |
| 6.4 (b) | Icon/Action Plus |
| 6.5 | Neil Tingle/Action Plus |
| 6.6 | Steve Bardens/Action Plus |
| 6.7 | Glyn Kirk/Action Plus |
| 6.8 | Mark Thompson /Allsport/Getty Imagex |
| 6.9 | Franck Faugere/DPPI/Action Plus |
| 6.10 | Neil Tingle/Action Plus |
| 6.11 | Paul Williams/Action Plus |
| 7.4 | Matthew Clarke/Action Plus |
| 7.8 (a) & (b) | Neil Tingle/Action Plus |
| 7.8 (c) | Image Source/Corbis |
| 7.12 | Neil Tingle/Action Plus |
| 7.19 | Robert Laberge/Getty Images |
| 8.2 | Glyn Kirk/Action Plus |
| 8.3 | Matthew Impey/Action Plus |

| | |
|---|---|
| 8.4 | Glyn Kirk/Action Plus |
| 8.13 | Glyn Kirk/Action Plus |
| 8.14 | Neil Tingle/Action Plus |
| 8.16 (a) | Laurie Strachan/Alamy |
| 8.16 (b)&(c) | Neil Tingle/Action Plus |
| 8.16 (d) | Glyn Kirk/Action Plus |
| 8.17 (a) | MAKKU ULANDER/Rex Features |
| 8.17 (b) | China Photos/Getty Images |
| 9.3 | Glyn Kirk/Action Plus |
| 9.9 | Richard Francis/Action Plus |
| 9.12 | Neil Tingle/Action Plus |
| 10.2 | Chris Brown/Action Plus |
| 13.3 | Corbis Super RF/Alamy |
| 13.4 | Glyn Kirk/Action Plus |
| 13.5 | David Sacks/Stone/Getty Images |
| 13.6 (a) | Neil Tingle/Action Plus |
| 13.6 (b) | © Daniel Garcia/AFP/Getty Images |
| 13.6 (c) | © Mark Ralston/AFP/Getty Images |
| 14.1 | Action Plus |
| 14.5 | Action Plus |
| 14.6 | www.gerardbrown.co.uk /Alamy |
| 14.9 | Bongarts/Getty Images |
| 14.10 | Mike King/Action Plus |
| 14.11 | Sean Aidan; Eye Ubiquitous/Corbis |
| 14.12 | Marcus Mok /Getty Images |
| 14.14 | Neil Tingle/Action Plus |
| 14.15 | JUPITERIMAGES/BananaStock/Alamy |
| 14.16 | LLUIS GENE/AFP/Getty Images |
| 14.17 | Glyn Kirk/Action Plus |
| 14.19 | Reuters/Corbis |
| 14.20 | Pete Saloutos/Corbis |
| 14.21 | JUPITERIMAGES/BananaStock/Alamy |
| 14.22 | China Photos/Getty Images |

# What does 'the expert choice' mean for you?

**We work with more examiners and experts than any other publisher**

- Because we work with more experts and examiners than any other publisher, the very latest curriculum requirements are built into this course and there is a perfect match between your course and the resources that you need to succeed. We make it easier for you to gain the skills and knowledge that you need for the best results.
- We have chosen the best team of experts – including the people who mark the exams – to give you the very best chance of success. Look out for their advice throughout this book – this is content that you can trust.

# Welcome to Dynamic Learning

Dynamic Learning is a simple and powerful way of integrating this text with digital resources to help you succeed, by bringing learning to life. Whatever your learning style, Dynamic Learning will help boost your understanding. And our Dynamic Learning content is updated online so your book will never be out of date.

- Searchable glossary to locate and explain complex anatomical and physiological terminology
- Easy access to the book's key photographs, charts and diagrams so that you can use them in your studies

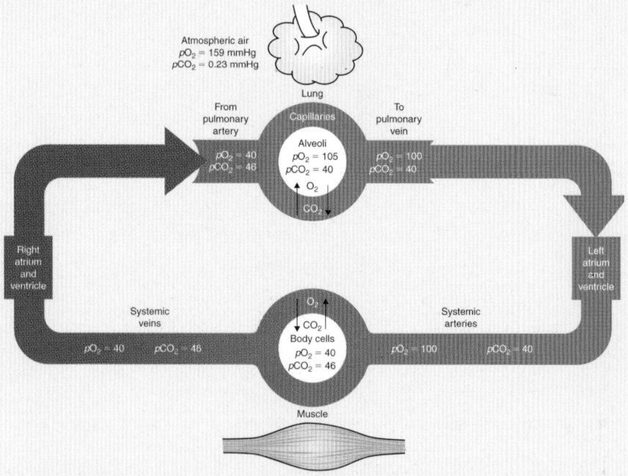


- Boost your understanding through interactive activities, quizzes and from support in additional Word and PowerPoint files

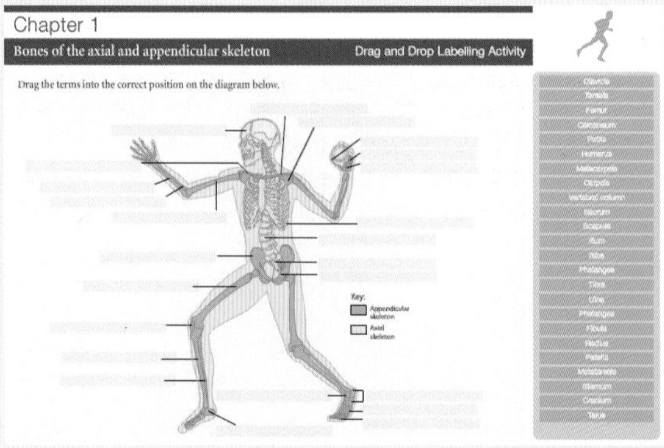

**More direct contact with teachers and students than any other publisher**

- We talk with more than 100 000 students every year through our student conferences, run by Philip Allan Updates. We hear at first hand what you need to make a success of your A-level studies and build what we learn into every new course. Learn more about our conferences at **www.philipallan.co.uk**
- Our new materials are trialled in classrooms as we develop them, and the feedback built into every new book or resource that we publish. You can be part of that. If you have comments that you would like to make about this book, please email us at: **feedback@hodder.co.uk**

**More collaboration with Subject Associations than any other publisher**

- Subject Associations sit at the heart of education. We work closely with more Associations than any other publisher. This means that our resources support the most creative teaching and learning, using the skills of the best teachers in their field to create resources for you.

**More opportunities for your teachers to stay ahead than with any other publisher**

- Through our Philip Allan Updates Conferences, we offer teachers access to Continuing Professional Development. Our focused and practical conferences ensure that your teachers have access to the best presenters, teaching materials and training resources. Our presenters include experienced teachers, Chief and Principal Examiners, leading educationalists, authors and consultants. This course is built on all of this expertise.

- Easy-to-use PowerPoint presentations show you what each chapter is going to deliver for you, and help you to check your understanding once you have worked through the section

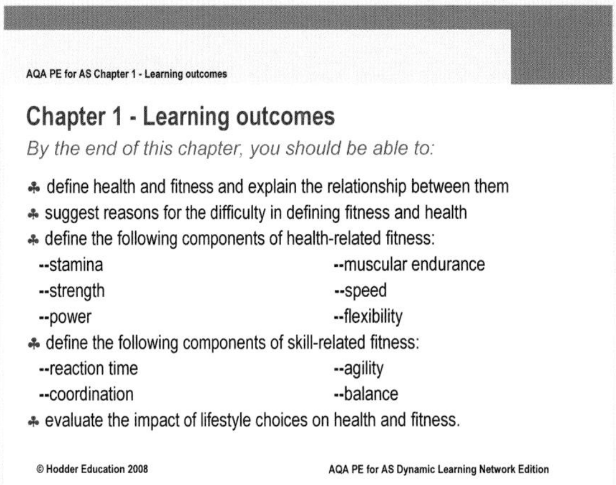

AQA PE for AS Chapter 1 - Learning outcomes
Chapter 1 - Learning outcomes
By the end of this chapter, you should be able to:
define health and fitness and explain the relationship between them
suggest reasons for the difficulty in defining fitness and health
define the following components of health-related fitness:
--stamina
--muscular endurance
--strength
--speed
--power
--flexibility
define the following components of skill-related fitness:
--reaction time
--agility
--coordination
--balance
evaluate the impact of lifestyle choices on health and fitness.
© Hodder Education 2008
AQA PE for AS Dynamic Learning Network Edition


To start up Dynamic Learning now, make sure that your computer has an active broadband connection to the internet and insert the disk into your CD ROM drive. Dynamic Learning should run automatically if you have 'Auto Run' enabled. Full installation instructions are printed on the disk label.

Basic system requirements for your Student Edition: **PC** Windows 2000 (SP4), XP SP2 (Home & Pro), Vista; **PC (Server)** Windows 2000 and 2003; **Mac** Mac OS X 10.3 or 10.4; G4, G5 or Intel processor. Dynamic Learning is not currently Leopard-compatible: see the website for latest details. Up to 1.4Gb hard disc space per title. Minimum screen resolution 1024 x 768. Sound card. A fast processor (PC, 1GHz; Mac, 1.25 GHz) and good graphics card.
Copyright restrictions mean that some materials may not be accessible from within the Dynamic Learning edition. Full details of your single-user licence can be found on the disk under 'Contents'.

**You can find out more at www.dynamic-learning.co.uk**

# Introduction

Welcome to the new edition of *AQA PE for AS*.

This book has been written specifically to support those students following the AQA AS specification in physical education. It has been designed to follow the exact requirements of the specification and, in doing so, to prepare you for both the written and coursework units of the qualification.

The book is divided into two parts – one for each area of study:

- Part 1: Opportunities for and the effects of leading a healthy and active livestyle (Unit 1);
- Part 2: Analysis and evaluation of physical activity as a performer and/or in adopted roles (Unit 2).

## How will each part be assessed?

| **Unit 1 – Opportunities for and the effects of leading a healthy and active lifestyle** | | |
|---|---|---|
| 2-hour written examination | 84 marks available | 60% AS marks<br>30% A Level marks |
| Section A (72 marks)<br>This section requires the candidates to answer 6 structured questions of:<br>2 questions each on:<br>• Applied exercise physiology<br>• Skill acquisition<br>• Opportunities for participation | Section B (12 marks)<br>One extended question on the application of theoretical knowledge to a practical situation | |

| **Unit 2 – Analysis and evaluation of physical activity as a performer and/or in adopted roles**<br>*Candidates are assessed on their ability to perform, analyse and evaluate the execution of core skills/techniques in isolation and in structured practice as either:*<br>*A player/performer and in an adopted role* **or** *in two adopted roles:* | | |
|---|---|---|
| Internal assessment with external moderation | 100 marks available | 40% AS marks<br>20% A Level marks |
| Section A<br>• Assessment of your ability in a choice of 2 from 3 roles (performer, coach or official) | Section B<br>The application of theoretical factors which improve performance. You are assessed on this element through the Section B question on the Unit 1 paper | |

## Features and symbols

Look out for the feature boxes and symbols which appear throughout the text. There are a number of different features, which are designed to give you all the information you need to be successful and to help reinforce your learning. A brief overview of each feature is given below:

- Key terms: definitions of significant words or phrases that are required knowledge.
- In context: real-life case studies which demonstrate the application of theoretical knowledge to sporting situations.
- Activities: opportunities to apply and reinforce your knowledge through a range of student-centred tasks.
- Examiner's tips: helpful hints on examination technique and revision tips from real examiners.
- What you need to know: a summary of key points at the end of each chapter which can be used as a quick progress check and a useful revision tool.
- Exam-style questions: apply your knowledge to the sorts of questions you can expect in your written examination.
- Review questions: check your progress with questions that address the important aspects of each chapter.

## Themes

There are several main themes that underpin this course and it is really important that you reflect on these when completing assessment activities.

Throughout the course you must relate and apply knowledge to lifelong involvement in an active and healthy lifestyle. You will already be aware that physical education is a multifaceted discipline which encompasses a number of theoretical areas. In part 1, for example, you will study three main theory topics:

1 applied exercise physiology;
2 skill acquisiton;
3 opportunities for participation.

It is imperative that you reflect on the impact of each area on lifelong participation and the contribution of each to the promotion of a healthy lifestyle.

You will be required to engage in higher-order thinking, and this text will help you to develop the necessary skills of critical evaluation and analysis.

# Higher-order thinking

Higher-order thinking skills require you to do more than simply show your knowledge and understanding. To be successful on this course, you must show your abilities of application, analysis, synthesis and evaluation.

| | What is involved? | What could I do? | Question cues |
|---|---|---|---|
| **Application** | Making use of your knowledge in a particular situation | Use your knowledge in a sporting context<br>Problem solving<br>(e.g. illustrate the pattern of heart rate during a game of netball) | Apply, demonstrate, illustrate, examine |
| **Analysis** | Taking something apart or breaking it down | Look at the effect that individual components have on the 'whole'<br>(e.g. break a skill down into its component parts and identify strengths and weaknesses of each part) | Explain, classify, compare |
| **Synthesis** | Pulling ideas together, rebuilding and solving problems | Formulate an action plan or development plan for improvement<br>(e.g. suggest how a coach can improve the skills of a performer) | Create, design, compose, formulate |
| **Evaluation** | Judging the value of material or methods as they might be applied in a particular situation | Reflect on the impact of methods or an action plan<br>Give recommendations<br>(e.g. judge the relative benefits of exercise compared to any negative aspects) | Assess, measure, recommend, convince, judge |

# Opportunities for and the effects of leading a healthy and active lifestyle (Unit 1)

# PART 1

# Applied Exercise Physiology

SECTION A

# CHAPTER 1

# Fitness and health

## Learning outcomes

**By the end of this chapter you should be able to:**

- define health and fitness and explain the relationship between them;
- suggest reasons for the difficulty in defining fitness and health;
- define the following components of health-related fitness: stamina, muscular endurance, strength, speed, power and flexibility;
- define the following components of skill-related fitness: reaction time, agility, co-ordination and balance;
- evaluate the impact of lifestyle choices on health and fitness.

## CHAPTER INTRODUCTION

Exercise physiology is the study of how the body's structures and functions adapt in response to exercise, and in particular how training can enhance the athlete's performance. Fundamental to sports physiology is knowledge of health, fitness and training. This chapter explores the dimensions of fitness relevant to a range of sports performers, as well as discussing the complexities involved in defining both health and fitness. Of course, our levels of fitness and health are affected by the lifestyle choices we make and we will conclude this chapter by considering the impact of lifestyle choices on leading a balanced, active and healthy lifestyle.

## Definitions of fitness

The term 'fitness' is difficult to define, since it means many different things to different people. For example, one individual may see himself as being 'fit' if he can run for the bus without getting too out of breath, whereas a physically active person may see a quick heart rate recovery following a distance run as a measure of fitness. However, in the search for an acceptable definition that encompasses most individuals, Dick (1989) has defined fitness as

> **'... the successful adaptation to the stressors of one's lifestyle ...'**

This suggests therefore that all of us must look closely at the stressors of our everyday activities and see how well we cope with those stressors if we are to gauge our fitness levels satisfactorily.

Another frequently quoted definition is

> **'... the ability to undertake everyday activities without undue fatigue ...'**

This once again is a very generic definition which encompasses everybody – athletes and non-athletes alike. The everyday activities undertaken by an athlete in heavy training for a major competition are obviously going to be very different from those experienced by a non-athlete.

When considering physical activity, however, it would not be acceptable to rely solely upon this definition, since the fitness requirements of various activities differ dramatically from each other. We therefore need to be a little more specific in our definitions. For example, consider the different fitness requirements of a 100m sprint and a marathon run:

- The sprint requires a tremendous amount of power, strength and speed in order to travel a relatively short distance in the quickest time possible. It also requires the muscles to work in the absence of oxygen and as such the composition of the muscle tissue will need to be specialised to accommodate this.
- The marathon run requires the body to work for an extended period of time and therefore relies upon the endurance capabilities of the cardiovascular and muscular systems. Oxygen consumption is essential in this instance and similarly the body will have become adapted to take in, transport and utilise as much oxygen as possible during the run.

## A definition of health

Fitness and health are not the same thing. It is possible for a sports performer to be fit yet unhealthy. Athletes may meet the necessary fitness requirements of a particular activity yet have an ongoing illness or make lifestyle choices that can make them unhealthy. No one can argue against the brilliance of George Best on a football pitch, for example, yet he paid the ultimate price with his health due to his heavy drinking throughout his career.

Health is therefore defined as

**'... a state of physical, social and mental well-being, where we are free from disease...'.**

In striving for optimal performance, a performer must therefore seek to maximise both their fitness and their health.

### Key terms

**Fitness:** The ability to undertake everyday activities without undue fatigue.
**Health:** A state of physical, social and mental well being, where we are free from disease.

### EXAMINER'S TIP

Make sure you can explain the difference between fitness and health in your exam.

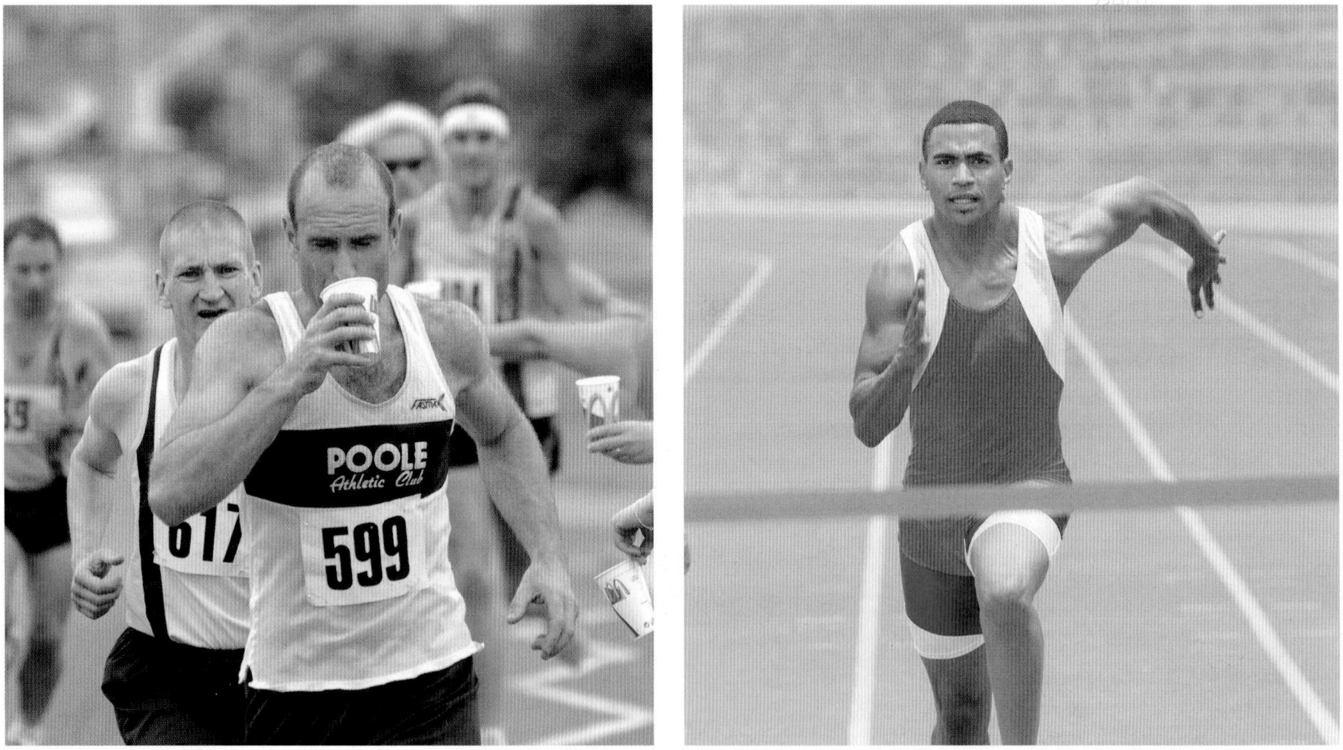


**Figure 1.1** The fitness demands of a distance runner (a) are very different to those of a sprinter (b)

# The components of fitness

The components of fitness relate to the requirements of a given sporting activity, and can help to explain success or failure in sport.

A distinction can be made between components which are generally considered to be health-related (health benefits may be gained through improvements in these components) and those that are skill-related, although both will affect performance in sport.

Health-related factors are physiologically based and determine the ability of an individual to meet the physical demands of the activity; the skill-related factors are based upon the neuromuscular system and determine how successfully a person can perform a specific skill. Both are required in all activities, but the relative importance of each dimension may differ. For example, a person may be physically suited to tennis, possessing the necessary speed, endurance and strength requirements, but may not possess the hand–eye co-ordination needed to strike the ball successfully. In this instance the individual may be best advised to switch to an activity that requires fewer skill-related components, such as distance running.

**Key terms**

**Health-related components of fitness:** Those dimensions of fitness that are physiologically based and determine how well a performer can meet the physical demands of an activity.

**Skill-related components of fitness:** Those elements of fitness that involve the neuro-muscular system and determine how successfully a performer can complete a specific task.

## Exam-style questions

1 Explain the division of fitness into health-related and skill-related components (4 marks).

## Health-related components of fitness

### Stamina or cardio-respiratory endurance

Cardio-respiratory endurance is dependent upon the ability of the cardiovascular system to transport and utilise oxygen during sustained exercise. It can be defined as:

**the ability to provide and sustain energy aerobically.**

Cardio-respiratory endurance is the component of fitness that underpins all aerobic activities, which include long-distance running, cycling or swimming, as well as being a contributory factor to many other sporting situations.

### Maximal oxygen uptake ($VO_2$max)

A key component of stamina is maximal oxygen uptake or $VO_2$max, which can be defined as:

**the maximal amount of oxygen that can be taken in, transported and consumed by the working muscles per minute.**

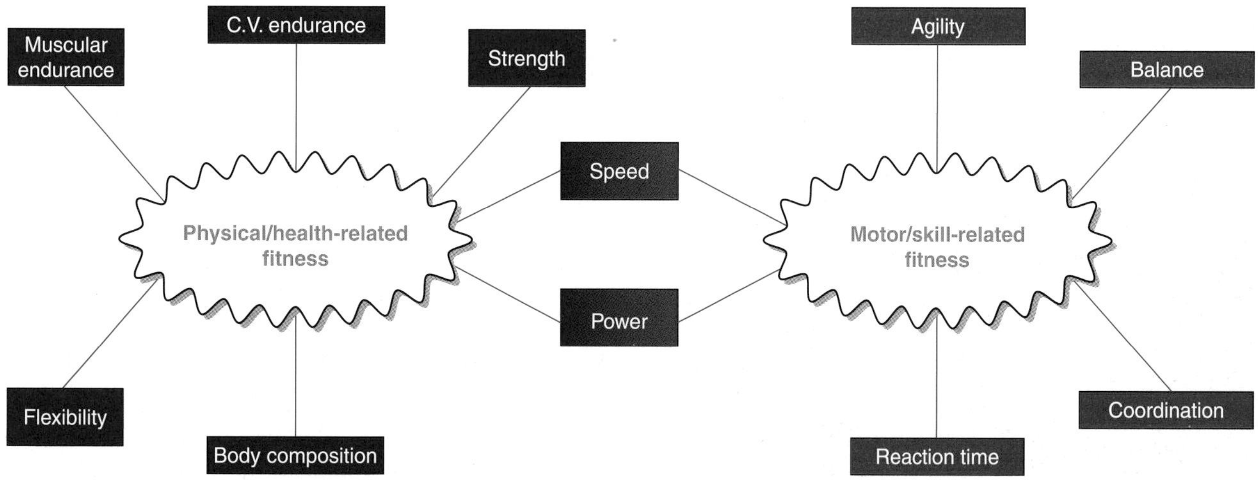


Figure 1.2

## Factors affecting stamina or cardio-respiratory endurance

Physiological factors that determine aerobic performance include the possession of a large proportion of **slow twitch muscle fibres**, a proliferation of **mitochondria** and large **myoglobin** stores. These help in the production of large amounts of energy via the aerobic pathway. Perhaps the major influencing factor of cardio-respiratory performance is the maximum volume of oxygen an individual can consume (VO2 max). This has a very large genetic component and is influenced little by training. Factors affecting cardio-respiratory endurance are summarised in Table 1.1.

Stamina can be assessed using the multi-stage fitness test or the PWC170 test. Refer to Chapter 6 for an outline of the testing protocols for these and other fitness tests.

**Key terms**

**Mitochondria:** The site of energy production under aerobic conditions (when oxygen is present).
**Myoglobin:** A respiratory pigment that acts as a store of oxygen within the muscle cell.
**Slow twitch muscle fibres (Type 1):** Muscle fibres designed to produce energy using oxygen over a long period of time.

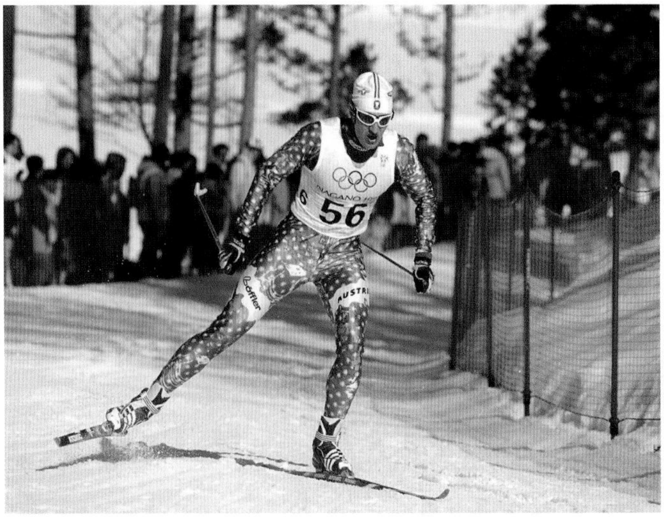


**Figure 1.3** A cross-country skier requires exceptionally high levels of stamina

# Strength

Strength relates to the ability of the body to apply a force. The recognised definition of strength is

> **the maximum force that can be developed in a muscle or group of muscles during a single maximal contraction.**

However, it is how we apply strength that is important when analysing sporting activity. Three dimensions of strength have been identified:

## Activity 1

For each of the activities shown, give approximate values of $VO_2$max for both male and female participants.

- a midfielder in hockey;
- a 100m sprinter;
- a male gymnast;
- an Olympic canoeist;
- a hammer thrower.

Using pictures and photographs from a range of sports compile a continuum of relative $VO_2$max.

**Table 1.1** A summary of the factors that determine aerobic capacities

| | |
|---|---|
| **Genetics** | Although there is some contention as to exactly how much genetics affects $VO_2$max, there is no doubt that it is significant. Some studies have suggested as much as 93 per cent! |
| **Age** | After the age of 25, $VO_2$max is thought to decrease at about 1 per cent per year. Regular physical activity, however, can offset some of this decline. |
| **Training** | Undertaking the right training can improve $VO_2$max by 10–20 per cent. |
| **Gender** | Women tend to have $VO_2$max scores that are about 15–30 per cent lower than men of the same group. As a simple rule subtract 10ml from the equivalent male score. |

Table 1.1 continued

| | |
|---|---|
| **Body composition** | Research suggests that $VO_2$max decreases as body fat percentage increases. This could contribute to some of the differences in $VO_2$max between males and females. |
| **Lifestyle** | Obviously a lifestyle that involves smoking and having a poor diet will have an adverse effect upon $VO_2$max. |
| **Exercise mode** | Care should be taken to select the most appropriate mode of testing $VO_2$max for when testing an athlete. A swimmer should have their $VO_2$max test conducted while swimming, a runner on a treadmill, and a cyclist on a cycle ergometer! Treadmill tests seem to produce the highest rating. |

- maximum strength
- elastic strength
- strength endurance.

An athlete who requires a very large force to overcome a resistance in a single contraction, such as we see in weight lifting, or performing a throw in judo, will require **maximum strength**. An athlete who needs to overcome a resistance rapidly yet prepare the muscle quickly for a sequential contraction of equal force will require elastic **strength**. This can be seen in explosive events such as sprinting, triple jumping or in a gymnast performing tumbles in a floor routine. Finally, an athlete who is required to undergo repeated contractions and withstand fatigue, such as a rower or swimmer, will view **strength endurance** as a vital determining factor to performance.

## Factors affecting strength

Strength is directly related to the cross-sectional area of the muscle tissue as well as the type of muscle fibre within the muscle. Fast twitch (white fibres) can generate greater forces than slow twitch (red fibres).

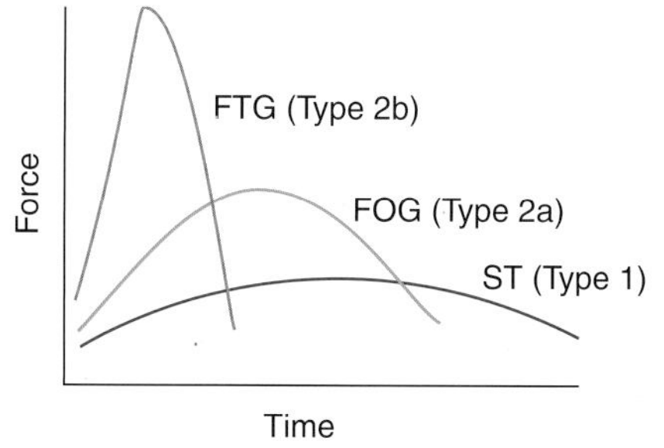


Figure 1.4 Muscle fibre twitch response: fast-twitch muscle fibres generate higher forces for a shorter space of time when compared to slow-twitch

The optimum age to develop strength appears to be in the early to mid-twenties. As the body ages, less protein becomes available in the body for muscle growth, and the stress and anaerobic nature of strength training also make it an inappropriate method of training during old age.

### EXAMINER'S TIP

Make sure you can distinguish between the different types of strength and apply each type to sporting activity.

In this age of gender equality it is highly appropriate to dismiss the notion of a weaker sex. In fact, relative to cross-sectional area of pure muscle tissue, men and women are equal in terms of strength. It is the greater fat content of women and the higher testosterone levels in men that can create the difference in the cross-sectional area of muscles and therefore strength, to the advantage of males.

### Key terms

**Fast twitch muscle fibres (Type 2):** Muscle fibres suited to high intensity anaerobic work. Type 2b fibres are recruited for activities of greatest intensity but fatigue rapidly whilst type 2a fibres are engaged in activities that require large forces and yet offer greater resistance to fatigue than type 2b fibres.

Strength can be assessed using a handgrip dynamometer or the 1 rep max test. Refer to Chapter 6 for an outline of the testing protocols for these and other fitness tests.

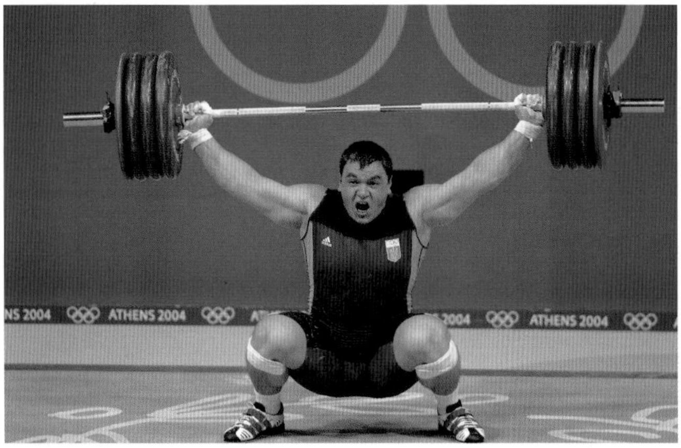

Figure 1.5 A weight lifter – maximum strength is vital to successful performance

## Muscular (strength) endurance

Muscular (strength) endurance is the ability of a muscle or group of muscles to sustain repeated contractions against a resistance for an extended period of time and withstands fatigue.

Slow twitch muscle fibres will ensure they receive a rich supply of blood to enable the most efficient production of aerobic energy. This enables the muscles to contract repeatedly without experiencing the fatigue due to the build-up of the lactic acid. Activities that require muscular endurance are numerous but can best be highlighted by using the example of rowing. Individual muscle groups are required to contract at high intensity for a period of approximately 5 minutes (or as long as it takes to complete the 2000m course!). Muscular endurance relies upon the efficiency of the body to produce energy under both anaerobic and aerobic conditions, together with its ability to deal with and '**buffer**' the lactic acid.

**Key terms**

**Buffering:** The body's method of maintaining acceptable levels of blood acidity and reducing the effects of lactic acid.

Muscular endurance can be assessed using the abdominal conditioning test. Refer to Chapter 6 for an outline of the testing protocols for these and other fitness tests.

# Flexibility

Flexibility can be defined as

**the range of movement possible at a joint.**

It is determined by the elasticity of ligaments and tendons, the strength and opposition of surrounding muscles (including antagonists) and the shape of the articulating bones. Although flexibility is most commonly associated with activities such as trampolining and gymnastics, it is in fact a requirement in all sports since the development of flexibility can lead to an increase in both speed and power of muscle contraction.

Table 1.2 A summary of the main factors that determine strength

| | |
|---|---|
| **Type of muscle fibre** | Fast twitch fibres can produce high levels of force (strength) over a short period of time. Slow twitch fibres on the other hand can only produce lower levels of force but over a longer period of time. |
| **Age** | Although strength can be gained at any age, the rate of strength gain appears to be greatest from your teenage years to your early twenties. We are at our strongest at this point. |
| **Gender** | Although men's and women's muscle tissue are characteristically the same, men generally have more muscle tissue than women due to the effect of testosterone. So although gender does not affect the quality of the muscle it does the quantity! |
| **Limb and muscle length** | The length of limbs determine the body's leverage systems. People with shorter limbs tend to be able to lift heavier weights due to their more advantageous lever systems. In the same way people who have developed longer muscles will have a greater potential for developing size and therefore strength! |
| **Other factors include ...** | Point of tendon insertion, lifting technique |

## Factors affecting flexibility

Often the degree of movement is determined by the type of joint, since joints are designed either for stability or mobility. The knee joint, for example, is a hinge joint and has been designed with stability in mind. It is only truly capable of movement in one plane of direction (it is uniaxial), allowing flexion and extension of the lower leg. This is due to the intricate network of ligaments surrounding the joint, which restricts movement. The shoulder joint, meanwhile, is a ball and socket joint and allows movement in many planes (it is polyaxial) since few ligaments cross the joint. However, the free movement at the joint comes at a price, as the shoulder joint can easily become dislocated. Flexibility training is even more important for athletes, since there is a distinct reduction in mobility from the age of 8 years, and following periods of inactivity. A summary of all the factors affecting flexibility can be seen in Table 1.3.

Flexibility can be assessed using the sit and reach test or a goniometer. Refer to Chapter 6 for an outline of the testing protocols for these and other fitness tests.

# Speed

Speed is

> **the ability to put body parts into motion quickly, or the maximum rate that a person can move over a specific distance.**

It is a major factor in many high-intensity, explosive activities such as sprinting, vaulting in gymnastics or fast bowling in cricket. However, speed is not simply concerned with the rate at which a person can move their body from point A to point B. Although this may be important during sprinting or when running down the wing in rugby, other sports require the athlete to put their limbs into action rapidly, such as when throwing the javelin.

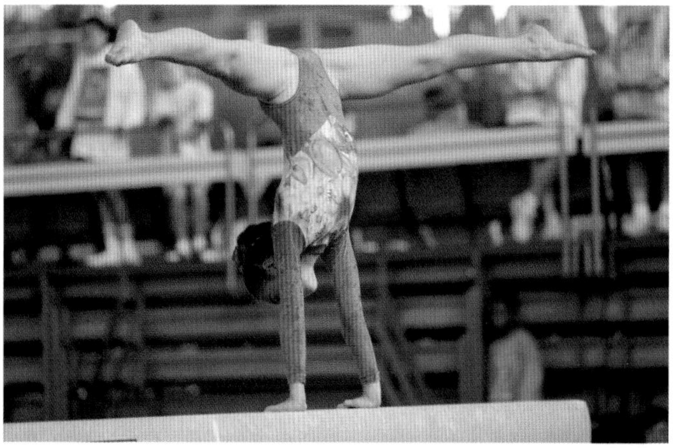

Figure 1.6 A gymnast performing the splits requires a high degree of flexibility at the hip joint

Our definition of speed therefore encompasses both aspects of speed. A fast bowler in cricket, for example, does not necessarily need to run at maximum pace but must be able to put his arm into action rapidly to achieve an effective outcome.

Speed tends to be genetically determined due to the physiological make-up of the muscle, and as such is least affected by training and can take some time to develop. Once again, fast twitch (FTG) muscle fibres tend to be beneficial in activities where speed is essential, since they can release energy for muscular contraction very rapidly. There are many physiological factors that help to determine speed, which include the ability to select motor units accurately, the elasticity of muscle tissue, and the availability of energy supply (**i.e. the ATP-PC system**). However, the role of body mechanics and the efficiency of the body's lever systems are also integral in determining speed of

**Key terms**

**ATP-PC system:** The method by which the body provides the energy required to perform activities that are of very high intensity (such as a 100m sprint).

Table 1.3 A summary of the many factors that determine flexibility

| Internal factors | External factors |
|---|---|
| The type of joint | The temperature of the local environment |
| Bony structures which limit movement (e.g. a deep socket) | Age |
| The elasticity of the muscle tissue | Gender |
| The elasticity of the surrounding tendons and ligaments | Restrictions of clothing |
| The temperature of the joint and associated tissues | Injury |
| Strength of the opposing muscle group | Activity level |

the body or body part, and in this way developing appropriate technique is essential.

Speed can be assessed using the 30m sprint test. Refer to Chapter 6 for an outline of the testing protocol for this and other fitness tests.

## Power

Power is

> **the amount of work done per unit of time; the product of strength and speed.**

It can also be thought of as explosive strength where the ability to exert a large force over a short period of time is paramount. It relies on the interaction of the neuro-muscular system to recruit fast twitch fibres as rapidly as possible.

Power can be assessed using the sergeant jump or standing broad jump. Refer to Chapter 6 for an outline of the testing protocols for these and other fitness tests.

# Skill-related components of fitness

### Agility

Agility is defined as:

> **the ability to move and change direction and position of the body quickly and effectively while under control.**

With reference to this definition we can see that many factors are involved in agility, including balance, co-ordination, speed and flexibility. However, agility is required in a range of sporting activities, from tumbling in gymnastics to retrieving balls in volleyball. Although activities can be undertaken to improve agility, development of this skill-related component is limited.

Agility can be assessed using the Illinois agility run or the zig-zag test. Refer to Chapter 6 for an outline of the testing protocols for these and other fitness tests.

### Balance

Balance is defined as:

> **the maintenance of the centre of mass over the base of support. This can be while the body is static (stationary) or dynamic (moving).**

Balance is an integral component in the effective performance of most activities. In gymnastics, for example, it may be necessary to maintain a balanced position when performing a handstand. This is static balance. However, in games such as netball, players must maintain balance while moving, for example when side-stepping or dodging – this is known as dynamic balance.

Again balance can be improved only slightly through training, but one effective method involves the maintenance of balance on a 'wobble' or balance board.

Balance can be assessed using the standing stork test or a balance board.

**Key terms**

**Centre of mass (COM):** The point in the body where all the weight tends to be concentrated, signifying that the body is balanced in all directions. In the human body the COM is not fixed and can change depending upon the relative positions of the limbs and body parts.

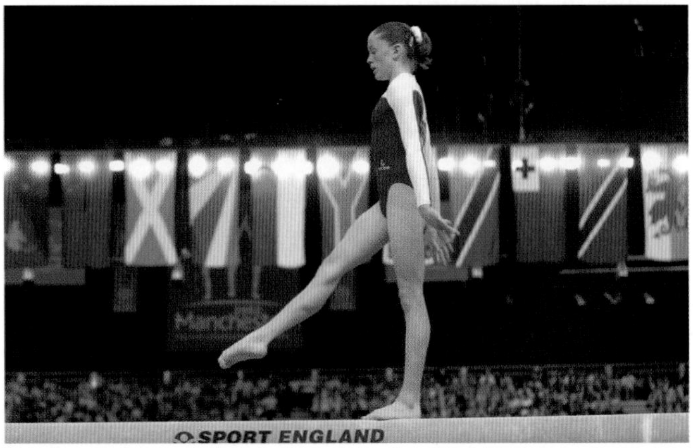


**Figure 1.7** A gymnast on a beam requires both static and dynamic balance

### Co-ordination

Co-ordination is defined as:

> **the interaction of the motor and nervous systems and is the ability to perform motor tasks accurately, and effectively.**

When serving in squash, for example, the player must co-ordinate the toss of the ball with one hand with the striking of the ball with the racket head in the other hand. This requires co-ordination. A swimmer performing breaststroke must co-ordinate the pull of the arms with the strong kick phase to ensure effective performance.

Co-ordination can be assessed using the alternate hand ball toss test. Refer to Chapter 6 for an outline of the testing protocol for this and other fitness tests.

## Reaction time

Reaction time can be defined as:

> **the time taken to initiate a response to a given stimulus.**

This stimulus may be visual, for example in responding to a serve in tennis, or aural, in responding to a gun in athletics or verbal guidance from players and coaches. Colin Jackson, one of the fastest starters in the world in the 1990s, explained his success by 'going on the "B" of the Bang'. Reaction time is dependent upon the ability of an individual to process information and initiate a response by the neuro-muscular system. Reaction time can be improved through training.

Reaction time can be assessed using reaction time computer software or the stick drop test. Refer to Chapter 6 for an outline of the testing protocols for these and other fitness tests.

### Activity 2

Copy out Table 1.4 and for each activity tick the two components of fitness that you think are the most important.

Table 1.4 Components of fitness for different activities

| Activity | Speed | Strength | Cardio-vascular endurance | Muscular endurance | Flexibility | Power | Reaction time | Agility | Balance | Co-ordination | Body composition |
|---|---|---|---|---|---|---|---|---|---|---|---|
| swimming | | | | | | | | | | | |
| squash | | | | | | | | | | | |
| marathon | | | | | | | | | | | |
| tennis | | | | | | | | | | | |
| cycling | | | | | | | | | | | |
| rugby | | | | | | | | | | | |
| sprinting | | | | | | | | | | | |
| x-country skiing | | | | | | | | | | | |
| aerobics | | | | | | | | | | | |
| basketball | | | | | | | | | | | |
| judo | | | | | | | | | | | |
| gymnastics vault | | | | | | | | | | | |
| badminton | | | | | | | | | | | |
| netball | | | | | | | | | | | |
| cricket | | | | | | | | | | | |

## Exam-style questions

1 Identify and define two main components of fitness required by a cricket player. (2 marks)

2 Name and define two main components of fitness required by a high jumper. Explain how these components are used in this event. (4 marks)

# The effect of lifestyle choices on health and fitness

We all have to make decisions when it comes to the search for a healthy lifestyle. Factors such as alcohol consumption, eating junk food, smoking, using recreational drugs and being tied to our games consoles can tempt even the most determined athlete and before long fitness levels can fall and health issues emerge. In fact, a recent study from Cambridge University found that by leading a healthy lifestyle your life expectancy can be increased by up to 14 years. The study looked at the effects of 4 'healthy' behaviours: taking regular exercise, eating 5 portions of fruit and vegetables per day, abstaining from smoking, and drinking moderate levels of alcohol (1–14 units per week). Subjects who followed all four healthy behaviours were found to live an additional 14 years compared with those who followed none of them.

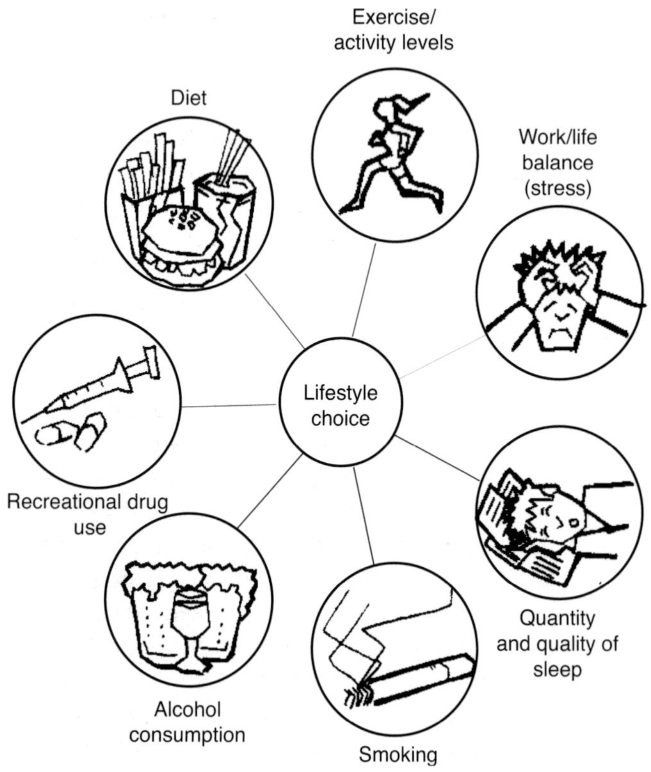


Figure 1.8 The pursuit of a healthy lifestyle is dependent upon certain lifestyle choices

This study looked at only 4 'healthy' behaviours:

- smoking;
- exercise/activity levels;
- diet;
- alcohol consumption.

There are, however, several other lifestyle choices we must make:

- work/life balance;
- recreational drug use;
- quality and quantity of sleep.

# Examples of lifestyle choices and their effect upon health and fitness

## Physical activity/inactivity

It is a well-known fact that exercise can contribute to a healthy and fulfilling lifestyle. There is now consistent evidence that people with higher levels of physical activity have a reduced risk of cardiovascular disease and some cancers. According to the World Health Organisation, currently more than 60 per cent of the global population are not sufficiently active, a pattern that is mirrored in the UK where only 35 per cent of men and 24 per cent of women are meeting the government guidelines of 30 minutes of moderate physical activity on at least five days a week. Moreover, despite increasing levels of exercise since 1997, 21 per cent of men and 26 per cent of women in the UK are still doing less than one session of at least 30 minutes of continuous physical activity every four weeks.

Physical activity can lead to longevity. Exercise even at an older age can significantly reduce the risk of obesity and cardiovascular diseases such as coronary heart disease, diabetes and hypertension. According to World Health Organisation research, doing as little as 150 minutes of exercise that is of moderate intensity or 60 minutes of vigorous physical activity per week reduces the risk of coronary heart disease by approximately 30 per cent.

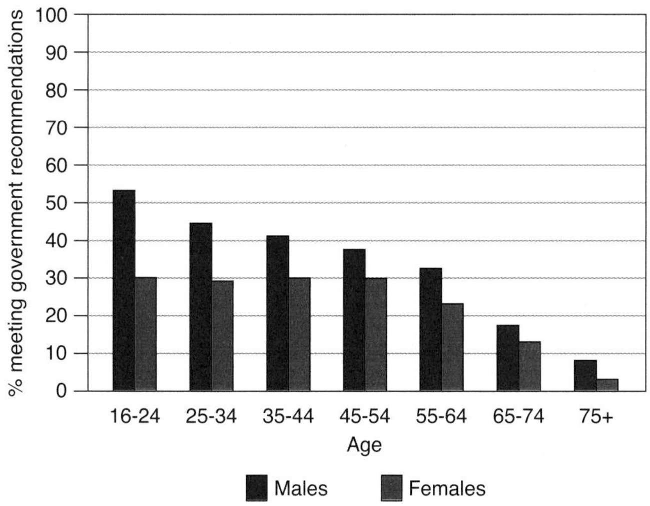


**Figure 1.9** Percentage of adults in England meeting government recommendations on physical activity, by age and sex, 2003

*Source*: Department of Health

## Activity 3

Figure 1.10 illustrates the time spent seated each week by people aged 18 years and above in selected countries. What factors have contributed to this increasingly sedentary lifestyle?

## Activity 4

Undertake some research on the following topic and draw up your conclusions: Critically evaluate the role of exercise in the prevention of cardiovascular diseases.

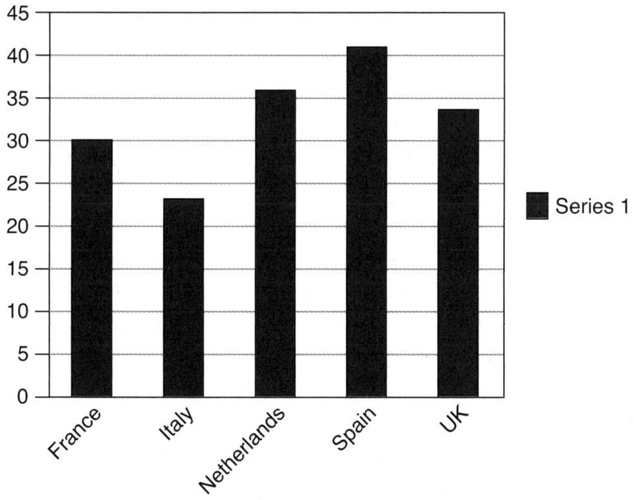


**Figure 1.10** Time spent seated each week by adults 18 years and above in selected European countries

# Smoking

A ban on smoking in enclosed spaces in Britain came fully into effect on 1 July 2007. Smoking can reduce levels of fitness, particularly aerobic fitness, which relies upon the effective transport and utilisation of oxygen by the body. Smoking primarily reduces the amount of oxygen available in the body, which hinders significantly physical performance.

The chief culprit for the reduced availability of oxygen to the tissues is the carbon monoxide contained in cigarette smoke. You will recall that once it leaves the lungs, oxygen is transported in the blood by attaching to the haemoglobin within red blood cells. Oxygen has a high affinity for haemoglobin. However, carbon monoxide's affinity for haemoglobin is about 250 times greater than that of oxygen and so binds preferentially to haemoglobin. Therefore as the levels of carbon monoxide increase in the blood, the level of oxygen transport and release decreases significantly. The net effect of this is to cause the heart to work harder in an attempt to compensate for the lack of oxygen reaching the muscles.

This condition is prominent with the carbon monoxide accumulation that results from smoking.

The case for not smoking due to respiratory complications is two-fold:

1 Impaired transport of oxygen in the blood
High levels of carbon monoxide found in cigarette smoke reduce the amount of oxygen absorbed into the blood from the lungs and the amount released to the tissues from the blood. This factor alone reduces physical endurance capacities and can reduce $VO_2$max by up to 10 per cent.
2 Greater airway resistance through the narrowing of the air passages. The act of inhaling cigarette smoke can increase resistance of the airways immediately by causing swelling of the mucous membranes that line them. Tar contained within cigarettes can also coat the airways and lungs, reducing the elasticity of the alveoli and hampering gaseous exchange, resulting in reduced lung volumes and less oxygen reaching the blood stream. Pollutants from cigarettes (and there are at least 400 toxic substances within them) can irritate the bronchial tubes and lungs, causing increased mucous secretion, phlegm and coughing – a problem that is only exacerbated when exercising.

If you want to maintain a healthy lifestyle and have a lifelong participation in sport and physical activity, the message is quite clear – DO NOT SMOKE!

**IN CONTEXT**

**People who smoke usually cannot compete with their non-smoking peers. This is because of the associated physical effects of smoking such as a rapid heartbeat, impaired circulation, and shortness of breath – which impair sports performance. Smoking also affects the body's ability to produce collagen, so common sports injuries, such as tendon and ligament damage, will take longer to heal in smokers than in non-smokers.**

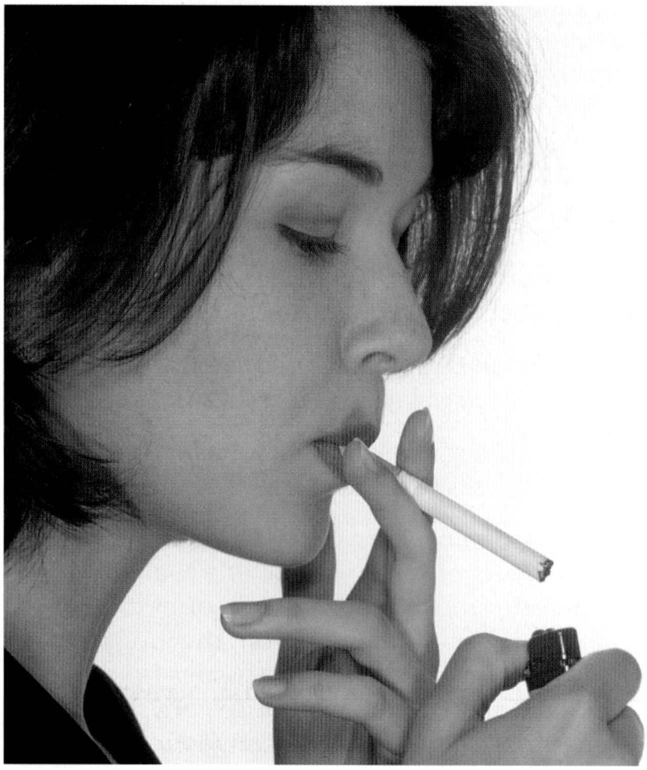

**Figure 1.11** Smoking can reduce the effectiveness of oxygen transport in the body, shortness of breathe and impaired circulation

## Diet

The adage 'you are what you eat' is certainly appropriate in any discussion on the benefits of a healthy diet and the consequences of a poor one. Scientific research has clearly demonstrated that what and how much we eat greatly affects growth, development, ageing, and the ability to enjoy life to its fullest. A healthy diet can make us feel great and full of life while a poor diet can lead to all kinds of medical conditions, from cancers to obesity and its associated health problems. This comes at a time when obesity is a problem reaching epic proportions around the world. In Chapter 2 the implications of obesity are discussed at length. Our discussion will now turn to the steps we can take to improve our diet.

The Food Standards Agency's education programme has developed the eat-well plate, which is based on the five food groups:

- bread, rice, potatoes, pasta and other starchy foods;
- fruit and vegetables;
- milk and dairy foods;
- meat, fish, eggs, beans and other non-dairy sources of protein;
- foods and drinks high in fat and/or sugar.

The eat-well plate encourages you to choose different foods from the first four groups every day. This will help to ensure that you are receiving a wide range of nutrients, allowing your body to function properly and perform at its best. The plate in Figure 1.12 indicates the amount each food group should contribute to your diet for it to be considered healthy.

Choosing a variety of foods from each group will add to the range of nutrients you consume. Foods in the fifth group, that is foods and drinks that are high in fat and/or sugar, are not essential to a healthy diet but can be consumed on occasion in moderation.

## Stress

Stress is the emotional and physical strain caused by our response to pressure from the outside world. It is almost impossible to live without some stress – we all have demands put upon us, such as deadlines to meet and exams to sit. Stress forms part of the biological defence mechanism – our '**fight or flight response**', which serves to protect us in the presence of danger or threatening situations. If we allow stress to get out of control it can get the better of us and have a negative impact on our health and enjoyment of life. What is therefore a key factor in any discussion on stress is our stress coping mechanism. Before we investigate this, let us briefly look at some of the main causes of stress and the health implications of these.

# The eatwell plate

Use the eatwell plate to help you get the balance right. It shows how much of what you eat should come from each food group.

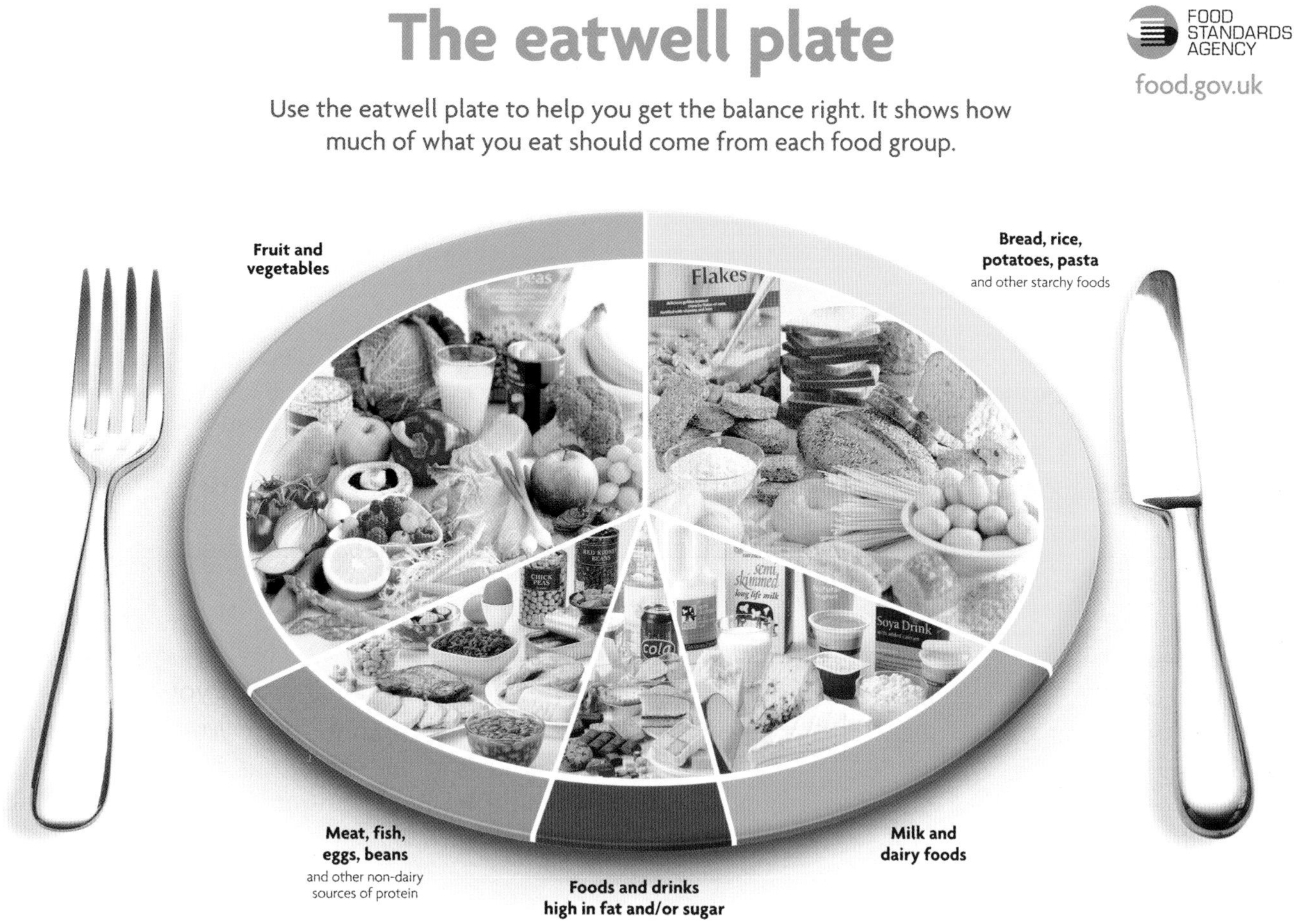

**Figure 1.12** The eatwell plate
*Source:* Food Standards Agency

---

**Key term**

**Fight or flight response:** The biological response of the body that prepares us for emergency action. Faced with danger the body is flooded with the hormones adrenaline, noradrenaline and cortisol, gearing us up to either run away from the situation or stand and fight.

## Causes of stress

The causes of stress are numerous and particular to individuals. The causes of stress or anxiety for one person may be the source of excitement and pleasure for others. What you consider to be a stressful situation will largely depend upon your personality type. Some personality types are more easily stressed out than others. Table 1.5 identifies some external and internal causes of stress.

**Table 1.5** Common causes of stress

| External stressors | Internal stressors |
|---|---|
| ● Work stressors<br>● Relationship stressors<br>● Social stressors<br>● Environmental stressors | ● Unrealistic expectations<br>● Low self-esteem<br>● Pessimism<br>● Uncertainty or worries<br>● A feeling that you are unable to meet the demands of the environment |

**Key term**

**Stressors:** Situations that are considered stress-provoking.

## The impact of stress on health

Any doctor will tell you that the root cause of many illnesses is stress and anxiety. The inability to cope with stress can lead to suppression of the immune system and a whole host of cardio-vascular diseases. In addition, enduring stress can alter the neural pathways in the brain which can lead to mental health problems. Table 1.6 identifies some physical and emotional health conditions that can result from severe stress.

**Table 1.6** Physical and emotional conditions associated with stress

| Physical health effects | Emotional health effects |
|---|---|
| • Coronary heart disease<br>• Hypertension (high blood pressure)<br>• Irritable bowel syndrome<br>• Obesity<br>• Ulcers<br>• Infertility<br>• Dermatological conditions | • Depression<br>• Anxiety<br>• Eating disorders<br>• Substance abuse |

## Combating stress

As we have seen it is impossible to live without stress; stress is part and parcel of everyday life. Just by making a few minor adjustments to our lifestyles, however, it may be possible to live and cope with the causes of our stress more positively. When you are feeling a little stressed out, try following some of the tips outlined below.

- Be aware and acknowledge the stressors in your life.
- There is nothing like a bit of aerobic exercise to eliminate stress.
- Try some relaxation techniques: imagery, controlled breathing exercises, progressive muscular relaxation.
- Make sure you get a good night's sleep.
- Eat healthily.
- Initiate a time management plan and stick to it.
- Learn to prioritise your time – do what needs to be done first, leaving other things for tomorrow.
- Goal setting can enhance motivation and the feelgood factor. Identify your **SMARTER goals** and work towards them.
- Surround yourself with a support network to rely on and sound off to in times of need.
- When stress arises, do not procrastinate – take immediate and direct action.

**Key term**

**Smarter goals:** Goals we set should be: Specific, Measurable, Agreed, Realistic, Time-framed, Exciting and Recorded.

Many of the lifestyle choices discussed above are also contributory factors in the development and progression of cardiovascular diseases.

## Cardiovascular disease

Cardiovascular disease is the main cause of dealth in the industrialised nations of Western civilisation, and accounts for an estimated 40 per cent of all deaths in the United Kingdom. There are several forms of cardiovascular disease, which include:

- atherosclerosis – a laying down of fatty deposits in the arteries
- coronary heart disease – may lead to angina pectoris (coronary thrombosis) or a myocardial infarction (heart attack)
- cerebral infarction (stroke)
- hypertension – constant elevated blood pressure.

Atherosclerosis is a degenerative disease. It is typified by a thickening and hardening of the arterial walls, as a result of atheroma or plaque being deposited.

By the laying down of atheroma, the Lumen of the vessel is decreased in diameter. This is further narrowed by the formation of blood clots on the rough edges of the plaque. With continual deposition of atheroma, the walls of the arteries harden and lose their elasticity; this reduces their ability to vasoconstrict and vasodilate – two important mechanisms in regulating blood pressure. Consequently, blood pressure rises permanently as the resistance to blood flow has increased – the body suffers hypertension. This is clinically defined as blood pressure consistently above 160/100 mmHg, and can increase the risk of stroke, heart attack and kidney failure.

When atherosclerosis occurs mainly in the cornonary arteries (which supply the myocardium with blood), parts of the heart become deprived of oxygen and a myocardial infarction or heart attack may ensue. For severe cases of coronary heart disease, a heart bypass operation may be required which enables blood to bypass the blocked part of the vessel and reach the oxygen deprived tissue. Similarly, severe blockages of the cerebral arteries supplying the brain may cause oxygen deprivation, resulting in a cerebral infarction or stroke.

The incidence and severity of the disease is linked to the following independent and dependent risk factors.

**Key terms**

**Coronary heart disease:** A narrowing of the small blood vessels that supply blood and oxygen to the heart (coronary arteries). The narrowing reduces the blood supply to the heart muscles and causes pain known as angina.
**Angina pectoris:** Angina pectoris is recurring acute chest pain or discomfort, resulting from decreased blood supply to the heart muscle.
**Arteriosclerosis:** A chronic disease in which thickening, hardening and loss of elasticity of the arterial walls results in impaired blood circulation.
**Atherosclerosis:** A process of progressive thickening and hardening of the walls of the arteries as a result of the deposition of fatty deposits on their inner lining.
**Hypertension:** Constantly elevated blood pressure – usually where systolic pressure exceeds 140mmHg and diastolic pressure exceeds 90mmHg.

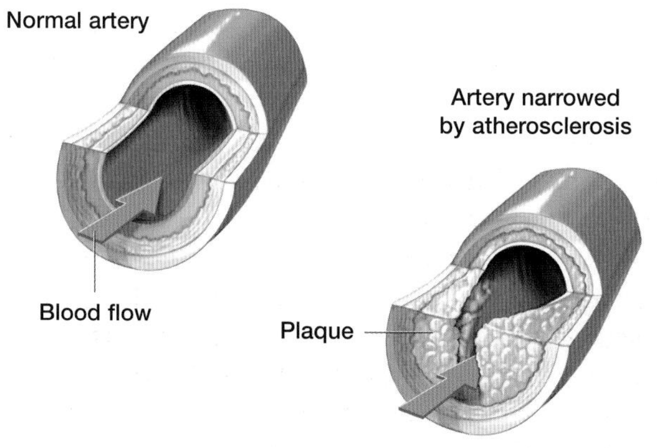


Figure 1.13 The development of atherosclerosis

## Independent risk factors

Independent or primary risk factors are so called because the presence of any one of them can cause the development of such vascular diseases. These include smoking and a high fat intake.

1 Smoking increases the risk up to 20 times, and is a dose-related factor: the more you smoke the more the risk. However, ceasing smoking can reduce this risk greatly within a few years.
2 A high fat diet can cause an increased risk, due to the deposition of cholesterol in the arteries.

Cholesterol is used by the body to form cell membranes and hormones. It is transported in the bood by protein molecules called lipoproteins. Generally a high level of blood cholesterol is associated with an increased risk of coronary heart disease.

More important, however, is the *type* of lipoprotein that carries the cholesterol. The inflated risk is largely linked to a high proportion of *low* density lipoproteins (LDL) to *high* density lipoproteins (HDL). The quantity of low density lipoproteins is increased when a diet high in saturated fats is followed. These lipoproteins have a tendency to deposit cholesterol in the arteries, whereas high density lipoproteins act as waste disposal units – they remove cholesterol from the arterial wall and carry it to the liver where it can be metabolised.

Consequently, a high proportion of high density lipoproteins to low density lipoproteins can substantially reduce the risk of atherosclerosis onset.

## Dependent risk factors

Dependent risk factors are those which do not necessarily cause CVD alone, but when in combination with other factors, may substantially increase the risk.

1 Heredity: there appears to be a genetic link in the development of cardiovascular diseases. The easiest way to determine if this factor is of concern is to look back at your family history for the incidence of this disease.
2 Personality or stress is also widely accepted as a contributing factor. Although almost everybody will experience stress, how the individual deals and copes with that stress is the vital point. Type A personalities (characteristics of impatience, aggression and ambitions) have a higher risk than type B individuals with the opposite characteristics.

3 Lack of exercise: studies show that people who habitually exercise at an intensity of 70 per cent of their predicted maximum heart rate have a much lower risk of heart and vascular diseases.
4 Other factors that are uncontrollable yet increase the risk are increasing age (due to the progressive narrowing of arteries through atherosclerosis) and gender (men historically have higher incidences of CVD than women, but this gap is closing).

Atherosclerosis is not confined to the middle age. Research had found that fatty steaks can start appearing in the arteries of early teenage children: by the mid-twenties these may develop into fibrous plaques and by the early forties, severe blockages of the artieries can start to occur. The rate at which the disease progresses is largely determined by the heredity factor and the lifestyles that individuals choose to enjoy.

## The role of exercise in the prevention of cardiovascular disease

Numerous studies have been conducted into how exercise can prevent cardiovascular diseases. The commencement of an exercise programme together with the cessation of smoking can go some way in the prevention of such diseases. The following factors help to justify the benefits of exercise:

- Exercise tends to reduce the overall risk of developing some form of cardiovascular disease by about 30 per cent, largely due to the adaption of the cardiovascular system. By exercising, improvements occur in the contractility of and blood supply to the heart. By causing blood vessels to vasoconstrict and dilate regularly, exercise can prevent the arteries from hardening and losing their elasticity, and so ward off the effects of

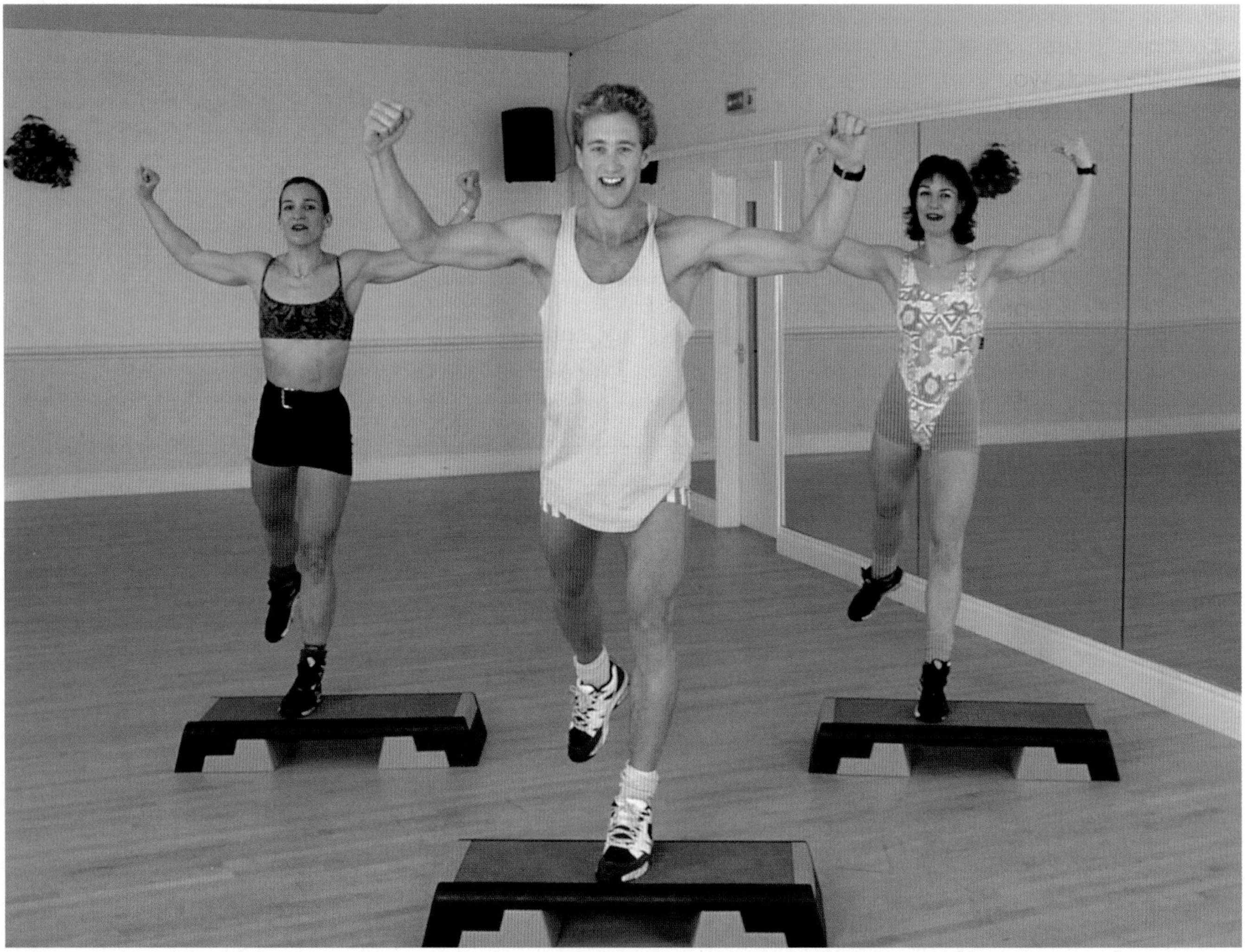

**Figure 1.14** Exercise can help to maintain a healthy lifestyle and prevent the onset of cardiovascular diseases such as atherosclerosis and coronary heart disease

atherosclerosis. This will also prevent hypertension and its associated dangers.

- Exercise can also reduce the level of fatty deposits in the blood and increase the proportion of HDL:LDL, as well as reducing overall cholesterol levels. The laying down of fatty deposits in the arteries is therefore significantly reduced.
- Exercise can also reduce body fat and reduce the strain upon the circulatory system.
- The increased breakdown of blood glucose as a result of exercise, reduces blood sugar content and decreases the incidence of adult onset diabetes.
- Vigorous activity can also have a cathartic effect, reducing stress and generally instilling the 'feel good factor'.

## Quantity and quality of sleep

The ever-increasing hectic lifestyles of modern society mean that we often forgo our sleep and most people seem to be accruing a certain degree of sleep debt. It would appear that lack of sleep through a choice of late nights and sleep that is of poor quality is endemic in our society – athletes included. In a recent national sleep survey (reported by *Peak Performance* magazine), 18 per cent of people reported that they did not get sufficient sleep most nights, while 60 per cent felt that they were deprived of sleep on one or more nights during the week.

Not only is the amount of time spent in bed important, but so is the quality of sleep. Sleep disturbances such as fidgeting and snoring can contribute to sleep debt, which is also cumulative.

### Effects of sleep debt on athletic performance

It would appear therefore that sleep deprivation is on the rise and is a problem that can significantly impair athletic performance. Below are a few consequences of sleep deprivation:

- increased blood pressure and heart rate;
- long-term deprivation can increase risk of cardiovascular disease (SLEEP 2007);
- weight gain due to increased appetite;
- impaired motor function including reaction times;
- mood swings that can influence levels of motivation to train;
- higher perceived exertion rates for a given work load;
- impaired memory function.

### Improving your sleep

As the quantity of sleep is largely a direct result of the choices an individual makes, it may be necessary to improve time management, prioritise tasks and activities that need to be completed during the day or even make some sacrifices. Below are a few guidelines that can be followed to enhance the quality of sleep:

- Avoid alcoholic drinks and caffeine near bedtime.
- Don't eat a heavy meal within three hours of bedtime.
- Try some exercise such as aerobics or a brisk walk earlier in the day.
- Don't be tempted to have a snooze during the day.
- Try relaxation techniques or meditation.
- Keep bed a place for sleep, not watching TV!
- Eat foods high in magnesium. Magnesium deficiency can lead to sleep disturbances.
- Supplement your diet with magnesium-rich foods such as nuts, cereals and green leafy vegetables.

**EXAMINER'S TIP**

In your exam you will need to comment upon the role of exercise in the pursuit of a healthy and fulfilling lifestyle.

**Activity 6**

You have been asked to prescribe a 10-week exercise programme for a group of middle-aged men who have been relatively inactive for some years.

1 What factors do you need to consider in preparing the programme?
2 State the type of exercises you would include and give reasons for your choices.

## Exam-style questions

**1** What is coronary heart disease? (1 mark)

**2** Give four major factors associated with increased risk of coronary heart disease. (4 marks)

**3** How might changes in lifestyle go some way towards preventing coronary heart disease? (6 marks)

## What you need to know

* Fitness is the ability to carry out everyday activities without undue fatigue.
* Health is the state of physical, social and mental well-being, where we are free from disease.
* Fitness is difficult to define as everybody has different ideas of what it means to be 'fit'.
* Fitness requirements differ tremendously between athletes and activities.
* Health-related components of fitness are largely physiologically based and include strength, speed, cardiorespiratory endurance, muscular endurance, flexibility and body composition.
* Skill-related components of fitness include agility, balance, co-ordination, reaction time and power and are dependent upon the interaction of the nervous system with the muscular system.
* Maximal oxygen uptake of $VO_2$ max is the maximum amount of oxygen that can be taken in, transported and consumed by the working muscles per minute. It is the best predictor of aerobic capacity and can only increase through training by 10–20 per cent since it has a 93 per cent genetic component.
* There are 3 dimensions of strength, maximum strength, elastic strength and strength endurance.
* The lifestyle choices we make will have an impact upon our health and fitness.
* Lifestyle choices include: exercise/activity levels; smoking; diet; alcohol consumption; work/life balance and quantity/quality of sleep.
* Making poor lifestyle choices such as smoking, inactivity, consuming a diet high in fat and getting the work/life balance wrong can lead to one of more cardiovascular diseases.
* Cardiovascular disease is the main cause of death in Western society and comes in many guises including: coronary heart disease, atherosclerosis and hypertension.

* Exercise can play a key role in preventing cardio-vascular disease:
  - reduces blood pressure
  - maintains elasticity of the blood vessels
  - promotes the production of HDLs which prevent the laying down of fatty deposits
  - Instills the feel-good factor and reduces stress.

## Review Questions

1 Identify two physical fitness components and two motor fitness components that will be required in **a)** sprint running, and **b)** gymnastics. Give details of when each component will be needed within the activity.

2 Identify two tests to assess each of: **a)** muscular endurance, **b)** aerobic capacity. State how each can be evaluated.

3 Explain the division of physical fitness into general fitness and specific fitness.

4 What physiological factors contribute to aerobic capacity of an individual?

5 The structure of the female cardiorespiratory system differs from that of the male. What effects does this have on the endurance performance of a female when compared with that of a male?

6 Outline the factors that determine the flexibility of an individual.

7 Explain when a gymnast might use each of the 3 dimensions of strength.

8 What physiological factors determine the speed of a performer?

9 What impact does smoking have on the health and fitness of an individual?

10 Briefly outline the factors that can contribute to the development of cardio-vascular disease.

11 How does exercise limit the progress of cardiovascular disease?

# CHAPTER 2

# Nutrition and performance

## Learning outcomes

**By the end of this chapter you should be able to:**

- name the seven classes of nutrient and for each state their role in exercise;
- explain the concept of a balanced diet;
- compare the different dietary requirements of an endurance performer and a power athlete;
- define obesity and identify the problems associated with its definition;
- show the relationship between weight control and the energy balance of food and exercise;
- assess measures of nutritional suitability and body composition.

## CHAPTER INTRODUCTION

In addition to following a well-planned and organised training programme, it is widely recognised that diet and nutrition are vital to successful performance. Many athletes now employ the services of nutritional experts in striving to be at the peak of their physical capacities.

Since the physical demands of training and competition on the athlete are high, much research has been undertaken concerning the extent to which diet can ease these demands. This chapter will explore the dietary requirements of the high-level performer, and the use of diet as an ergogenic performance-enhancing aid (through supplementation and diet manipulation).

## Nutritional effects upon performance

Whatever the sport or activity, nutrition is of great importance. A well-balanced diet is essential for optimum performance in both training and during competition. Athletes place enormous demands on their bodies when competing at the highest level, and to enable the body to function at its peak during the daily training regimes, an adequate diet is needed. Not only should the athlete's diet be designed to provide the energy required during exercise, but it should also provide the necessary nutrients for tissue growth and repair and those needed to keep the human machine functioning at its optimal level.

**Key terms**

**Ergogenic aid:** Any substance, method or object used by a sports performer with the aim of improving athletic performance.

Essentially there are seven groups of nutrients that should be included in the athlete's diet:

1 Carbohydrate
2 Fat
3 Protein
4 Vitamins
5 Minerals
6 Water
7 Dietary fibre.

## Carbohydrate

Carbohydrate comes in various forms, including:

- simple sugars (glucose, fructose)
- complex starches (rice, pasta, potatoes).

Carbohydrate is vital to the athlete since it is the primary energy fuel (particularly during high-intensity exercise), it is essential for the nervous system to function properly and also determines fat metabolism in the body. Intake should comprise approximately 65 per cent of the athlete's diet.

Carbohydrate is stored in the muscles and liver as glycogen, but the amount that can be stored here is limited (approximately 450g which is sufficient for 90 minutes of exercise) and therefore regular refuelling is needed. Excellent sources of carbohydrate include cereals, fruit and vegetables and confectionery – the latter should be included in the athlete's diet only in moderation.

Carbohydrates are absorbed by the body at different rates. The glycaemic index (GI) is an indication of the absorption rates of different foodstuffs. Foods with a high glycaemic index are absorbed and used rapidly by the body and can cause blood glucose levels to fall very quickly. Consuming an energy bar or fizzy drink just prior to exercise may give you an immediate energy buzz, but this will be short-lived. Foods with a low glycaemic index, however, are absorbed at a much slower rate and break down to release energy more steadily, so that blood glucose levels are maintained for longer. Foods with a low GI include porridge, beans, pulses and nuts. An understanding of the glycaemic index of foods is therefore vital to the coach since it ensures that the athlete has consumed and stored adequate energy reserves.

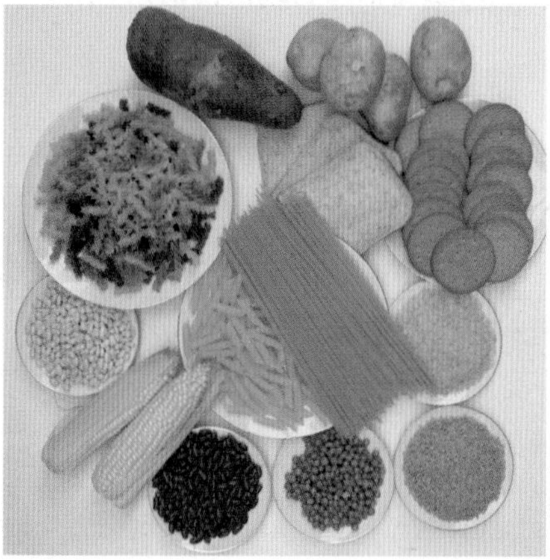

**Figure 2.1** Good sources of carbohydrate include brown bread, wholewheat pasta and some fruit and vegetables

**Key terms**

**Glycogen:** The stored form of carbohydrate in the body – usually in the muscles and liver. Glycogen is initially converted to glucose to release energy for athletic performance.
**Glycaemic index (GI):** A measure of the effect different foods have on blood glucose levels. Foods with a high GI produce a rapid rise in blood glucose, while those with a low GI release glucose more gradually into the bloodstream.

## Fat

Fat is also a major source of energy in the body, particularly during low-intensity exercise such as endurance activities. Up to 70 per cent of our energy is derived from fat during our resting state.

Typically fat exists in the body as:

- triglycerides (the stored form of fat); or
- fatty acids (the usable form of fat for energy production).

When sufficient oxygen is available to the muscle cell, fatty acids constitute the favoured fuel for energy production, as the body tries to spare the limited stores of glycogen for higher intensity bouts of exercise which can delay the effects of fatigue. This is known as glycogen sparing. Through training, the body adapts by increasing its ability to use fat as a fuel. The body, however, cannot use fat as its sole fuel source, due to its low solubility in the blood. This means that transportation of fat to the muscle cell is slow and so energy production in the muscle is usually fuelled by a combination of glycogen and fat.

One explanation for marathon runners 'hitting the wall' is that glycogen stores are completely depleted and the body attempts to supply all the energy required by metabolising fat alone. The hydrophobic (low water solubility) quality of fat, however, inhibits this metabolism, energy production is slow and the muscles fail to contract. Furthermore, fat requires approximately 15 per cent more oxygen to metabolise than carbohydrates.

Eating fat alone does not improve the muscle's ability to use it as a fuel source and the problems associated with excessive fat consumption are well documented.

It is recommended, therefore, that the athlete should keep the consumption of fatty foods low (at a maximum of 30 per cent of total calories consumed), which will ensure adequate energy stores, good health and a greater proportion of calorie intake to be supplied by carbohydrate.

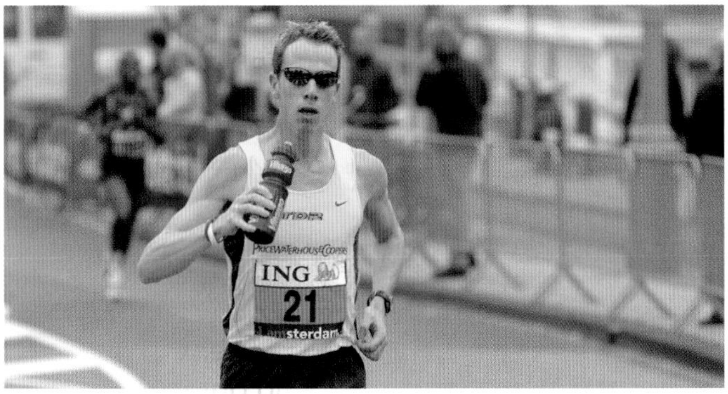


Figure 2.2 Glycogen and fats form the preferred fuel during endurance activity

**Key term**

**Fatty acids:** The body's preferred fuel during endurance-based activity, where there is an abundance of oxygen available.

## Protein

Proteins are chemical compounds composed of chains of amino acids. They provide the building blocks for tissue growth and repair (including muscle tissue), produce enzymes, hormones and haemoglobin, and can provide energy when glycogen and fat stores are low.

Typically protein should constitute approximately 15 per cent of total calorie intake or approximately 1.5g protein/kg of body weight per day should be sufficient for most sportspeople. Good sources include meat, fish, poultry, dairy products and beans and pulses.

The value of protein supplementation as an ergogenic aid remains unclear, but it is generally thought that sufficient protein can be gained from the athlete's diet. Excessive protein consumption may in fact pose some health risks, as the kidneys may become overworked in excreting any unused amino acids.

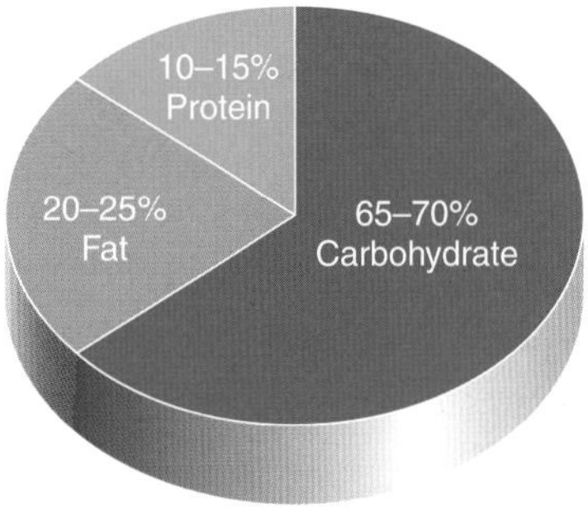


Figure 2.3 The recommended proportion of energy providing nutrients in an athlete's diet

## Vitamins

Vitamins are chemical compounds required in only small amounts by the body. However, they perform a vital role in energy production and metabolism.

Generally the body can gain the required amounts of vitamins through a well-balanced diet. Vitamins are largely found in fresh fruit and vegetables and wholegrain cereals, although some athletes believe that supplementation will enhance energy production and subsequently lead to improved athletic performance. Taking a multivitamin pill may prove useful as a precaution for some athletes, but megadoses of up to 100 times the recommended daily allowance are definitely not necessary and may in fact cause some health problems.

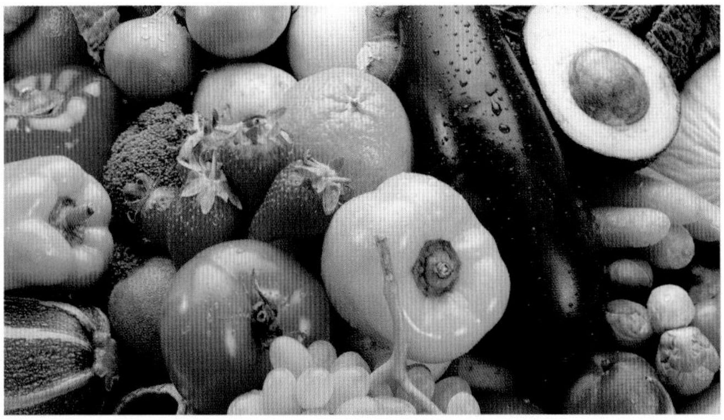

Figure 2.4 Many of our vitamins can be gained through consuming at least 5 portions of fruit and vegetables a day

## Minerals

These nutrients are also required in relatively small amounts by the body, but are vital for tissue functioning. Many of the minerals are dissolved by the body as ions and are called electrolytes. These have the important function of maintaining the permeability of the cell. They also aid the transmission of nerve impulses and enable effective muscle contraction.

Many minerals may be lost through sweating during exercise. These must be replaced quickly and there is now a vast array of fluid replacement products on the market designed for just that purpose.

**Key term**

**Electrolytes:** Mineral ions in the body which maintain the electrical charge of cell membranes. This maintains the effectiveness of muscle contraction and firing of nerve impulses. Electrolytes can be lost from the body through sweat and must therefore be replaced by drinking isotonic sports drinks.

## Water

Water is a nutrient whose importance is sometimes neglected. It is essential for the sportsperson, as it carries nutrients to and removes waste products from the body's cells, and helps to control body temperature. Water makes up about 50–60 per cent of a young person's body weight, up to a third of which is contained in the blood plasma. Plasma carries oxygen via the red blood cells to the working muscles, transports nutrients such as glucose and fatty acids, transports hormones vital to metabolism and removes waste products such as $CO_2$ and lactic acid.

Water loss through sweating is accelerated during prolonged exercise and in hot conditions, and it is essential that this fluid is replaced in order to maintain a good state of hydration. Dehydration of as little as 2 per cent of body weight will have a detrimental effect on performance. Even small losses of water can impair performance and adversely affect work capacity in a number of ways. These include:

- reducing the efficiency of the circulatory functioning, largely by a drop in blood pressure, which reduces blood flow to the active muscles;

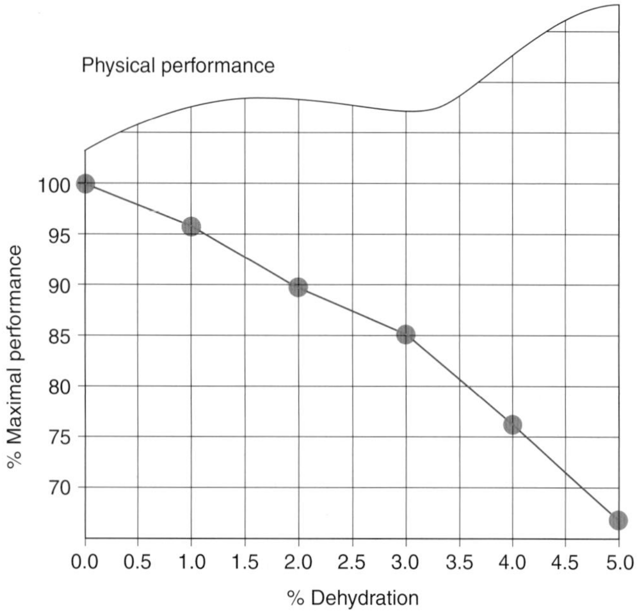


**Figure 2.5** Dehydration index

- inhibiting the thermoregulatory centre, which can lead to problems such as heat stroke;
- the loss of electrolytes such as sodium, chloride and potassium. Although it was once believed that this loss may induce muscle cramps, it is still an area of contention; many studies show that such losses may not have a direct effect on performance.

In order to maintain optimal performance, rehydration is essential. Drinks with a carbohydrate content of more than 6 per cent can be consumed before and following exercise to top up the body's energy and fluid stores, while drinks with a carbohydrate content of less than 6 per cent can be consumed during exercise to prevent dehydration. Sports drinks have been developed

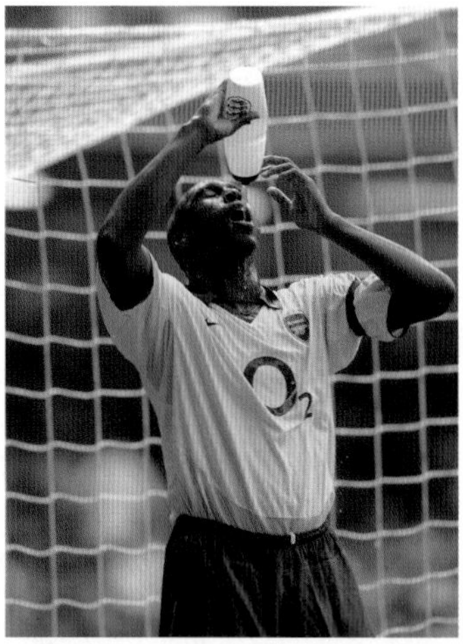

**Figure 2.6** Rehydration is essential to maintain effective performance

to cater for the needs of specific athletes. Isotonic drinks, such as Lucozade Sport, replace fluids and electrolytes lost through sweating and can boost glucose levels in the blood. Hypertonic drinks have a much greater concentration of carbohydrate and are normally used following exercise to increase glycogen stores.

## Dietary fibre

Dietary fibre, or roughage, should be an essential part of every athlete's diet. Fibre is found in all plant cells and is part of a plant that cannot be entirely digested. As such it causes a bulk in the intestine, absorbing many times its weight in water and helping the whole digestion and excretion process. Good sources of fibre include nuts, vegetables, beans and pulses.

**Table 2.1** The role of nutrients in exercise

| **Category of nutrient** | **Exercise-related role** |
|---|---|
| Carbohydrate | The principal role of carbohydrates during exercise is to maintain a constant supply of energy to the muscles which will enable them to contract throughout the duration of the exercise period. |
| Fat | Fats are the major source of energy during low-intensity exercise. They will be used in conjunction with carbohydrates to sustain muscle contraction. By absorbing fat-soluble vitamins such as Vitamin A, D, E and K, which help to form enzymes, fats can also contribute to energy release. When exercising in colder environments, adipose tissue (the layer of fat underneath the skin) can offer some insulation and barrier against the cold. |
| Protein | The major function of protein really starts once exercise has been completed. The growth and repair of tissues for example can really occur only inbetween training sessions. Protein's secondary role as an energy provider, however, will certainly occur during exercise. Up to 10 per cent of energy is supplied by protein during endurance activities such as an iron-man triathlon. A further role of protein in energy production is its contribution to the manufacture of enzymes and hormones responsible for energy release. Furthermore, proteins also contribute to oxygen transportation in the body as they provide the amino acids necessary for the production of haemoglobin and myoglobin – our oxygen transporters. |
| Vitamins | Vitamins perform a vital role in energy production as they help to manufacture energy-releasing enzymes. Vitamins also contribute to the maintenance of a robust immune system, which enables a performer to train maximally and recover quickly between training sessions. |
| Minerals | Minerals contribute to successful exercise performance in many ways. Iron, for example, is the main constituent of haemoglobin and myoglobin, which both help to transport oxygen around the body, while sodium, potassium and chloride are electrolytes of the body and provide the energy for life itself. Electrolytes maintain the electrical charge of cell membranes, which enables them to perform their normal functions such as allowing nerve cells to control muscle contraction. Another mineral, calcium, facilitates muscle contraction and nerve transmission, while phosphorous helps to create a continuous supply of energy by helping to maintain levels of the body's energy store adenosine triphosphate and creatine phosphate. |
| Water | As the body's major component, water is an essential ingredient for successful exercise performance. As the main constituent of the blood, water provides the means of transport in the body for all that is required to produce energy such as oxygen, nutrients, hormones and enzymes. Similarly, water makes the disposal of harmful waste products and toxins resulting from exercise possible. Water is also fundamental in the maintenance and regulation of the core temperature of the body – particularly important when exercising in warm environments. |
| Dietary fibre | A diet high in fibre can help maintain blood glucose levels by reducing the rate of glucose take-up as well as reducing the body's absorption of fat and cholesterol, thereby reducing the risk of vascular diseases and promoting health. |

## Activity 1

Make a list of everything you eat during one day. Try to work out the relative percentages of carbohydrate, fat and protein you consume. How does this compare with the expected values for an athlete?

# The balanced diet

A diet that contains a variety of foodstuffs is likely to contain all the essential nutrients a performer needs rather than one which focuses on just one or two different food groups. No single food group will provide all the essential nutrients the body needs to maintain health and function optimally. So it should be the aim of each performer to eat a variety of foods from each category in order to train, compete and recover effectively – it is just a matter of getting the balance right.

The nutrition pyramid has been developed to help athletes plan their diets. Food groups towards the base of the pyramid should be a major component of the diet, while those towards the top should feature less often. The nutrition pyramid is illustrated in Figure 2.7.

### Key terms

**Balanced diet:** A diet which contains all seven of the essential nutrients. For a diet to be balanced it needs to be varied, and the more varied your diet, the more likely you are to benefit from all the nutrients you need to optimise performance.

# The athlete's diet

What you eat before, during and after exercise will have a direct effect on how you perform, either in training or in competition. There is no one-size-fits-all diet for all sports performers; rather, the performer's diet must be specifically developed according to the demands of their particular sporting activity.

Undoubtedly the chief ingredient in every athlete's diet will be carbohydrate, which is stored in the body as glycogen. However consumption of all 7 nutrients is essential for effective performance (outlined in Table 2.1).

Not only is the content of the diet important for the athlete but also its organisation. Research points to the athlete having 4–6 small meals a day rather than 2–3 larger ones. This ensures that muscle and liver glycogen stores are kept topped up throughout the day.

On the day of competition or if there is going to be a particularly hard training session, the athlete should eat a meal high in carbohydrate 3–4 hours before competing, to keep blood glucose levels high for the duration of the competition.

For those involved in heats or bouts of work over the day, it will be necessary to top up glycogen stores by consuming small amounts of carbohydrate through snacks such as dried fruit or one of the many carbohydrate drinks on the market. Fluids such as water should also be taken during competition to prevent dehydration.

Table 2.2 Getting the balance right – A guide to what and how much to eat

| Category of food | Examples of foodstuffs | Portions per day |
|---|---|---|
| Vegetables | Broccoli, carrots, green beans | 3–5 |
| Fruit | Bananas, apples, cherries | 2–4 |
| Carbohydrate-rich foods | Whole wheat pasta, baked potato | 4–6 |
| Protein-rich foods | Fish, lean red meat, quorn, beans and pulses | 2–4 |
| Calcium-rich foods | Cheese, milk | 2–4 |
| Healthy fats | Avocados, olive oil, oily fish | 1–2 |
| Junk food | Cakes, biscuits | 1 |

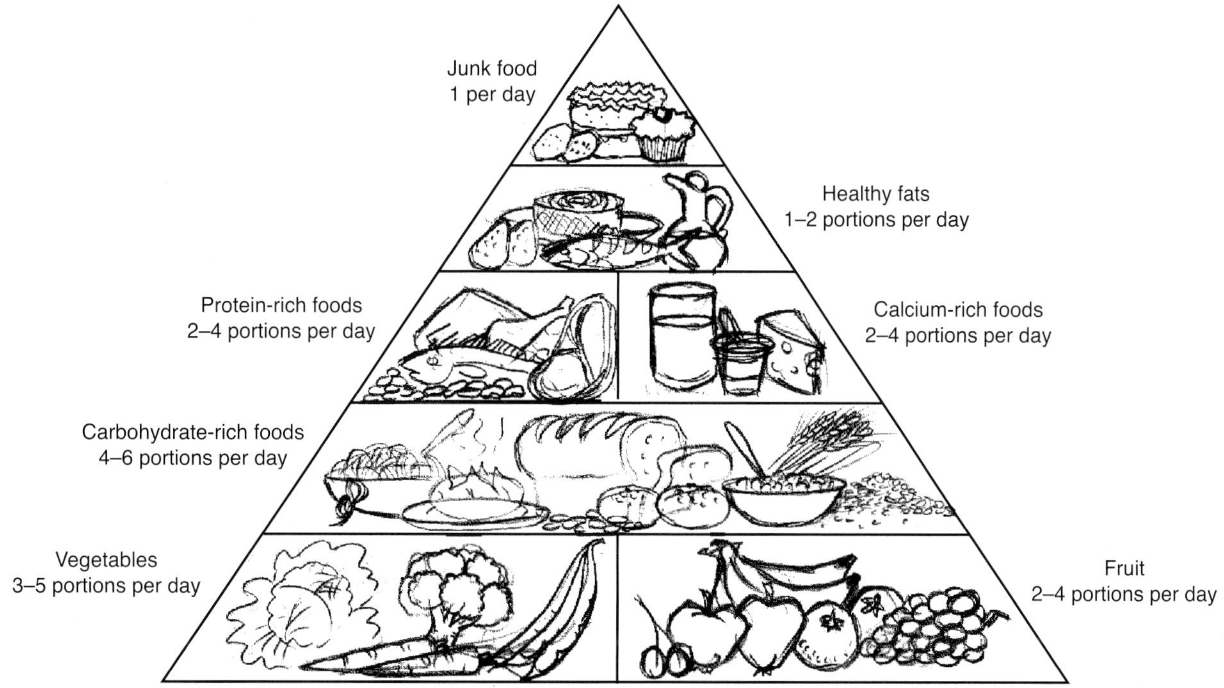


**Figure 2.7** The nutrition pyramid

**Table 2.3** A recommended carbohydrate loading regiment

| | |
|---|---|
| Day 1 | moderately long exercise bout (should not be exhaustive) |
| Day 2 | mixed diet; moderate carbohydrate intake; tapering exercise |
| Day 3 | mixed diet; moderate carbohydrate intake; tapering exercise |
| Day 4 | mixed diet; moderate carbohydrate intake; tapering exercise |
| Day 5 | high-carbohydrate diet; tapering exercise |
| Day 6 | high-carbohydrate diet; tapering exercise or rest |
| Day 7 | high-carbohydrate diet; tapering exercise or rest |
| Day 8 | competition |

Note: the moderate carbohydrate intake should approximate 200–300g of carbohydrate per day; the high carbohydrate intake should approximate 500–600g of carbohydrate per day.

*Source*: Williams, 1989

Following the competition or training, it is necessary to refuel the body as soon as possible in order to resynthesise muscle and liver glycogen stores. A high-carbohydrate meal should be eaten within 45–60 minutes of the cessation of the exercise to start this refuelling process. Intake of protein-rich foods will also help tissue repair. Water and isotonic supplements should also be taken to replenish what has been lost through sweating and aid in rehydration.

When planning their diet the sports performer must take into account many factors, such as the amount of training they do; in this way they can ensure that they are eating the best foods for fuelling their performance and promoting their recovery effectively. To this end we might expect the dietary requirements of an endurance performer to be very different to that of a power athlete.

## The endurance athlete

Athletes undertaking daily endurance training sessions need a very high energy intake through eating carbohydrate-rich foods, which should form up to 60–70 per cent of total energy intake.

The marathon runner will often seek to manipulate dietary intake before competition in order to optimise performance. One method of doing this is by glycogen loading or supercompensation. This process involves depleting the glycogen levels 7 days prior to the event through endurance-based training, then starving the body of carbohydrate over the following three days. For the remaining days leading up to competition the athlete will consume high-carbohydrate meals to boost muscle glycogen stores up to twice that normally stored.

This method of manipulation is widely practised in endurance events and maximises energy production via the aerobic pathway. Recent research has shown, however, that total depletion of glycogen may not be necessary for trained athletes. The three days of carbohydrate starvation will cause great fatigue, and lead to an increased risk of injury and possible kidney problems. Simply resting for three days prior to competition and eating high-carbohydrate meals may maximise glycogen stores. It is important to point out, however, that storage of glycogen requires a greater ingestion of water and so water intake must increase accordingly. This will obviously be of use anyhow to the athlete, since it will help prevent dehydration during the endurance race.

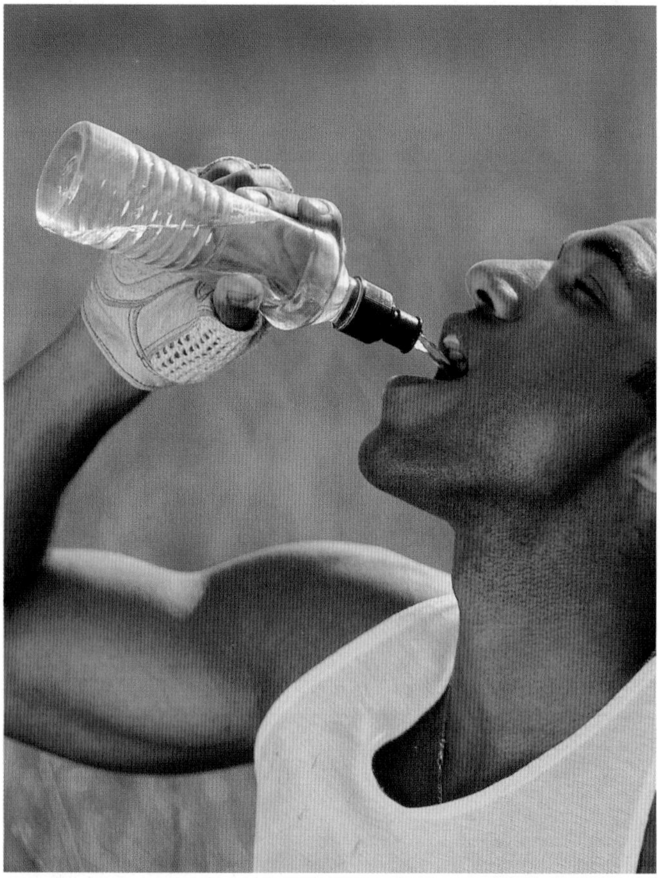

Figure 2.8 Athletes who typically compete for over 90 minutes may need to boost their muscle glycogen stores through glycogen loading

In fact, endurance athletes should take on board between 150–200ml of fluid every 15–20 minutes during the exercise period to remain hydrated and help replace the electrolytes lost through sweating.

**Key terms**

**Glycogen loading:** The manipulation of an athlete's intake of carbohydrate prior to competition so that muscle glycogen stores increase over and above that which can normally be stored. Glycogen loading is typically followed by endurance performers who exercise in excess of 90 minutes.

### Advantages

- increased glycogen synthesis
- increased muscle stores of glycogen
- increased endurance capacity
- delays fatigue and enhances endurance performance.

### Disadvantages

- water retention and bloating
- weight increase
- muscle stiffness, fatigue and tiredness
- depression and irritability during the depletion phase.

A suggested glycogen loading regime is outlined in Table 2.3

## The power athlete

As power athletes train at high intensities several times a day, glycogen remains the preferred fuel during the training session and so they too need a diet that is high in carbohydrates in order to maintain levels of muscle glycogen. However, due to the explosive nature of power events, sprinters

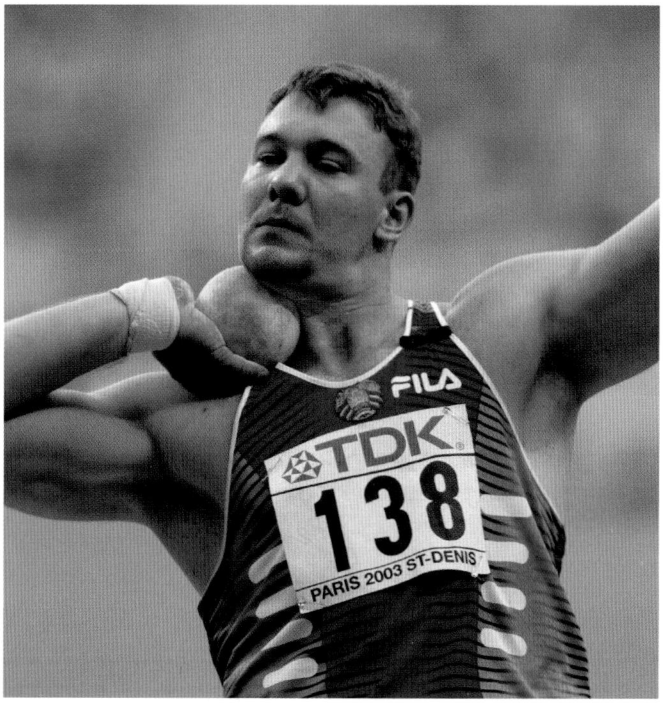


Figure 2.9 Power athletes such as shot-putters need to ensure their diet contains sufficient protein to optimise the growth and repair of muscle tissue

and shot-putters will need to ensure that they are consuming sufficient quantities of protein, which will be used to help the body recover from the high-intensity training sessions and competition.

Power-based training can cause damage to muscle and the surrounding connective tissues, so a high-protein diet is required to promote the growth and repair of the damaged tissues. Power athletes also rely on the high-energy compound creatine phosphate to provide energy during activities that are explosive and of high intensity. These performers will therefore wish to include in their diet foodstuffs that are high in natural sources of creatine (such as lean red meat, eggs and fish) in order sustain all-out activity for longer and speed up the recovery process.

**Key terms**

**Creatine:** A high-energy compound found naturally in the body that provides the body's energy during explosive events such as sprinting. Some athletes seek to enhance the natural sources of creatine found in some foods through creatine monohydrate supplementation.

## Exam-style questions

1. In what ways should the diet of a triathlete differ from that of a shot-putter? Give reasons for your answer. (3 marks)
2. A well-balanced diet will include minerals such as calcium and iron. What are the physiological benefits to the sports performer of a diet rich in calcium and iron? (3 marks)
3. In what form is carbohydrate stored in the body and where is it stored? (2 marks)
4. What are the principles of carbo-loading and how should a performer follow a carbo-loading regime? (4 marks)

# Obesity and weight control – getting the energy balance right

## Obesity and weight control

Obesity is a condition which accompanies a sedentary or inactive lifestyle, and is an excessive increase in the body's total quantity of fat.

One method frequently used to estimate the extent of obesity is the Body Mass Index (BMI). This does not solely consider a person's weight, but also takes into account body composition. A person's BMI can be calculated by dividing body weight in kilograms by the square of body height in metres. It is assumed that the higher the BMI, the greater the level of 'adiposity' or fat. Critical values of BMI are 27.8 for males and 27.3 for females, and scores above these figures assume a person is overweight or if it exceeds 30kg/m$^2$, obese. For example:

- A man weighing 110 kg and measuring 1.83 m in height will have a BMI of 33 kg/m$^2$.

**EXAMINER'S TIP**

A BMI of 30 or above defines obesity.

**Activity 2**

1 Calculate your body mass index.
2 Compare it with results from the rest of your group and comment upon your findings.

BMI figures published by the Obesity Resource information show that over the past 20 years incidence of obesity has trebeled in the UK population and now lies at 21.5% of the population.

Obesity can lead to an increased risk of cardiovascular diseases such as atherosclerosis, hypertension, heart disease and strokes. Other complications may include the development of gall bladder disease and diabetes. This is characterised by increased blood sugar levels, resulting from insufficient insulin production from the pancreas. Furthermore, the obese person now has the psychological problems of dealing with the social stigma of an unacceptable body shape and size and this in turn can lead to a poor self-image and depression.

We do, however need to be a little careful when using BMI as a measure of obesity as it does not distinguish between fat-mass and fat-free mass (muscle and bones). Consequently, a very muscular rugby player may be classed as obese even if he has very low body fat!

## The control of body weight

The rate at which the body uses energy is termed the metabolic rate, and is an important factor in weight control. At rest the body still requires energy; the rate of energy expenditure at rest is known as the basal metabolic rate and may vary from 1,200–2,400 Kcal per day.

The amount of food required by an individual above that which is required for the body's essential physiological functions, is dependent upon the amount of physical activity in which the individual is engaged throughout the day.

For body weight to remain constant, energy *input* via food must equal energy *expenditure*. This is the basis of weight control and is known as the energy equation. Too much food consumed for energy requirement will lead to a positive energy balance and a gain in weight. Conversely, if energy expenditure is greater than the energy derived from the food consumed, a negative energy balance occurs, the body will draw upon its energy stores in the form of fat, and a decrease in weight will be seen.

In order to cure obesity, it is necessary to shift the energy balance from a positive to a negative one, so that energy expenditure is greater than energy input. The body will then draw upon its fat stores for the missing calories; as fat mobilisation and consumption occurs, body weight decreases. The formation of a negative energy balance is best achieved by a combination of decreased calorie intake and increased activity.

Other benefits of performing exercise as part of a weight control programme include the suppression of appetite, and an increase in the resting metabolic rate, which assumes that more calories are used up in the body even if exercise is not taking place!

The best type of exercise to perform in order to lose weight would be aerobic exercise, using large muscle groups that continues for a minimum of 30 minutes. It is also ideal to prescribe non- or partial-weight bearing activities such as swimming or cycling for the overweight individual, since this will prevent undue stress being placed on the joints.

**Table 2.4** Energy expenditure in different sports

| Sport | Duration | Energy expenditure |
|---|---|---|
| Swimming | 60 mins | 5/25 kcal/min |
| Jogging | 30 mins | 7–9 kcal/min |
| Soccer | 90 mins | 9 kcal/min |
| Rugby | 80 mins | 6–9 kcal/min |
| Tennis | 60 mins | 6–9 kcal/min |
| Sprinting | 15 secs | 90 kcal/min |

**Key terms**

**Obesity:** A condition which accompanies over-consumption and an inactive lifestyle. An imbalance between energy intake and expenditure exists which results in an excessive increase in the body's total quantity of fat. A person is classed as obese when their BMI exceeds 30.

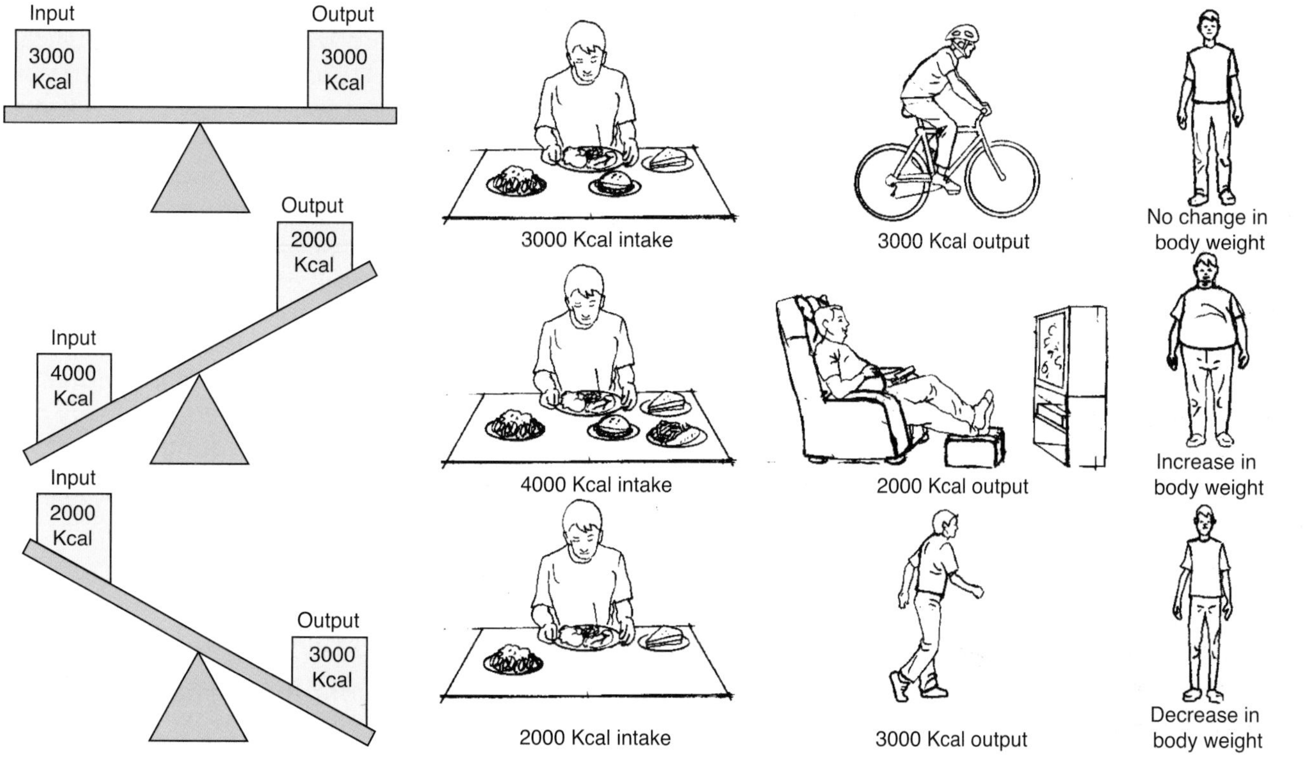


**Figure 2.10** The energy equation

# Assessing body composition

## Body composition

Body composition is concerned with the physiological make-up of the body with regard to the relative amounts and distribution of muscle and fat. Body composition is commonly defined as:

> **'...the component parts of the body in terms of the relative amounts of body fat compared to lean body mass...'**

For an average 18 year old, men range from 14–17 per cent fat, while women range from 24–29 per cent. Body composition has an important role for elite athletes and more generally in health and well-being. Excessive body fat can lead to obesity and the associated complications such as cardiovascular diseases. For the athlete, high body fat can result in a reduction in muscle efficiency and contributes to greater energy expenditure, since more weight requires more energy to move around and a consequent increase in oxygen consumption. Body composition requirements vary with different sports, but generally the less fat the better. Muscle mass is desirable for those activities or sports that require muscular strength, power and endurance.

The relative shape of the body or somatotype can also be mentioned at this point. Somatotyping is a method used to measure body shape. Three extremes exist:

1 Endomorphy – the relative fatness or pear-shapeness of the body.
2 Mesomorphy – the muscularity of the body.
3 Ectomorphy – the linearity or leanness of the body.

The characteristics of a performer's body can be categorised according to these somatotypes and plotted on the delta-shaped graph.

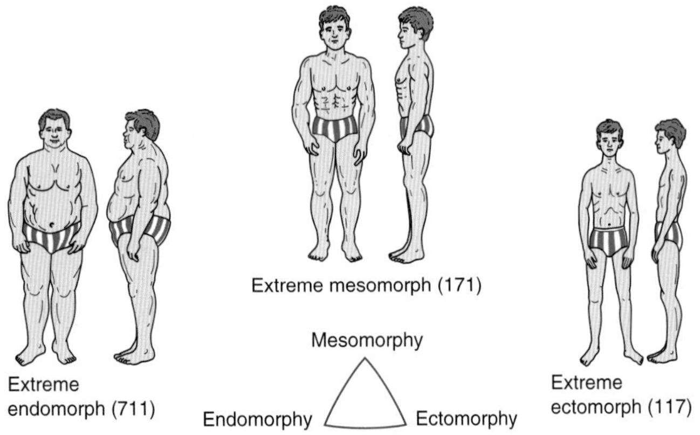


**Figure 2.11** Somatotyping: the three extremes of body type

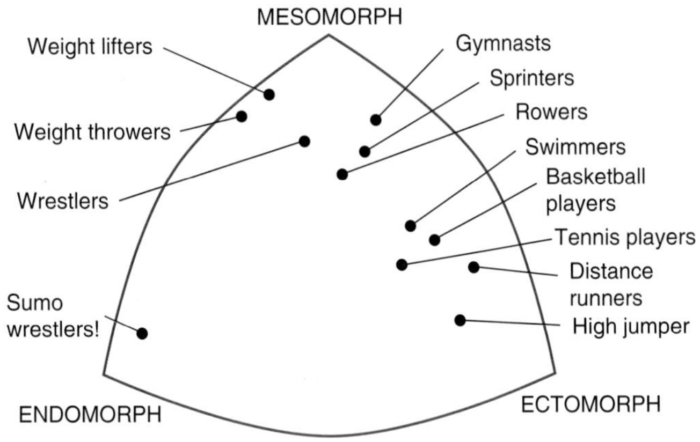


**Figure 2.12** Somatotyping relates body composition to sporting activity

It is rare that an individual would be classed as an extreme endo, meso or ectomorph at the apex of the delta. More realistically they would possess characteristics of all three, but the relative contributions of each somatotype would differ depending upon the activity. For example, rowers tend to be very lean yet very muscular, with little body fat, and are placed accordingly (see Figure 2.12).

## Measuring body composition

Body composition is measured in a variety of ways:

1 Hydrostatic weighing considers water displacement when the body is submerged in water, but requires a large hydrostatic weighing tank, and a knowledge of the subject's residual volume is required for the calculation.

2 Bioelectrical impedance is another popular objective measure whereby a small electrical current is passed through the body from wrist to ankle. As fat restricts the flow of the current, the greater the current needed, the greater the percentage of body fat. Although this test requires specialist equipment, it is becoming more accessible with the introduction of simple scales which transmit an electrical current.

3 The most common and simplest measure of body fat is made through the Body Mass Index (BMI). Through calculation of an individual's BMI, body fat can be predicted. The body mass index is calculated by measuring the body mass of the subject (weight in kg) divided by the height (in metres) of the individual squared, i.e.:

$$\text{BMI} = \frac{\text{weight in kg}}{\text{height in m}^2}$$

The higher the score, the greater the levels of body fat.

| | |
|---|---|
| healthy | 20–25 |
| overweight | 25–29 |
| obese | +30 |

Although this test is very quick and a prediction can be made instantaneously, it can obviously be inaccurate since it does not make a difference between fat mass and muscle mass. So large, lean muscular athletes may well fall into the wrong category.

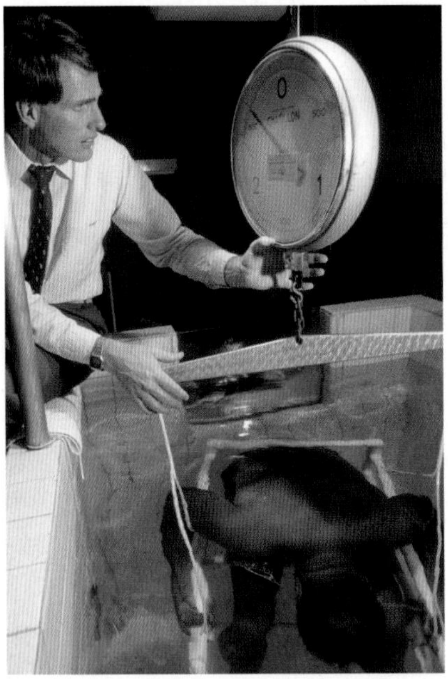

**Figure 2.13** A body composition assessment through hydrostatic weighing

4 Skinfold measures using callipers is by far the simplest measure. On the left side of the body, take measures at the following sites: You may wish to refer to Figure 2.14 to locate the sites.

- biceps brachii
- triceps brachi
- subscapular
- supra iliac.

Add together the totals in millimetres and record your results.

At this stage, you may wish to make some other anthropometrical measures such as length of bones and overall height, muscle girths or circumferences, and condyle measures at the joints.

## Key terms

**Body mass index:** A measure of body composition and a widely used indicator of obesity. It is calculated using the following formula:

$$\frac{\text{Weight in kg}}{\text{Height in m}^2}$$

Obesity is assumed in subjects with a BMI of 30 kg/m$^2$ or more.

**Biolectric impedance:** A test to assess body composition which measures the resistance to an electrical current passed through the body. The higher the reading, the higher the level of body fat as fat does conduct the current particularly effectively. This test is now used widely by coaches and athletes as it is simple and the equipment is relatively cheap.

## Exam-style questions

**1** What are the principles behind weight control? What types of exercise would promote fat metabolism and therefore be useful in a weight-control programme? (5 marks)

1. **Triceps brachii**
With the pupil's arm hanging loosely, a vertical fold is raised at the back of the arm, midway along a line connecting the acromion (shoulder) and olecranon (elbow) processes.

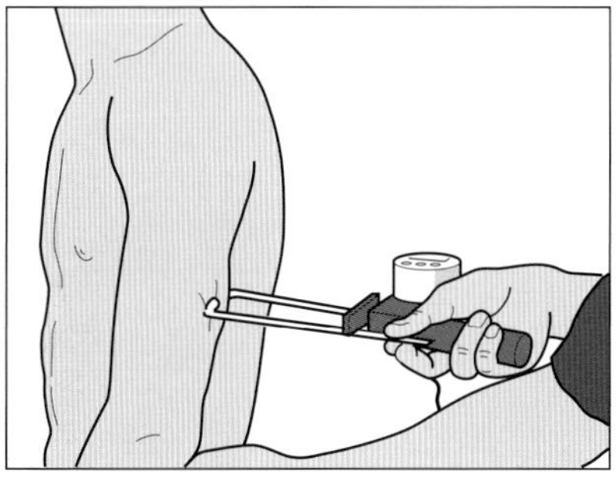

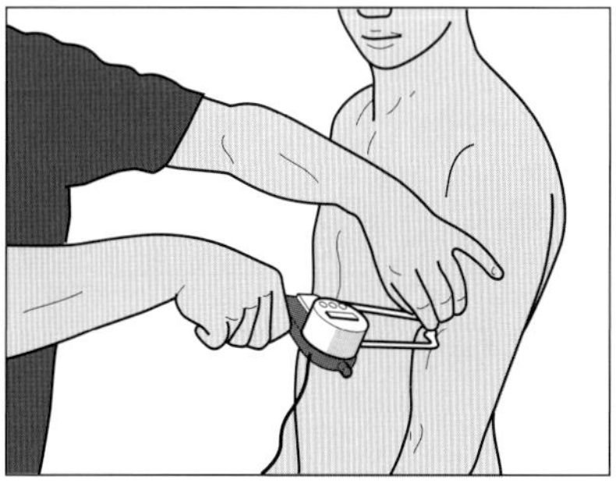

2. **Biceps brachii**
A vertical fold is raised at the front of the arm, opposite to the triceps site. This should be directly above the centre of the cubital fossa (fold of the elbow).

3. **Subscapular**
A fold is raised just beneath the inferior angle of the scapula (bottom of the shoulder-blade). This fold should be at an angle of 45 degrees downwards and outwards.

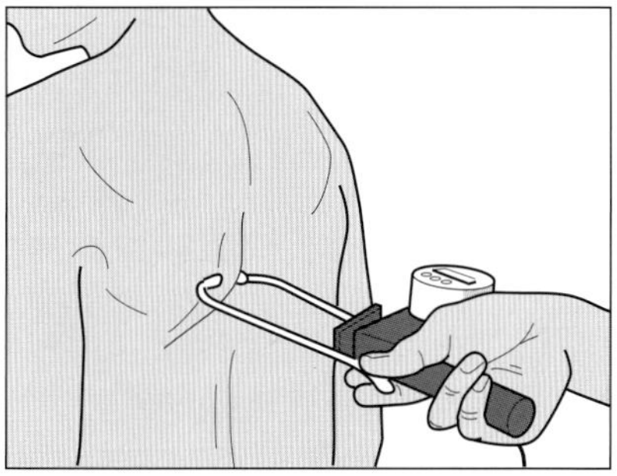

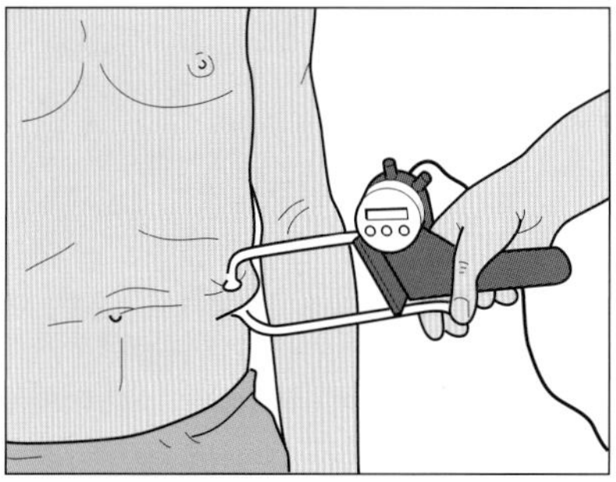

4. **Anterior suprailiac**
A fold is raised 5–7 cm above the spinale (pelvis), at a point in line the anterior axillary border (armpit). The fold should be in line with the natural folds downward and inwards at up to 45 degrees.

**Figure 2.14** Body fat measurements

## Activity 3

Study the table below, which shows a comparison of the rates of obesity worldwide. Using examples from the table, suggest reasons why the incidence of obesity varies so much from one country to another.

Percentage of people classified as obese

| | | % obese | |
|---|---|---|---|
| | | **female** | **male** |
| USA | 1999–2000 | 34 | 27.7 |
| Argentina | 1997 | 25.4 | 28.4 |
| Mexico | – | 25.1 | 14.9 |
| Russia | – | 25 | 10 |
| England | 2001 | 23.5 | 21.0 |
| Germany | 1991 | 19.3 | 17.2 |
| Finland | – | 19 | 20 |
| Spain | 1997 | 15.2 | 11.5 |
| Italy | 1999 | 9.9 | 9.5 |
| France | 1995–1996 | 7.0 | 8.0 |

NB: data are not necessarily directly comparable due to different years of survey and varying age ranges.

*Source*: Food Standards Agency

## What you need to know

* A well-balanced diet is essential for successful performance in sport both while training and in preparation for competition.
* Seven groups of nutrients should be included in an athlete's diet. These are carbohydrate, fat, protein, vitamins, minerals, water and dietary fibre.
* Carbohydrate in the form of sugars and starches is the main energy provider for the high-intensity athlete – it is stored in the muscles and the liver as glycogen.
* Fat is the major source of energy in the body and is mainly used during low-intensity, endurance-based activities. Stored fat is broken down into free fatty acids – its usable form. The body cannot use fat alone but uses a combination of fat and glycogen.

* Proteins are composed of amino acids, the body's building blocks. They are also an energy provider, but are used only when glycogen stores are very low.
* Vitamins can aid in the production of energy. Given a well-balanced diet there should be no need for supplementation.
* Minerals are vital for tissue functioning, transmission of nerve impulses and the enabling of effective muscle contraction.
* Water is an essential nutrient. Water loss during exercise can impair performance in a number of ways. It certainly contributes to heat stroke and can induce muscle cramps.
* Athletes should ensure that they receive adequate energy supplies. A high carbohydrate diet of approximately 60% of total energy intake is essential. Many small meals are better than two or three larger meals.
* Glycogen loading or super-compensation is a form of diet manipulation followed by endurance performers to ensure that glycogen stores of the body are at their greatest prior to a competition.
* Power-based performers will require a higher protein intake to promote recovery and enable the growth and repair of damaged muscle tissue
* Obesity is an excessive increase in the body's total quantity of fat:
  - A person is classed as obese when body fat exceeds 30%
  - Obesity can lead to an increased incidence of cardiovascular disease and obesity.
* The basis of weight control is the energy equation. A positive energy balance occurs when energy input exceeds energy output and results in an increase in weight. A negative energy balance occurs where energy input is less than energy output resulting in a decrease in weight
* Exercise increases energy output and so shifts towards a negative energy balance.
* Body composition can be defined as the component parts of the body in terms of the relative amounts of body fat compared to lean body mass.
* There are many tests of body composition, including bioelectric impedance, hydrostatic weighing, Body Mass Index (BMI), and skinfold measurement.

## Review Questions

1 What nutritional advice would you give to a triathlete both in training and preparing for competition?

2 Why might increased muscle glycogen stores increase performance? How would you increase the muscle glycogen stores of your athletes?

3 Explain how diet may be used as an ergogenic aid.

4 What are some of the effects on the body of dehydration? How does this affect performance in sport?

5 Why might consumption of sugary foods prior to competition lead to a decrease in performance?

6 What nutritional advice would you give to a hockey player, playing in a tournament that requires five or six games to be played in one day?

7 Outline the advantages and disadvantages of using fatty acids as a fuel during exercise.

8 With reference to exercise intensity, explain the fuel usage of a performer during an activity of varying intensity.

9 Summarize the role of each category of nutrient during exercise.

10 Evaluate the Body Mass Index as an assessment of obesity.

11 What do you understand by the energy equation? How does knowledge of the energy equation help the sports person?

12 What factors should be taken into account when designing an exercise programme for a person classed as obese?

CHAPTER

3

# Pulmonary function and the exchange of respiratory gases

## Learning outcomes

**By the end of this chapter you should be able to:**

- outline the structure of the respiratory system;
- describe the process of external respiration;
- explain the mechanics of breathing at rest and the respiratory muscles involved;
- describe the changes in the mechanics of breathing during physical activity and the respiratory muscles involved;
- explain how the respiratory control centre regulates the mechanics of breathing, at rest and during physical activity;
- outline the process of gaseous exchange that takes place between the alveoli and blood, and between the blood and tissue cells;
- explain the changes in gaseous exchange that take place between the alveoli and blood, and between the blood and tissue cells, as a direct result of participation in physical activity;
- give a critical evaluation of the impact of different types of physical activity on the respiratory system.

## CHAPTER INTRODUCTION

During exercise, the body requires oxygen to produce energy to fuel muscular contraction. It is the role of the respiratory system, in conjunction with the cardiovascular system, to ensure that sufficient oxygen is taken into the body and transferred to the body's tissues to satisfy the demand. Likewise, the respiratory system is also responsible for ensuring adequate removal of waste products such as carbon dioxide and lactic acid.

This chapter examines the structure and function of the respiratory system, with a particular focus on the changes that occur from rest to exercise. Featured areas of study include the mechanics of breathing, the regulation of breathing, and the gaseous exchange that takes place between the alveoli and blood, and between the blood and tissue cells.

# External respiration

External respiration involves the movement of gases into and out of the lungs. The exchange of gases between the lungs and the blood is known as pulmonary diffusion.

On its journey to the lungs, air drawn into the body passes through many structures, as outlined below and illustrated in Figure 3.1.

> **Key term**
>
> **External respiration:** The process of moving respiratory gases into and out of the lungs.

## Nasal passages

Air is drawn into the body via the nose. The nasal cavity is divided by a cartilaginous septum,

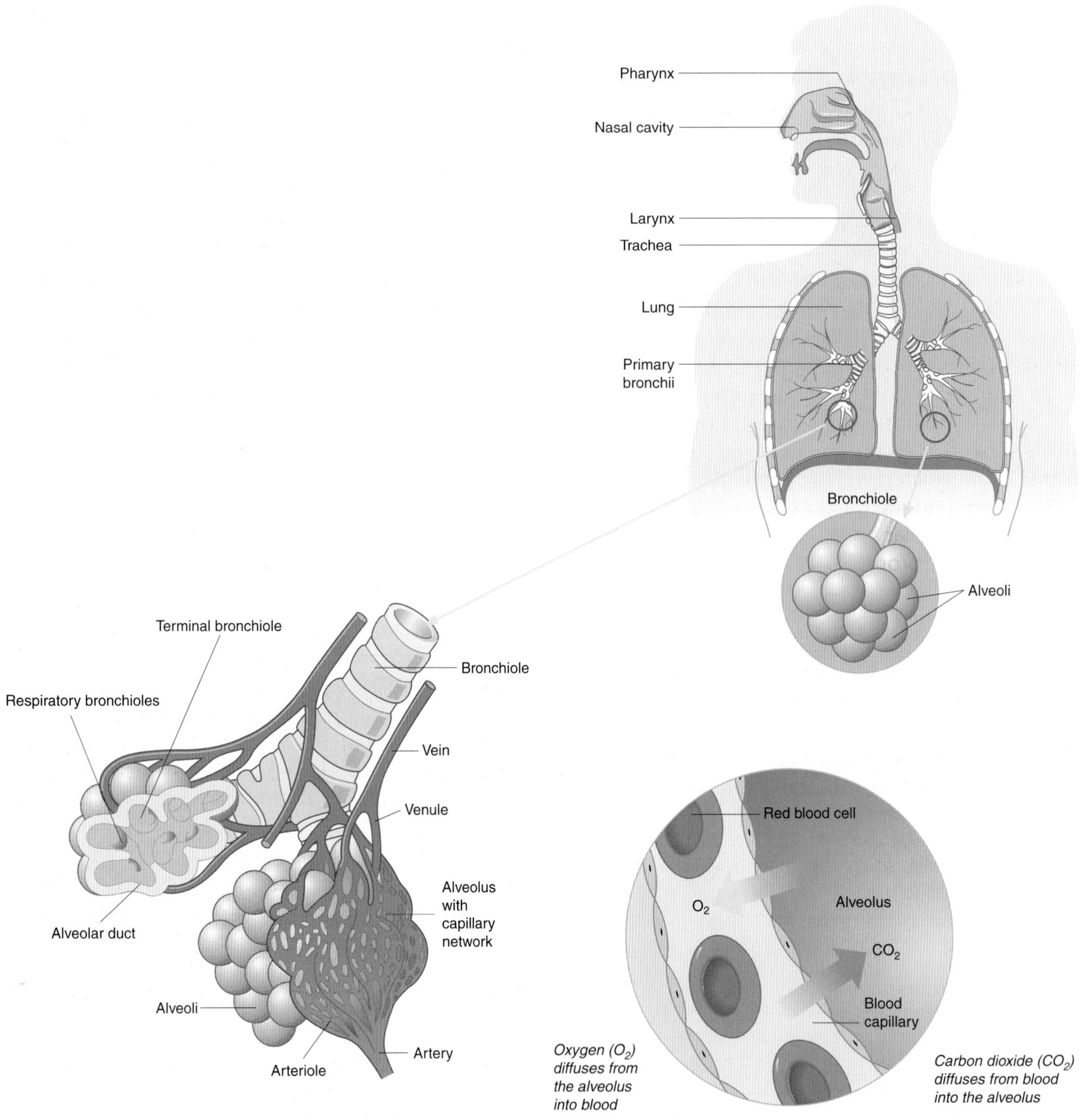


**Figure 3.1** The structure of the respiratory system

forming the nasal passages. The interior structures of the nose help the respiratory process by performing the following important functions:

1 The mucous membranes and blood capillaries moisten and warm the inspired air.
2 The ciliated epithelium filters and traps dust particles, which are moved to the throat for elimination.
3 The small bones known as chonchae increase the surface area of the cavity to make the process more efficient.

### The oral pharynx and larynx

The throat is shared by both the respiratory and alimentary tracts. Air entering the larynx passes over the vocal chords and into the trachea. In swallowing, the larynx is drawn upwards and forwards against the base of the epiglottis, thus preventing entry of food.

### The trachea

The trachea, or windpipe, is approximately 10cm in length and lies in front of the oesophagus. It is composed of 18 horseshoe-shaped rings of cartilage, which are also lined by a mucous membrane and ciliated cells, which provide the same protection against dust as in the nasal passageways. The trachea extends from the larynx and directs air into the right and left primary bronchi.

### The bronchi and bronchioles

The trachea divides into the right and left bronchi, which further subdivide into lobar bronchi (three feeding each lobe on the right, two feeding each lobe on the left). Further subdivision of these airways forms bronchioles, which in turn branch into the smaller terminal or respiratory bronchioles. The bronchioles enable the air to pass into the alveoli via the alveolar ducts, and it is here that pulmonary diffusion occurs.

### Alveoli

The alveoli are responsible for the exchange of gases between the lungs and the blood. The alveolar walls are extremely thin and are composed of epithelial cells, which are lined by a thin film of water, essential for dissolving oxygen from the inspired air.

Surrounding each alveolus is an extensive capillary network, which ensures a smooth passage of oxygen into the pulmonary capillaries. The tiny lumen of each capillary surrounding the alveoli ensures that red blood cells travel in single file, and that they are squeezed into a biconcave shape, increasing the surface area and enabling the greatest possible uptake of oxygen. It has been estimated that each lung contains up to 150 million alveoli, providing a tremendous surface area for the exchange of gases. The alveoli walls also contain elastic fibres, which further increase the surface during inspiration.

## The mechanics of breathing

The lungs are surrounded by pleural sacs containing pleural fluid, which reduces friction during respiration. These sacs are attached to both the lungs and the thoracic cage, which enables the lungs to inflate and deflate as the chest expands and flattens. The interrelationship between the lungs, the pleural sacs and the thoracic cage is central to an understanding of the respiratory processes of inspiration and expiration.

### Inspiration

The process of inspiration is an active one. It occurs as a result of the contraction of the respiratory muscles, namely the external intercostal muscles and the diaphragm.

The external intercostal muscles are attached to each rib. When they contract, they cause the ribcage to pivot about thoracic vertebral joints and move upwards and outwards, much like the handle of a bucket as it is lifted. The diaphragm, a dome-shaped muscle separating the abdominal and thoracic cavities, contracts downwards during inspiration, increasing the area of the thoracic cavity. As the chest expands through these muscular contractions, the surface tension created by the film of pleural fluid causes the lungs to be pulled outwards, along with the chest walls. This action causes the space within the lungs to increase and the air molecules within to move further apart.

As pressure is determined by the rate at which molecules strike a surface in a given time, the pressure within the lungs (intrapulmonary pressure) decreases and becomes less than that outside the body. Gases always move from areas of higher pressure to areas of lower pressure, so that air from outside the body rushes into the lungs via the respiratory tract. This process is known as inspiration.

During exercise, greater volumes of air can fill the lungs, since the sternocleidomastoid, pectoralis minor and scaleni muscles help increase the thoracic cavity still further.

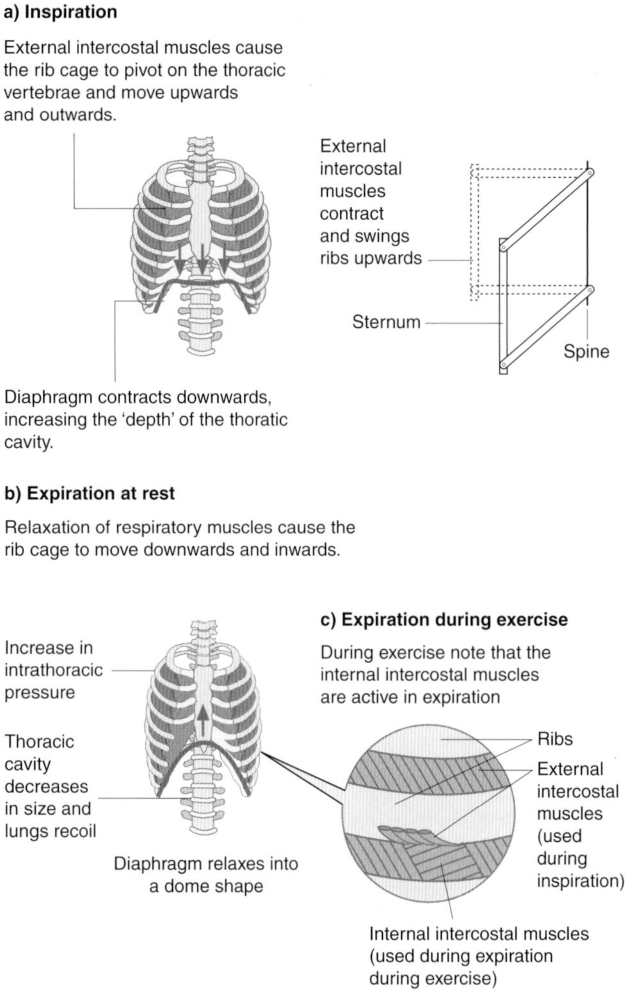
a) Inspiration
External intercostal muscles cause the rib cage to pivot on the thoracic vertebrae and move upwards and outwards.
External intercostal muscles contract and swings ribs upwards
Sternum
Spine
Diaphragm contracts downwards, increasing the 'depth' of the thoratic cavity.
b) Expiration at rest
Relaxation of respiratory muscles cause the rib cage to move downwards and inwards.
c) Expiration during exercise
During exercise note that the internal intercostal muscles are active in expiration
Increase in intrathoracic pressure
Thoracic cavity decreases in size and lungs recoil
Diaphragm relaxes into a dome shape
Ribs
External intercostal muscles (used during inspiration)
Internal intercostal muscles (used during expiration during exercise)

**Figure 3.2** Action of the ribcage during (a) inspiration, (b) expiration and (c) expiration during exercise

> **EXAMINER'S TIP**
>
> Gases always move from areas of higher pressures (or concentrations) to areas of lower pressures (or concentrations), until equilibrium is reached.

> **EXAMINER'S TIP**
>
> When determining which of the intercostal muscles are responsible for inspiration and expiration, think opposites: external intercostals are needed for inspiration, and internal intercostals are needed for expiration during exercise.

## Expiration

The process of expiration is generally a passive process, and occurs as a result of the relaxation of the respiratory muscles used in inspiration. As the external intercostal muscles relax, the ribcage is lowered into its resting position, and the diaphragm relaxes and domes up into the thoracic cavity. The area of the lungs is thus decreased, and intrapulmonary pressure increases to an extent where it is greater than atmospheric pressure. Air inside the lungs is forced out to equate the pressure inside and outside the body.

During exercise, the process of expiration becomes more active as the internal intercostal muscles pull the ribs downwards to help increase the ventilation rate. These muscles are ably assisted by the abdominals and the latissimus dorsi muscles. Take a moment to study Figure 3.2, which illustrates the process of inspiration and expiration.

> **EXAMINER'S TIP**
>
> Make sure you can state the respiratory muscles used in inspiration and expiration, at rest and during exercise.

### Activity 1

Read the section above on 'The mechanics of breathing', then copy and complete the table below, naming the muscles responsible for inspiration and expiration, at rest and during exercise.

| | Rest | Exercise |
|---|---|---|
| Inspiration | | |
| Expiration | | |

# Respiratory regulation – the respiratory control centre

Ventilation is controlled by the nervous system, and this enables us to alter breathing patterns without thinking about it consciously. The basic rhythm of respiration is governed and coordinated by the respiratory centre, situated in and around the medulla area of the brain. During inspiration, nerve impulses are generated and sent to the inspiratory muscles (external intercostals and diaphragm), causing them to contract. This lasts for approximately two seconds, after which the impulses cease and expiration occurs passively by elastic recoil of the lungs.

During exercise, however, when breathing rate is increased, the expiratory centre may send impulses to the expiratory muscles (internal intercostals), which speeds up the expiratory process.

## The role of carbon dioxide in regulating respiratory rate

It is the chemical composition of the blood, however, which largely influences respiration rates, particularly during exercise. The respiratory centre has a chemosensitive area, which is sensitive to changes in blood acidity. Chemoreceptors located in the aortic arch and carotid arteries assess the acidity of the blood and, in particular, the relative concentrations of $CO_2$ and $O_2$. If there is an increase in the concentration of $CO_2$ in the blood, the chemoreceptors detect this, and the respiratory centre sends nerve impulses to the respiratory muscles, which increase the rate of ventilation. This allows the body to expire the excess $CO_2$. Once blood acidity is lowered, fewer impulses are sent and respiration rates can decrease once again.

Other factors that help the control of breathing include:

- proprioceptors and mechanoreceptors, which inform the inspiratory centre that movement is taking place;
- thermoreceptors, which inform the respiratory centre that heat energy has been produced and the temperature of the blood increased;
- baroreceptors (located in the lungs), which send information to the expiratory centre concerning the state of lung inflation.

This regulation of breathing is aided by a series of stretch receptors in the lungs and bronchioles, which prevent overinflation of the lungs. If these are stretched excessively, the expiratory centre sends impulses to induce expiration – this is known as the Hering–Breur reflex.

Factors affecting the regulation of breathing are illustrated in Figure 3.3.

**Key term**

**Hering–Breur reflex:** A spontaneous response of the lungs that prevents overinflation.

**IN CONTEXT**

**When a swimmer such as Ian Thorpe prepares to race, the contraction of the external intercostal muscles and the diaphragm initiate inspiration, while expiration remains a passive process through the relaxation of these muscles, as the swimmer remains at rest on the poolside. During the swim, however, both the rate and depth of breathing need to increase. This is controlled by the respiratory control centre in the medulla oblongata of the brain. The inspiratory centre responds to changes in the chemical composition of the blood (most notably an increase in $CO_2$, and a decrease in $O_2$ and pH), increases in blood temperature, and increased movement at the joints and contraction of the muscles. Consequently, the inspiratory centre calls on additional muscles to help expand the thoracic cavity further. These additional muscles include the sternocleidomastoid, the scaleni and the pectoralis major.**

**In order to help increase the rate of breathing, the expiratory centre responds to information from stretch receptors in the lungs, and enrols the help of the internal intercostal muscles and the abdominals to pull the ribcage down more quickly. In doing so, the process of gaseous exchange is facilitated and more oxygen can enter the swimmer's body, and more carbon dioxide can be expelled.**

### Activity 2

1. Explain the process of increased breathing rates during exercise.
2. Why do breathing rates remain high following exercise, even though exercise has ceased?

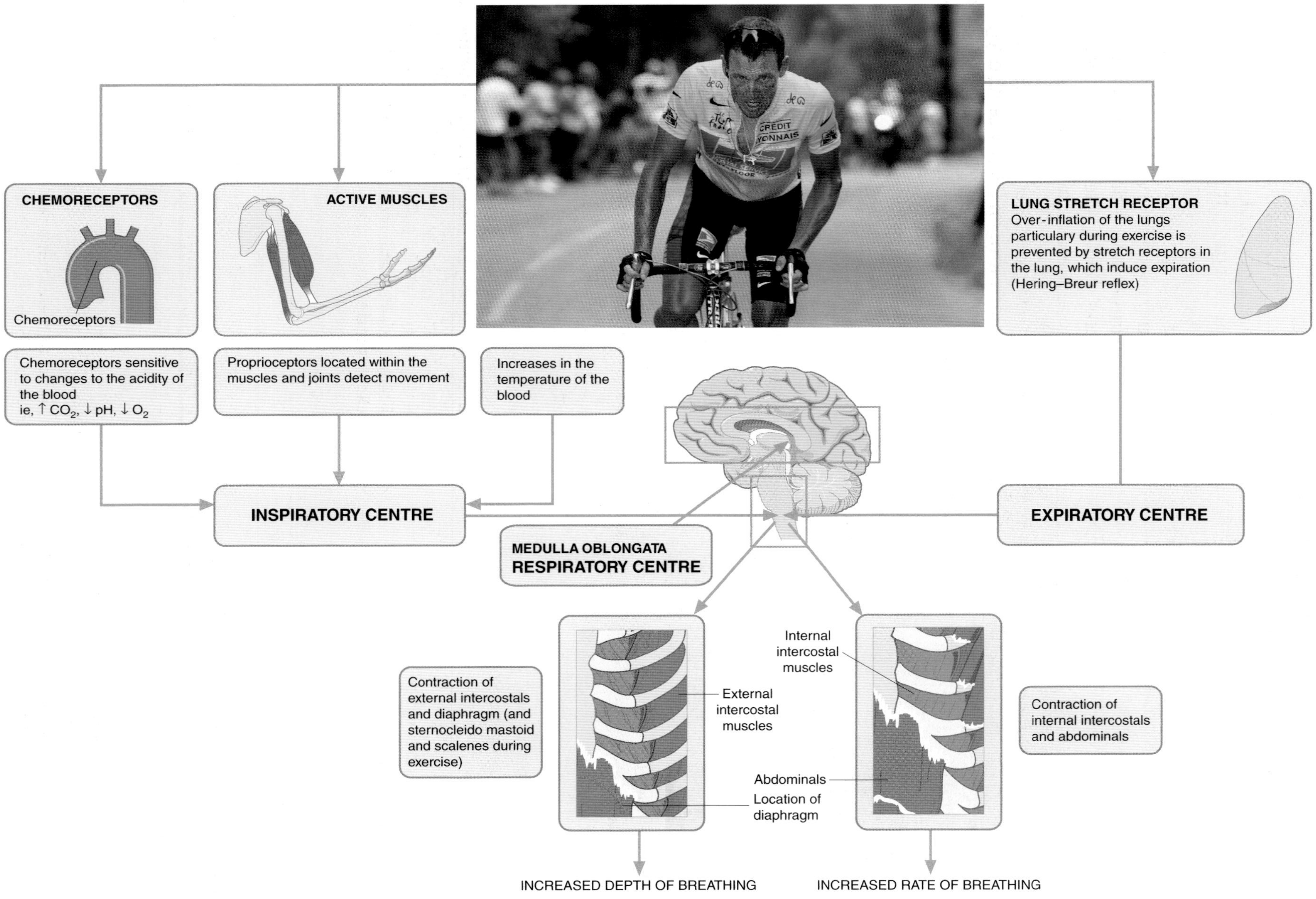
CHEMORECEPTORS
Chemoreceptors
ACTIVE MUSCLES
CREDIT LYONNAIS
LUNG STRETCH RECEPTOR
Over-inflation of the lungs particulary during exercise is prevented by stretch receptors in the lung, which induce expiration (Hering–Breur reflex)
Chemoreceptors sensitive to changes to the acidity of the blood ie, ↑ $CO_2$, ↓ pH, ↓ $O_2$
Proprioceptors located within the muscles and joints detect movement
Increases in the temperature of the blood
INSPIRATORY CENTRE
EXPIRATORY CENTRE
MEDULLA OBLONGATA
RESPIRATORY CENTRE
Contraction of external intercostals and diaphragm (and sternocleido mastoid and scalenes during exercise)
External intercostal muscles
Internal intercostal muscles
Abdominals
Location of diaphragm
Contraction of internal intercostals and abdominals
INCREASED DEPTH OF BREATHING
INCREASED RATE OF BREATHING

Figure 3.3 Respiratory regulation during exercise

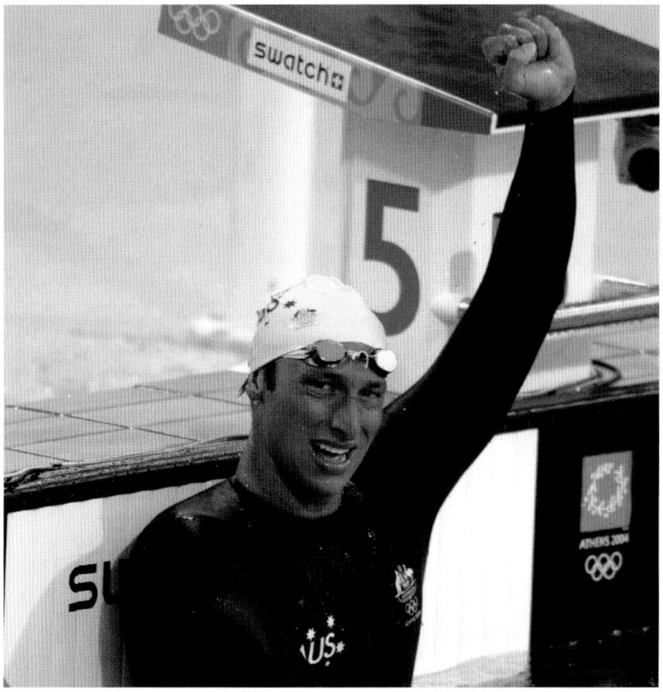


Figure 3.4 Respiratory regulation enables a performer such as Ian Thorpe to remove excess carbon dioxide and supply the muscles with the necessary oxygen

## Exam-style questions

**1** With reference to the mechanics of breathing explain how a swimmer can inspire greater volumes of oxygen during a training session. (3 marks)

**2** (a) Explain the role played by carbon dioxide in the regulation of breathing during the swim. (2 marks)

(b) What other regulatory factors help ensure that sufficient oxygen enters the swimmer's body? (3 marks)

# Pulmonary diffusion – gaseous exchange at the lungs

Pulmonary diffusion is the term used to explain the process of gaseous exchange in the lungs. It has two major functions:

1 to replenish the blood with oxygen where it can, then be transported to the tissues and muscles;
2 to remove carbon dioxide from the blood which has resulted from metabolic processes in the tissues.

## Partial pressure of gases

Central to the understanding of gaseous exchange is the concept of partial pressure. The partial pressure of a gas is the individual pressure that the gas exerts when it occurs in a mixture of gases. The gas will exert a pressure proportional to its concentration within the whole gas. Thus the partial pressures of each individual gas within a mixture of gases should, when added together, be equal to the total pressure of the gas.

For example, the air we breathe is composed of three main gases: nitrogen (79 per cent), oxygen (20.9 per cent) and carbon dioxide (0.03 per cent). The percentages show the relative concentrations of each gas in atmospheric air.

At sea level, total atmospheric pressure is 769mmHg, which reflects the pressure that atmospheric air exerts. For example:

- The concentration of $O_2$ (oxygen) in the atmosphere is approximately 21 per cent.
- The concentration of nitrogen in the air is approximately 79 per cent.
- Together they exert a pressure of 760mmHg at sea level. Therefore, the $pO_2$ (partial pressure of oxygen) is calculated as:

$$pO_2 = \text{Barometric pressure} \times \text{Fractional concentration}$$
$$= 760 \times 0.21$$
$$= 159.6\text{mmHg}$$

Partial pressure of gases explains the movement of gases within the body, and accounts for the processes of gas exchange between the alveoli and the blood, and between the blood and the muscle, or tissue.

**Key terms**

**Partial pressure:** The pressure exerted by an individual gas when it exists within a mixture of gases.
**Diffusion:** The movement of respiratory gases from areas of higher partial pressure to areas of lower partial pressure, until equilibrium is reached.

**EXAMINER'S TIP**

The units of measurement of pressure are millimetres of mercury (mmHg).

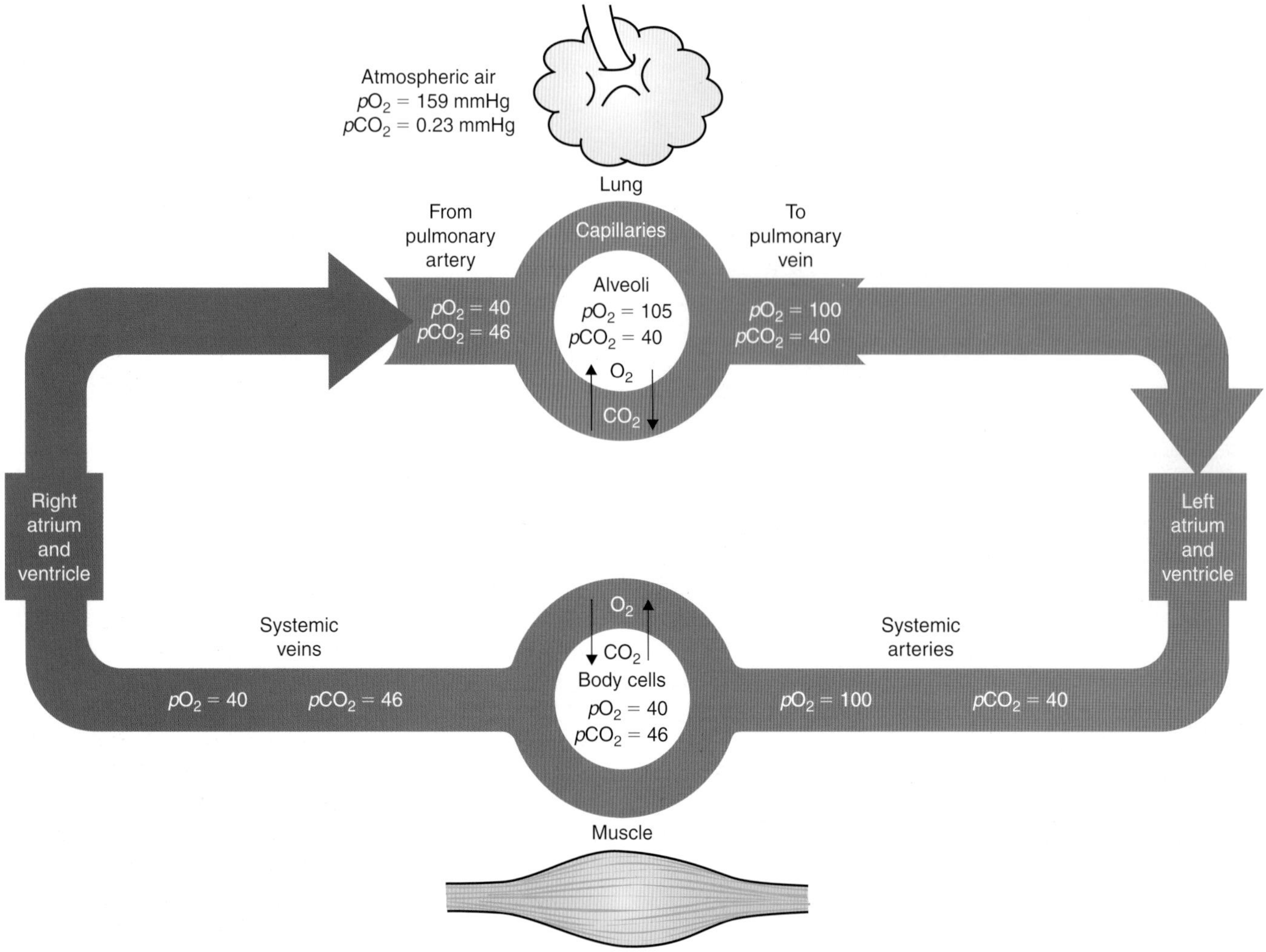


**Figure 3.5** Partial pressures of oxygen and carbon dioxide at various sites in the body

## Activity 3

Calculate the partial pressure in the atmosphere of:

- carbon dioxide ($pCO_2$);
- nitrogen ($pN_2$).

## Gaseous exchange at the lungs

It is the imbalance between gases in the alveoli and the blood that causes a pressure gradient, which results in a movement of gases across the respiratory membrane (which facilitates this movement by being extremely thin, measuring only 0.5mm). This movement is two-way, with oxygen moving from the alveoli into the blood, and carbon dioxide diffusing from the blood into the alveoli. The partial pressure of oxygen ($pO_2$) in the atmosphere is approximately 159mmHg (0.21 × 760mmHg), which drops to 105mmHg in the alveoli, since the air combines with water vapour and carbon dioxide which is already present in the alveoli.

## The diffusion gradient

Blood in the pulmonary capillaries which surround the alveoli has a $pO_2$ of 45mmHg, since much of the oxygen has already been used by the working muscles. This results in a pressure gradient of approximately 60mmHg, which forces oxygen from the alveoli into the blood, until such time that the pressure is equal on each side of the membrane.

In the same way, carbon dioxide moves along a pressure gradient, from the pulmonary capillaries into the alveoli. With a $pCO_2$ of 45mmHg in the blood returning to the lungs, and a $pCO_2$ of 40mmHg in the alveolar air, a small pressure gradient of 5mmHg results. This causes $CO_2$ to move from the pulmonary blood into the alveoli, which is later expired. Although the pressure gradient is relatively small, the $CO_2$ can cross the respiratory membrane much more rapidly than oxygen, as its membrane solubility is 20 times greater.

Endurance athletes, with larger aerobic capacities, will have greater oxygen diffusion ability (the rate at which oxygen diffuses into the pulmonary blood from the alveoli) as a result of increased cardiac output, increased alveoli surface area and reduced resistance to diffusion.

### Activity 4

Discuss why the diffusion gradient of carbon dioxide and oxygen is relatively small at rest and increases during exercise.

### EXAMINER'S TIP

A diffusion gradient can be calculated by subtracting the partial pressure of the gas on one side of the respiratory membrane from the partial pressure of the gas on the other side of the respiratory membrane.

### Activity 5

1 Explain what is meant by the partial pressure of a gas.
2 State how this affects gaseous exchange around the body.
3 What happens to the partial pressure of oxygen ($pO_2$) and carbon dioxide ($pCO_2$) in the **muscle cell** during exercise?

### Exam-style questions

**1** Describe the process of gaseous exchange at the alveoli during exercise (5 marks)

**2** Describe the characteristics of the structure of the lungs and surrounding tissues that make gaseous exchange an efficient process (3 marks)

**3** Define partial pressure. Explain the significance of partial pressure to the process of gaseous exchange (3 marks)

### Activity 6

Draw diagrams to show how and why gases move between:

- the alveoli and the pulmonary capillaries;
- the systemic capillaries and the muscle.

### EXAMINER'S TIP

Don't forget that an increase in blood acidity amounts to a decrease in the pH of the blood.

## Gas exchange at the muscles and tissues

We have seen how oxygen is brought into the lungs and transported to the capillary beds on the muscles. We now need to turn our attention to how the oxygen can enter the muscle cell.

The process is similar to the exchange of gases at the lungs: the partial pressure of the gases in the blood and tissues determines the movement of oxygen and carbon dioxide into and out of the tissue cells. The high partial pressure of oxygen in the arterial blood, and the relatively low $pO_2$ in the muscles, causes a pressure gradient which enables oxygen to dissociate from haemoglobin and pass through the capillary wall and into the muscle cytoplasm. Conversely, the high $pCO_2$ in the tissues and low $pCO_2$ in the arterial blood causes a movement of carbon dioxide in the opposite direction. In fact, the production of carbon dioxide stimulates the dissociation of oxygen from haemoglobin and this, together with greater tissue demand for oxygen, increases the pressure gradients during exercise.

Once oxygen has entered the muscle cell, it immediately attaches to a substance called myoglobin, which is not dissimilar to haemoglobin and transports the oxygen to the mitochondria, where aerobic respiration can take place. The concentration of myoglobin is much higher in the cells of slow-twitch muscle fibres, as these are more suited to aerobic energy production. Myoglobin has a much higher affinity for oxygen than haemoglobin, and also acts as an oxygen reserve, so that when demand for oxygen is increased, as for example during exercise, there is a readily available supply.

**Key terms**

**Myoglobin:** A respiratory pigment that binds to oxygen in the muscle cell. As well as acting as an oxygen store, it transports oxygen to the mitochondria.

**Mitochondria:** Specialised cells in the body's tissues that use the inspired oxygen to produce energy.

**Aerobic respiration:** The process of energy creation through the oxidation of food fuels. As well as energy, carbon dioxide and water are produced.

# Lung volumes and capacities

## Lung volumes

During normal quiet breathing, we inspire approximately 500ml of air; the same amount is exhaled during the process of expiration. This volume of air inspired or expired is known as tidal volume. Of this 500ml, only about 350ml makes its way to the alveoli. The other 150ml remains in the passageways of the nose, throat and trachea and is known as dead space. The volume of air which is inspired or expired in one minute is called minute ventilation and is calculated by multiplying tidal volume by the number of breaths taken per minute. On average we breathe 12 to 15 times per minute, so our resting minute ventilation can be calculated as follows:

$$\text{minute ventilation} = \text{tidal volume} \times \text{frequency (breaths/min)}$$

$$VE = TV \times f$$

$$= 500\text{ml} \times 15$$

$$= 7{,}500\text{ml/min}$$

However, at rest we can still inspire much more air than our normal tidal volume. This excess volume of air inspired is the inspiratory reserve volume. It can be defined as the maximum volume of air inspired following normal inspiration, and measures approximately 3,300ml. Following normal expiration at rest we can also expire more air; this volume is known as the expiratory reserve volume and measures approximately 1,200ml. The lungs can never completely expel all the air they contain. Approximately 1,200ml remains in the alveoli to keep them slightly inflated and regulate pressure; this volume is called the reserve volume.

**Key terms**

**Minute ventilation:** The total volume of air taken into the lungs per minute. It is the product of tidal volume and the number of breaths taken per minute. At rest, this volume should be between 6,000 and 7,500ml per minute.

**EXAMINER'S TIP**

When asked to calculate minute ventilation, be sure to state the correct units – ml/min or L/min.

## Lung capacities

Lung capacities can be calculated by adding together different lung volumes. For example:

1 Inspiratory capacity is the sum of tidal volume and the inspiratory reserve volume, and amounts to 3,800ml.
2 Functional residual capacity is the sum of expiratory reserve volume and residual volume, and accounts for approximately 2,400ml.
3 Vital capacity is the amount of air that can be forcibly expired following maximal inspiration and is the sum of tidal volume, inspiratory reserve volume and expiratory reserve volume; this measures about 5,000ml.
4 Total lung capacity is the sum of all volumes and on average is approximately 6,000ml.

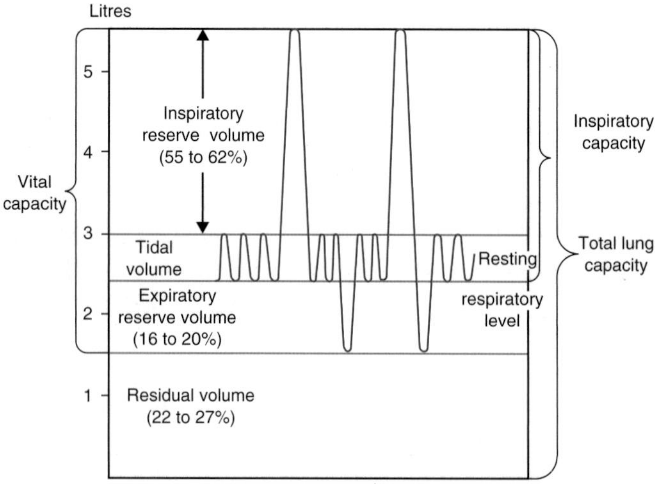


Figure 3.6 Lung volumes shown by a spirometer trace

The forced expiratory volume (FEV1) is the percentage of vital capacity that can be expired in one second. This is approximately 85 per cent and gives an indication of the overall efficiency of the airways. A low reading may assume that the airways are resisting the passage of air during expiration and consequently the efficiency of the gaseous exchange process at the lungs may decrease. A summary of lung volumes and capacities, their values and the effect of exercise is outlined in Table 3.1.

## Ventilation during exercise

During exercise, both the depth and rate of breathing increase. The tidal volume increases by utilising both the inspiratory reserve volume and the expiratory reserve volume. Consequently both these volumes decrease during exercise, while tidal volume may increase six-fold. Since both tidal volume and the frequency of breathing increase during exercise, minute ventilation increases dramatically – values up to 180L/min have been recorded for trained endurance athletes. This is shown in Table 3.2.

Changes in ventilation occur before, during and after exercise, as shown in Figure 3.8. Before exercise starts there is a slight increase in ventilation; this is called the anticipatory rise and is the result of hormones, such as adrenaline, stimulating the respiratory centre. Once exercise begins there is a rapid rise in ventilation caused by nervous stimulation. During submaximal exercise this sudden increase in ventilation begins to slow down and may plateau into what is known as the steady state. This assumes that the energy demands of the muscles are being met by the oxygen made available, and that the body is expelling carbon dioxide effectively. During maximal exercise, however, this steady state does not occur and ventilation continues to increase until the exercise is finished. This is thought to be due to the stimulation of the respiratory centre by carbon dioxide and lactic acid, and suggests that it is the body's need to expel these metabolites rather than its desire for oxygen which determines the pattern of breathing. If exercise intensity continues to increase to a point near the athlete's $\bar{V}O_2$ max (the maximum amount of oxygen that can be taken in, transported and utilised in one minute), then the amount of oxygen entering the body is not sufficient to meet the demands of the working muscles. Because the athlete is working at maximal levels they are unable to meet the body's requirements and the athlete may need to stop exercising, or at the very best, significantly reduce the intensity of the exercise. In this way oxygen supply can once again meet the demands imposed by the body.

### Key terms

**$\bar{V}O_2$ max. (maximal oxygen uptake):** The maximum volume of oxygen that can be taken in, transported and utilised by the working muscles per minute.

**Steady state:** The plateau demonstrated in pulmonary ventilation that represents a situation where oxygen demand is being met by oxygen supply.

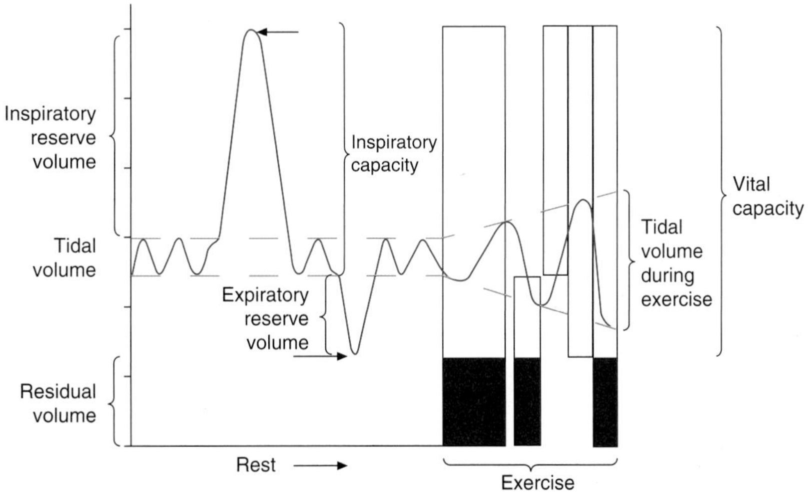


Figure 3.7 The effect of exercise on lung volumes

Table 3.1 Lung volumes and capacities defined; resting values and changes during exercise

| Lung volume or capacity | Definition | Approximate normal values (ml) | Changes during exercise |
|---|---|---|---|
| Tidal volume (TV) | Volume inspired *or* expired per breath | 500 | Increase up to 3–4 litres |
| Inspiratory reserve volume (IRV) | Maximal volume inspired from end-inspiration | 3,300 | Decrease |
| Expiratory reserve volume (ERV) | Maximal volume expired from end-expiration | 1,000–1,200 | Slight decrease |
| Residual volume (RV) | Volume remaining at end of maximal expiration | 1,200 | Slight increase |
| Total lung capacity (TLC) | Volume in lung at end of maximal inspiration | up to 8,000 | Slight decrease |
| Vital capacity (VC) | Maximal volume forcefully expired after maximal inspiration | 5,500 | Slight decrease |
| Inspiratory capacity (IC) | Maximal volume inspired from resting expiratory level | 3,800 | Increase |
| Functional residual capacity (FRC) | Volume in lungs at resting expiratory level | 2,400 | Slight increase |
| Dead space | Volume of air in the trachea/ bronchi etc. that does not take part in gaseous exchange | 150 | None |
| Minute ventilation | Volume of air inspired/expired per minute<br>$VE = TV \times F$<br>$= 500 \times 15$<br>$= 7{,}500$ml/min | 7,500 | Large increase (200 L/min) in trained athletes |

During recovery from exercise, ventilation drops rapidly at first, followed by a slower decrease. The more intense the preceding exercise, the longer the recovery period and the longer ventilation remains above the normal resting level. This is largely due to the removal of by-products of muscle metabolism such as lactic acid.

## Activity 7

With reference to Figure 3.7, state what the effect of exercise is upon:

- tidal volume;
- expiratory reserve volume;
- inspiratory reserve volume.

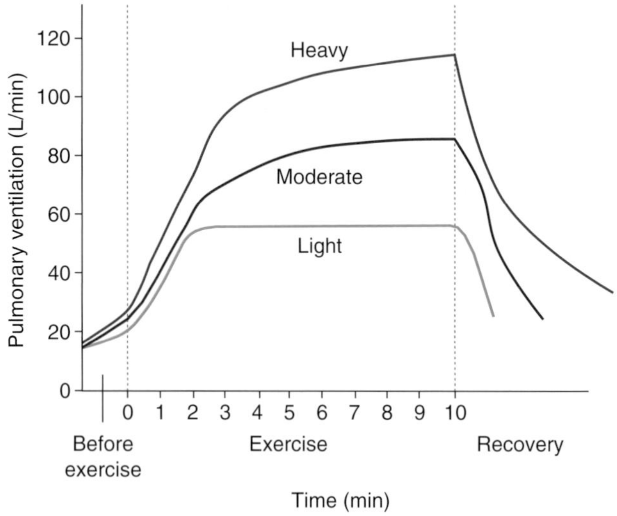


**Figure 3.8** Respiratory response to varying intensity of exercise
*Note*: Remember the anticipatory rise prior to exercise and the continual increase in ventilation during intense exercise

Table 3.2 Minute ventilaton at rest and durng maximal exercise

| | Tidal volume (TV) × Frequency (breaths/min) | = Minute ventilation |
|---|---|---|
| Rest | 500ml (0.5L) × 15 | = 7.5L/min |
| Maximal work | 4,000ml (4.0L) × 50 | = 200L/min |

## Exam-style questions

1 Sketch a graph to show the minute ventilation of a 1500m runner during a competitive race. On your graph identify the minute ventilation of the runner during the following stages:
- Immediately prior to the run
- During the run
- During a 10-minute recovery period following the run (4 marks)

2 During maximal exercise, minute ventilation can increase significantly. Define minute ventilation and give an approximate value for a performer at rest and during maximal exercise. (3 marks)

3 Describe what happens to the following lung volumes as an athlete moves from rest to exercise:
- Tidal volume
- Inspiratory volume
- Expiratory volume (3 marks)

4 Endurance training will cause changes to the structure and functioning of the body which helps to enhance performance. Describe these changes with reference to the respiratory system. (3 marks)

## Activity 8

You are going to carry out an investigation to estimate total lung capacity, using a handheld spirometer.

1 Take a deep breath and exhale.
2 Take another deep breath until you cannot take in any more air.
3 Place your mouth tightly around the spirometer and expel all air possible. (If you bend forwards slightly towards the end of exhalation, you will be able to force all air out of the lower area of the lungs. This represents your vital capacity (VC).)
4 Record your results.
5 Now calculate and record your residual volume:

Males: Residual volume = 0.24 × VC

Females: Residual volume = 0.27 × VC

6 If **Total lung capacity = Vital capacity + Residual volume,** calculate your total lung capacity.

## Activity 9

Copy and complete the table below, showing the responses of the respiratory system to exercise. The first factor has been completed for you.

| Factor | Increase/decrease | Explanation |
|---|---|---|
| Respiratory rate | Increase | The respiratory rate increases directly in proportion to exercise intensity. Initially, there is a rapid rise in the rate of breathing. This is largely due to proprioceptive feedback from skeletal muscles. There then follows a more gradual increase, or sometimes a plateau, in respiratory rate, depending on exercise intensity. This is determined by increases in $CO_2$ and the lactic acid content of arterial blood, as well as an increase in body temperature. |
| Expiratory reserve volume | | |
| Oxygen content of arteries | | |
| Minute ventilation | | |
| Tidal volume | | |
| Oxygen consumption | | |
| Max. oxygen consumption | | |
| a–$VO_2$ diff. | | |
| Action of respiratory muscles | | |
| Transport of carbon dioxide | | |

### EXAMINER'S TIP

Minute ventilation at rest is typically between 6,000 and 7,500ml per minute, and is dependent on age, sex, body size and levels of fitness.

### IN CONTEXT

**Peak flow is a measure of how fast you can expel air from your lungs. It measures how wide the respiratory airways are. Average measures for 16-year-olds range between 500 and 600L/min. Asthmatics will often use peak flow to assess the state or impact of their asthma on a particular day. In extreme cases, peak flow may reach levels as low as 70L/min.**

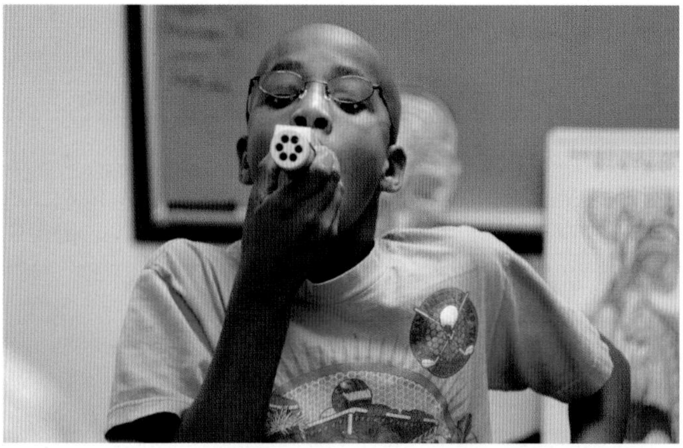

**Figure 3.9** Peak flow is used by asthmatics to determine the severity of asthma on any particular day

### Activity 10

Use a peak flow metre to measure your peak flow, and compare your score to others in your class. What reasons can you suggest for the individual differences in results?

## The adaptive responses of the respiratory system to training

Training signals an improvement in lung function. This is due to the following factors:

1 Small increases in lung volumes:
- Tidal volume remains unchanged at rest and during submaximal exercise, but does appear to increase during high-intensity, maximal exercise. This ensures as much oxygen as possible is being taken into the lungs with each breath, and as much carbon dioxide expelled.
- Vital capacity also increases slightly, which causes a small decrease in the residual volume.

These increases in lung volumes result from the increased strength of the respiratory muscles following training.

2 Improved transport of respiratory gases:
- Training can signal an increase in the total volume of the blood (primarily due to an increase in blood plasma volume), and an increase in the number of red blood cells (erythrocytes), which leads to an increase in the content of haemoglobin. These changes provide for increased oxygen delivery to the working muscles and improved removal of carbon dioxide.
- The increase in blood plasma volume also means that the viscosity of the blood is reduced. Reduced blood viscosity means that there is less resistance to blood flow, allowing the blood to flow more freely and improving the blood supply to the working muscles.

3 Enhanced gaseous exchange at the alveoli and the tissues:
- Capillary density surrounding the alveoli and muscle tissue increases substantially following endurance training, which provides for greater gaseous exchange. This therefore enhances the supply of oxygen to, and the removal of carbon dioxide from, the working muscle.
- Endurance athletes also appear to have enhanced blood flow to the lungs (pulmonary blood flow), which, together with an increase in maximal minute ventilation, causes a significant increase in pulmonary diffusion (i.e. gaseous exchange at the alveoli), once again ensuring maximum exchange of oxygen and carbon dioxide.

4 Greater uptake of oxygen by the muscles:
- Endurance training improves the ability of skeletal muscle to extract oxygen from the blood. This is largely the result of increased myoglobin and mitochondrial density within the muscle cell, which will cause an improvement in an athlete's maximum oxygen uptake, or $\bar{V}O_2$ max., by about 10–20 per cent.
- The enhanced oxygen extraction by skeletal muscle also causes an increase in the arterial–venous oxygen difference (a–$\bar{V}O_2$ diff.), which is a measure of the amount of oxygen actually consumed by the muscles.

**IN CONTEXT**

**Elite rowers, such as Matthew Pinsent and James Cracknell, are some of the fittest athletes around. Their bodies have adapted to cope with the demands of their excessive training regimes. Matthew Pinsent is reported to have a vital capacity of 8.5L, compared to the average male score of 5.5L. Not surprisingly, he is also reported to have one of the highest $\bar{V}O_2$ max. scores ever recorded in the UK, at 8.5L/min.**

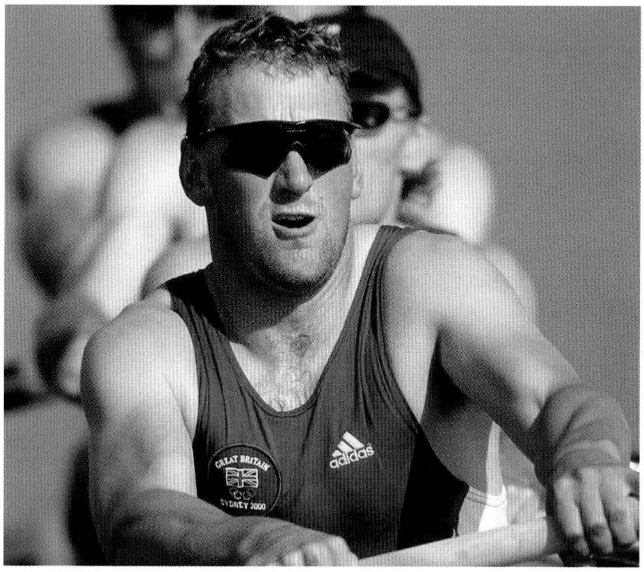

**Figure 3.10** Elite rowers, such as Matthew Pinsent, have some of the greatest aerobic capacities

## What you need to know

* Respiration can be divided into external and internal respiration.
* External respiration is the process of getting air into and out of the lungs.
* Inspiration occurs when the respiratory muscles contract, lifting the ribcage upwards and outwards, and lowering the diaphragm. The resultant pressure differential causes air to rush into the lungs.
* Expiration at rest is a passive process, simply a result of the intercostals and diaphragm relaxing. This causes a pressure differential and air is forced out of the lungs.
* Respiration is governed by various levels within the brain. The main regulatory mechanism is performed by chemoreceptors within the aortic arch and carotid arteries. These assess the concentration of carbon dioxide within the blood.
* Oxygen enters the bloodstream at the alveoli, through the process of diffusion.
* Diffusion of gases at the alveoli is facilitated by several structural features of the respiratory system:
  - The respiratory (alveolar-capillary) membrane is very thin, which means that the diffusion distance between the air in the alveoli and the blood is very short.
  - The numerous alveoli create a very large surface area over which diffusion can take place.
  - The alveoli are surrounded by a vast network of capillaries, which further provides a huge surface area for gaseous exchange.
  - The diameter of the capillaries is slightly narrower than the area of a red blood cell, which causes the blood cell to distort, increasing its surface area and ensuring the blood cells travel slowly in single file, maximising oxygen absorption.
* Gaseous exchange occurs as a result of differences in concentration of oxygen and carbon dioxide round the body.
* The partial pressure of a gas is the individual pressure the gas exerts when in a mixture of gases, and this explains the movement of gases in the body.
* During exercise, both the rate (frequency) and depth (tidal volume) of breathing increases in direct proportion to the intensity of the activity.
* The ventilatory response to exercise (including changes from submaximal exercise to maximal exercise) mirrors that of the heart.
* Training improves respiratory and lung function due to:
  - small increases in lung volumes and capacities;
  - improved transport of the respiratory gases;
  - more efficient gaseous exchange at the alveoli and tissues;
  - improved uptake of oxygen by the muscles.

## Review Questions

1 Trace the path of inspired air, outlining the structures it passes on its journey from the nasal cavity to the alveoli.

2 Identify the muscles used in respiration, at rest and during exercise.

3 Sketch a graph to show what happens to oxygen consumption ($VO_2$) during an exercise session that gets progressively harder (e.g. the multi-stage fitness test).

4 Identify and explain four factors that influence the efficiency of gaseous exchange between the lungs and the pulmonary capillaries.

5 Explain the importance of the partial pressure of gases in the respiratory process.

6 What factors influence the respiratory system during exercise?

7 How does the body combat increases in blood acidity resulting from intense exercise?

8 What factors account for the enhanced respiratory functioning that accompanies training?

9 Outline and explain the changes that occur to lung volumes and capacities during exercise.

10 Explain the role that carbon dioxide plays in the regulation of breathing rate.

CHAPTER

4

# Cardiac function and the transport of blood gases

## Learning outcomes

**By the end of this chapter you should be able to:**

- explain how the structure of the heart suits its function as a dual-action pump;
- explain the relationship between stroke volume, heart rate and cardiac output when resting, and the changes that occur during different intensities of exercise;
- describe the pattern of heart rate during maximal and submaximal exercise;
- relate the conduction system of the heart to the cardiac cycle;
- explain the regulation and control of the heart rate through neural, hormonal and intrinsic mechanisms;
- explain the transport of oxygen and carbon dioxide in the body;
- name and describe the structure of each of the different types of blood vessel, identifying their main features in relation to their respective functions;
- explain the five facets of the venous return mechanism;
- define and explain how blood pressure is regulated and its role in the redistribution of blood;
- describe the effects of training on cardiovascular functioning.

## CHAPTER INTRODUCTION

This chapter will examine the structure and function of the cardiovascular system, which includes the heart, blood and blood vessels. We will investigate the response of the cardiovascular system to exercise, looking in particular at the changes in heart rate, stroke volume, cardiac output and blood pressure.

We will learn how the heart, blood vessels and blood adapt in response to the demands of exercise, and you will see how the maintenance and control of the blood supply is the major determining factor in the effective and successful performance of aerobic or endurance-based exercise. The final section of this chapter will enable you to make a critical evaluation of the impact of different types of physical activity on the cardiovascular system in the prevention of health-related illness and disease, such as coronary heart disease, arteriosclerosis, atherosclerosis, angina and heart attack.

# The structure and function of the heart

The human body is an amazing machine, and at the centre of its operation is the heart. The heart is a muscular pump that beats continuously, over 100,000 times per day. Together with the blood vessels and the blood, the heart provides the tissues and cells with the essentials for life itself – oxygen and nutrients.

The heart lies behind the sternum (breastbone) and ribs, which offer protection. In adults, it is about the size of a clenched fist – although trained athletes often experience cardiac hypertrophy, which is an enlargement of the heart.

In terms of structure, the heart is composed of four chambers:

- The two chambers at the top or superior part of the heart are called the atria.
- The two lower or inferior chambers are termed ventricles.

The ventricles are much more muscular than the atria, since it is here that the pumping action of the heart occurs which circulates the blood all round the body.

As well as being divided into upper and lower portions, the heart can also be divided into left and right halves, due to a muscular partition called the septum. Study Figures 4.1 and 4.2 and get to know the structure of the heart.

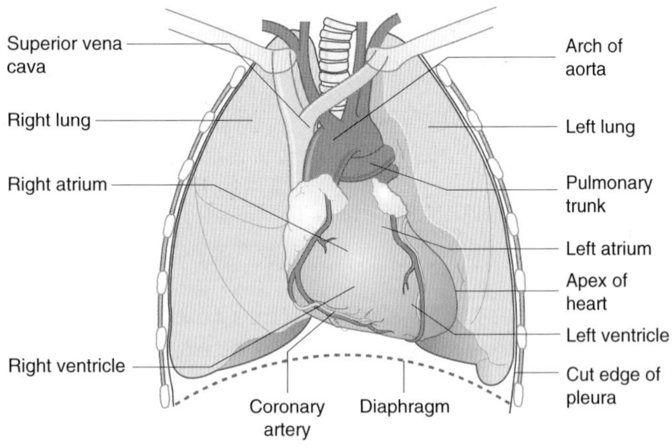


Figure 4.1 Position of the heart in the thoracic cavity

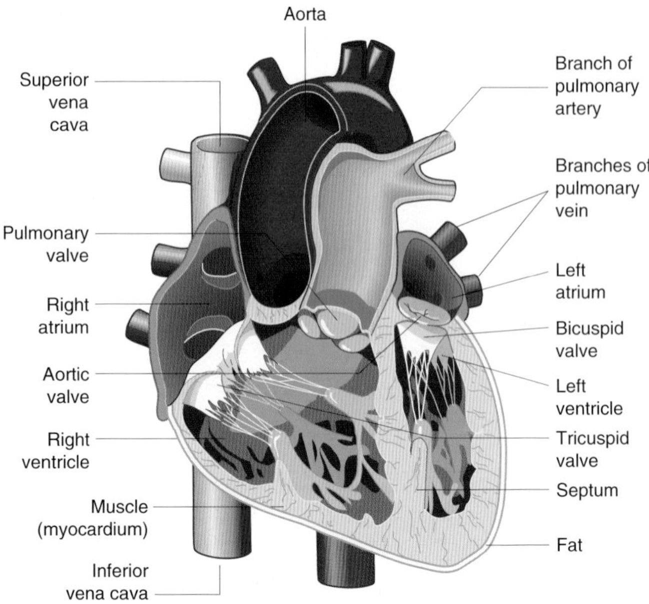


Figure 4.2 The structure of the heart

**EXAMINER'S TIP**

Don't forget that the left side of the heart is on the right as we look at it, and the right side of the heart is on the left.

## The heart as a dual-action pump

This separation into left and right is essential for the heart to carry out its function effectively, since each side has a slightly different role:

- The left side of the heart is responsible for circulating blood rich in oxygen throughout the entire body. This is known as systemic circulation.
- The right side is responsible for ensuring that oxygen-poor blood is pumped to the lungs, where it can be reoxygenated. This is known as pulmonary circulation.

**Key terms**

**Systemic circulation:** The component of the circulatory system which conducts oxygenated blood from the left ventricle to all the major muscles and organs of the body (excluding the lungs) and returns it to the right atrium via the venae cavae.

**Pulmonary circulation:** The component of the circulatory system which conducts blood between the heart and the lungs.

The major vessels act as entry and exit points for the blood to enter or leave the heart, and are all situated towards the top of the heart. To ensure a smooth passage of blood through the heart, a number of valves exist. These valves make sure that the blood only flows in one direction and prevent backflow of blood.

The thick muscular wall of the heart is called the myocardium and is composed of cardiac muscle fibres. It is this muscle that is responsible for the contraction of the heart and the subsequent ejection of blood from the heart.

Covering the exterior of the heart are coronary arteries, which feed the heart muscle with blood; being a muscle, it still requires fuel to keep the pump working continually. Blockages of these arteries are responsible for many problems of the heart, in particular cardiovascular diseases such as hypertension, angina pectoris and myocardial infarctions (heart attacks).

**Key term**

**Myocardium:** The muscular tissue of the heart. It is the contraction of the myocardium that is responsible for pumping blood round the body.

## Blood flow through the heart

To help you understand the anatomy of the heart, you will now be taken on a journey through it. Make a note of the key structures and their functions as you go.

- Blood low in oxygen returns from the body to the right atrium via the superior (upper body) and inferior (lower body) venae cavae.
- At the same time, oxygen-rich blood returns to the left atrium from the lungs via the pulmonary veins.
- The atria are the top two chambers of the heart. You will see from Figure 4.3 that they are separated by a thick muscular wall that runs through the middle of the heart, known as the septum. This enables the two pumps to function separately – thus enabling the heart to be dual-purpose.
- Blood will eventually start to enter the larger lower chambers of the heart, called the right and left ventricles.
- In doing so, it passes the atrioventricular (AV) valves. The right AV valve is the tricuspid valve, and the left AV valve is the bicuspid valve. The purpose of these valves is not merely to separate the atria from the ventricles, but also to ensure that the blood can only flow in one direction through the heart.
- When the ventricles contract, blood on the right side of the heart is forced through the semilunar pulmonary valve into the pulmonary artery, from where it travels towards the lungs.
- Meanwhile, blood from the left ventricle enters the aorta via the semilunar aortic valve.
- The aorta branches into many different arteries, which then transport the blood around the whole body.
- Once again, the semilunar valves ensure the unidirectional flow of blood, preventing backflow of blood into the heart.

As the left side of the heart is responsible for pumping blood round the whole body, the wall of cardiac tissue (myocardium) surrounding the left ventricle is much thicker than that on the right side of the heart.

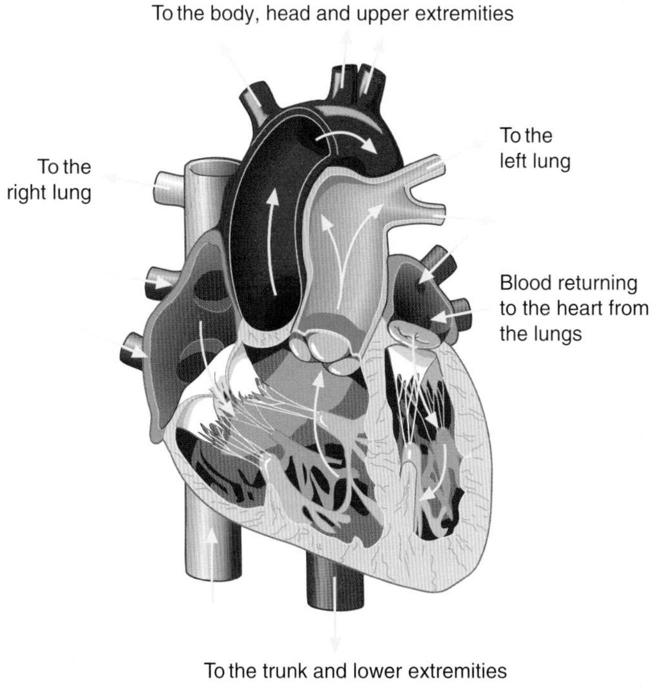


**Figure 4.3** The path of blood through the heart

*Source*: Tortora (1991) *Introduction to the Human Body: The Essentials of Anatomy and Physiology*, 2nd edn, HarperCollins

## Activity 1

1 Place the following terms in the correct sequential order to explain the flow of blood returning to the heart from the body, and its path through the heart:
- Aorta
- Pulmonary vein
- Lungs
- Pulmonary artery
- Tricuspid valve
- Left atrium
- Aortic valve
- Pulmonary valve
- Left ventricle
- Right atrium
- Right ventricle
- Bicuspid valve
- Venae cavae

2 Describe the location of the heart.

3 Draw a simple model to illustrate the dual role of the heart. Use red lines to highlight oxygen-rich blood and blue lines to show oxygen-poor blood.

# The conduction system – how the heart works

The heart produces impulses that spread and innervate specialised muscle fibres. Unlike skeletal muscle, the heart produces its own impulses (i.e. it is myogenic), and it is the conduction system of the heart that spreads the impulses throughout the heart and enables the heart to contract.

**Key term**

**Myogenic:** The capacity of the heart to generate its own impulses which cause the heart to contract.

From Figure 4.4 it can be seen that the electrical impulse begins at the pacemaker – a mass of cardiac muscle cells known as the sinoatrial node (SA node) located in the right atrial wall. It is the rate at which the SA node emits impulses that determines the heart rate. As an impulse is emitted, it spreads to the adjacent interconnecting fibres of the atrium, which spread the excitation extremely rapidly, causing the atria to contract. It then passes to another specialised mass of cells called the atrioventricular node (AV node). The AV node acts as a distributor and passes the action potential to the bundle of His, which, together with the branching Purkinje fibres, spreads the excitation throughout the ventricles.

There is a delay of about 0.1 seconds from the time when the AV node receives stimulation to when it distributes the action potential throughout the ventricles. This is crucial to allow completion of atrial contraction before ventricular systole begins, so that as much blood as possible is passed from the atria to the ventricles.

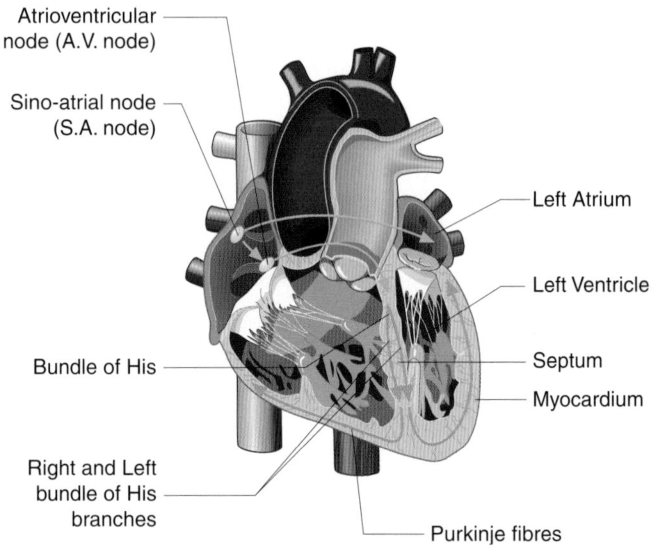


Figure 4.4 The conduction system of the heart

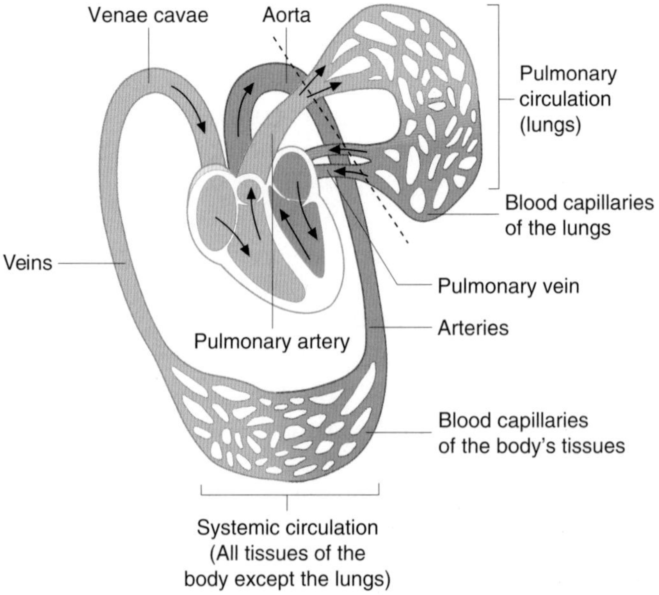


Figure 4.5 The heart as a dual-action pump

## The cardiac cycle

The cardiac cycle refers to the process of cardiac contraction and blood transportation through the heart. The cardiac cycle explains the sequence of events that takes place during one complete heartbeat. This includes the filling of the heart with blood (diastole phase) and the emptying of the blood into the arterial system (systole phase).

Each cycle takes approximately 0.8 seconds and occurs on average 72 times per minute. There are four stages to each heartbeat:

1 atrial diastole: } 0.5 sec.
2 ventricular diastole; }
3 atrial systole: } 0.3 sec.
4 ventricular systole. }

Each stage depends on whether the chambers of the heart are *filling* with blood while the heart is relaxing (diastole) or whether they are *emptying*, which occurs when the heart contracts (systole), forcing blood from one part of the heart to another, or into the arterial system, and subsequently to the lungs and the body.

**Key terms**

**Diastole:** The phase of the cardiac cycle that sees the heart relax and fill with blood.

**Systole:** The phase of the cardiac cycle when the heart contracts. During systole, blood is ejected from the heart or forced from one chamber of the heart to another.

The first stage of the cardiac cycle is atrial diastole. The upper chambers of the heart are filled with blood returning from:

- the body via the venae cavae to the right atrium;
- the lungs via the pulmonary vein to the left atrium.

At this time, the atrioventricular valves are shut, but as the atria fill with blood, atrial pressure overcomes ventricular pressure. Since blood always moves from areas of high pressure to areas of low pressure, the atrioventricular valves are forced open, and ventricular diastole now takes place. During this stage, the ventricles fill

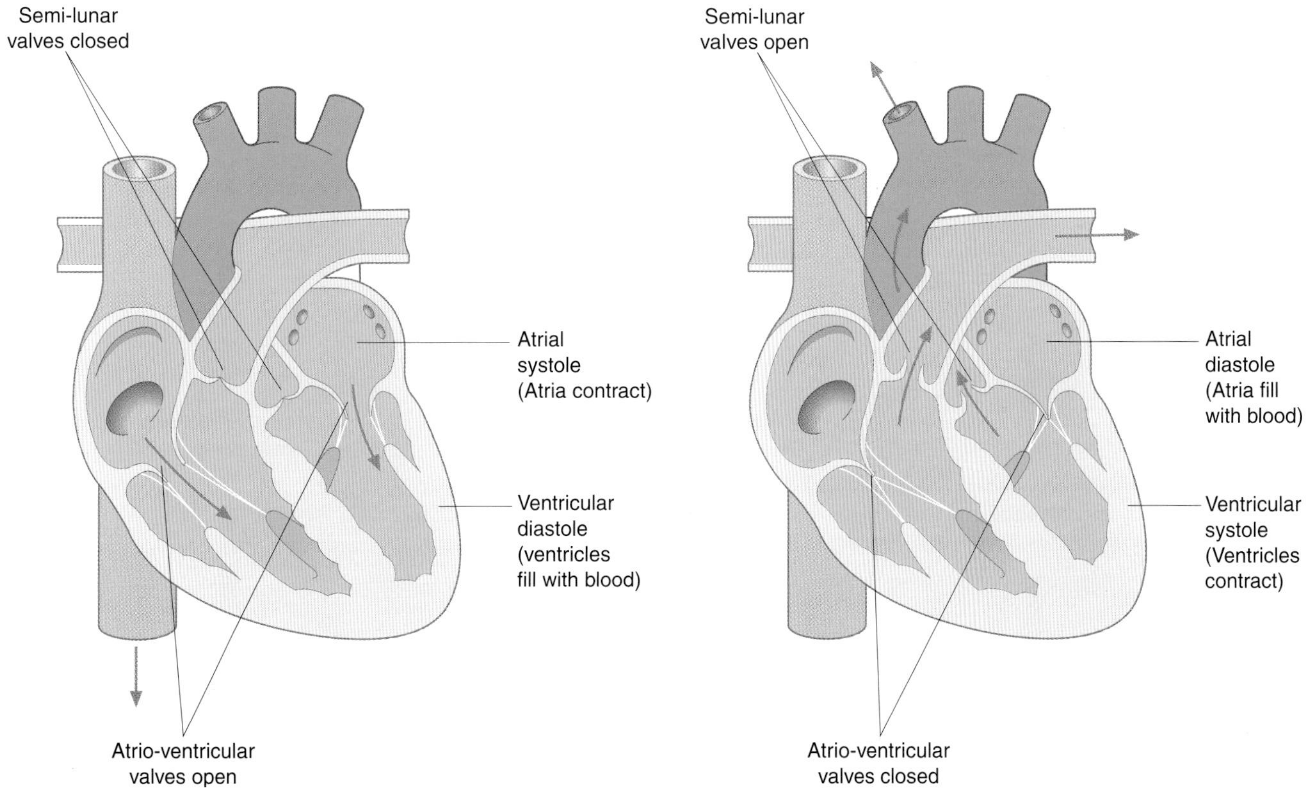


**Figure 4.6** Stages of the cardiac cycle

*Source*: Tortora (1991) *Introduction to the Human Body: The Essentials of Anatomy and Physiology*, 2nd edn, HarperCollins with blood and the semilunar valves remain closed. The atria now contract, causing atrial systole, which ensures that all the blood is ejected into the ventricles. As the ventricles continue going through diastole, the pressure increases, which causes the atrioventricular valves to close. Ultimately, the ventricular pressure overcomes that in the aorta and the pulmonary artery. The semilunar valves open and the ventricles contract, forcing all the blood from the right ventricle into the pulmonary artery, and the blood from the left ventricle into the aorta. This is ventricular systole, and, once this is completed, the semilunar valves snap shut. The cycle is now complete and ready to be repeated.

Generally, the complete diastolic phase takes approximately 0.5 seconds, and the complete systolic phase lasts 0.3 seconds. However, it is interesting to note that trained athletes have been reported to have a longer diastolic phase of the cardiac cycle, enabling a more complete filling of the heart. In this way, the trained athlete can increase venous return and therefore stroke volume (refer to Starling's law of the heart) during resting periods, which accounts for the decreased resting heart rate (known as bradycardia) often experienced by trained athletes. Take a moment to study Figure 4.6, which illustrates the stages of the cardiac cycle.

## Activity 2

You should appreciate by now that the conduction system of the heart and the cardiac cycle are inextricably linked. Figure 4.7 shows the link between the cardiac cycle and the conduction system of the heart, but the stages have been muddled up. Can you identify the correct sequence? Assume that the first box is correct.

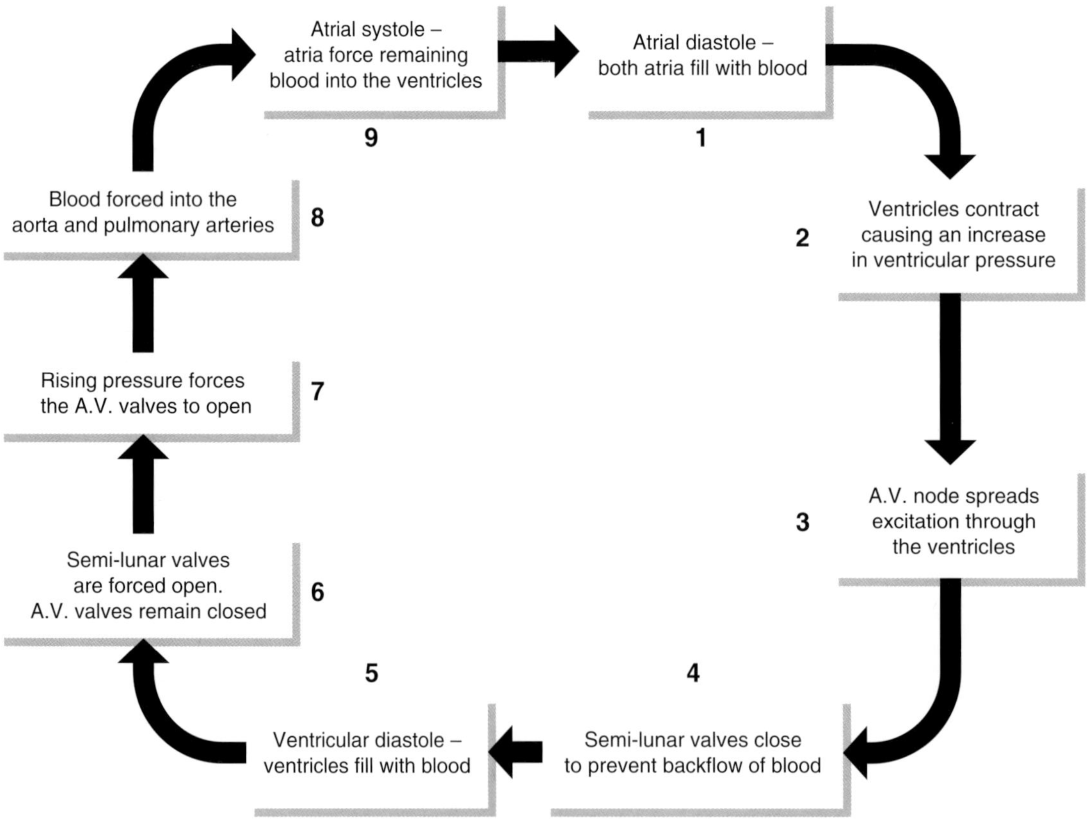


Figure 4.7 The interaction of the conduction system of the heart and the cardiac cycle

## Exam-style questions

1 Describe the stages of the cardiac cycle in relation to the conduction system of the heart. (6 marks)

2 During exercise a greater volume of blood can be ejected from the heart during ventricular systole. Explain how this happens and why this is beneficial to performance. (4 marks)

## Activity 3

1 Fill in the missing gaps:
The ___________ is a bundle of specialised cardiac muscle cells which generate action potentials and govern the heart rate. Impulses are spread across the atria and reach the ___________, which delays the action potentials from spreading through the ventricles.

2 Describe the structure and function of the heart's conducting system.

# Cardiac dynamics – the relationship between heart rate, stroke volume and cardiac output

The performance of the heart is largely dependent on two variables, which work together to optimise cardiac functioning:

- stroke volume;
- heart rate.

## Stroke volume

Stroke volume is the volume of blood pumped out of the heart per beat. It usually refers to the blood ejected from the left ventricle and is measured in millilitres (ml) or $cm^3$. A typical resting value of stroke volume is about 75ml, but this can increase significantly in a trained athlete.

Stroke volume is determined by several factors:

- Venous return – the volume of blood returning to the right atrium. The greater the venous return, the greater the stroke volume, since more blood is available to be pumped out.
- The elasticity of cardiac fibres (sometimes referred to as pre-load) – this refers to the degree of stretch of cardiac tissue just prior to contraction. The greater the stretch of the cardiac fibres, the greater the force of contraction, which can further increase the stroke volume. This is also known as the Frank-Starling mechanism (Starling's law).
- The contractility of cardiac tissue – with increased contractility, a greater force of contraction can occur, which can cause an increase in stroke volume. This is partly due to an increased ejection fraction. The ejection fraction is the percentage of blood actually pumped out of the left ventricle per contraction. It is determined by dividing the stroke volume by the end-diastolic volume and is expressed as a percentage. At rest, the ejection fraction is about 60 per cent (meaning that 40 per cent of blood that enters the heart remains in it), but this can increase to over 85 per cent during exercise.

## Heart rate

The heart rate represents the number of complete cardiac cycles, and therefore the number of times the left ventricle ejects blood into the aorta, per minute. The average resting heart rate of a human is 72 beats per minute, but this can vary tremendously depending on levels of fitness. We might expect an elite endurance athlete, for example, to have a resting heart rate of below 60 beats per minute. When this happens, bradycardia is said to have taken place.

It is possible to measure your heart rate by palpating your radial or carotid arteries. This is referred to as your pulse rate.

**IN CONTEXT**

**Five times winner of the Tour de France, Miguel Indurain, is reported to have a resting heart rate of 28 beats per minute, one of the lowest human rates ever recorded.**

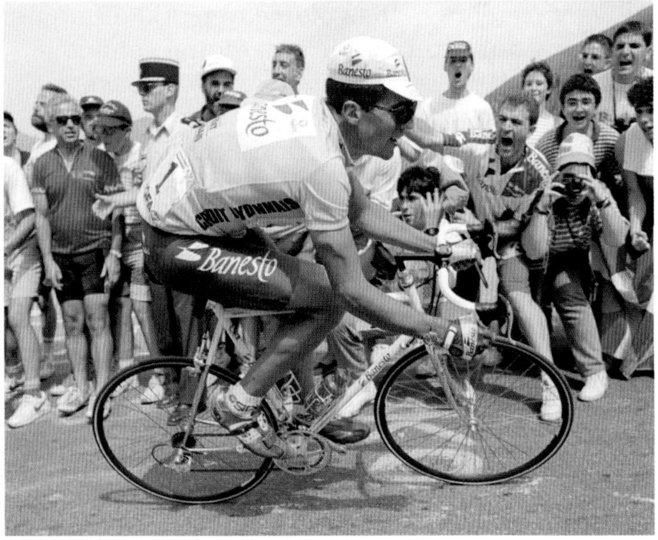


**Figure 4.8** Michael Indurain is reported to have a resting heart rate of 28 beats per minute

## Cardiac output

Cardiac output is the volume of blood that is pumped out of the heart, from one ventricle, per minute. Cardiac output is generally measured from the left ventricle, and is equal to the product of stroke volume and heart rate. The relationship between these variables is summarised below:

Cardiac output = Stroke volume × Heart rate
Q = SV × HR

- The stroke volume is the volume of blood ejected into the aorta in one beat.
- The heart rate reflects the number of times the heart beats per minute.

On average, the resting stroke volume is 75ml per beat, and the resting heart rate for a person is 72 beats per minute. Therefore, cardiac output at rest is:

Q = SV × HR
= 75ml × 72bpm
= 5,400ml/min (5.4L/min)

However, during exercise, cardiac output may rise to 30L/min – a sixfold increase!

# Cardiac dynamics during exercise

During exercise, the body's muscles demand more oxygen. Consequently, the heart must work harder in order to ensure that sufficient oxygen is delivered by the blood to the working muscles, and that waste products such as carbon dioxide and lactic acid are removed. We have just seen that:

Cardiac output (Q) = Stroke volume (SV) × Heart rate (HR)

It is now necessary to consider what happens to each of these variables during exercise.

## Heart rate response to exercise

You will be aware that when we exercise our heart rate increases, but the extent of the increase is largely dependent on exercise intensity. Typically, heart rate increases linearly, in direct proportion to exercise intensity, so that the harder you are working, the higher your heart rate will be. This proportional increase in heart rate will continue until you approach your maximum heart rate (you should recall that this can be calculated by subtracting your age from 220). However, we do not always perform exercise of increasing intensity. During submaximal exercise, where exercise is performed at constant intensity over a prolonged period of time, such as a 1,500m swim, you might expect heart rate to plateau into a steady state for much of the swim. This steady state represents the point where oxygen demand is being met by oxygen supply, and the exercise should therefore be relatively comfortable. Figure 4.10 (below) illustrates typical heart rate curves for maximal and submaximal exercise. Make sure that you are able to draw and label these curves. You will note that just prior to exercise, heart rate increases, even though the exercise has yet to commence. This phenomenon is known as the anticipatory rise and represents the heart's preparation for the forthcoming activity. It results from the release of

**Table 4.1** Stroke volume values at rest and during exercise for trained and untrained subjects

| | Resting stroke volume | Submaximal exercise | Maximal exercise |
|---|---|---|---|
| **Trained** | 80–110ml | 160–200ml | 160–200ml |
| **Untrained** | 60–80ml | 100–120ml | 100–120ml |

hormones such as adrenaline, which cause the SA node to increase the heart rate. You will also note that following exercise the heart rate takes a while to return to its resting level; this represents the body's recovery period. During this phase, the heart rate must remain slightly elevated in order to rid the body of waste products such as lactic acid.

## Stroke volume response to exercise

You will recall that stroke volume is the volume of blood pumped out of the heart with each contraction. As with heart rate, stroke volume increases linearly with increasing intensity, but only up to 40–60 per cent of maximum effort. After this point, stroke volume plateaus (see Figure 4.9 below). One reason for this is the shorter diastolic phase (ventricular filling) that results from the significantly increased heart rate near maximal effort.

Stroke volume is able to increase during exercise for two reasons:

- Increased venous return – this is the volume of blood that returns from the body to the right side of the heart. During exercise, the venous return significantly increases due to a mechanism called the muscle pump, where skeletal muscles squeeze blood back towards the heart. (This will be explained a little later in this chapter.)
- The Frank-Starling mechanism – this mechanism basically suggests that when the heart ventricles stretch more, they can contract with greater force and therefore pump more blood out of the heart. With increased venous return, more blood enters the ventricles during the diastolic phase, which causes them to stretch more and thus contract more forcefully. The reduced heart rate that is experienced by the trained athlete also allows greater time for the ventricles to fill with blood, increasing the degree of stretch by the cardiac tissue and therefore causing the stroke volume of these trained individuals to increase.

## Cardiac output response to exercise

We have seen that cardiac output is the volume of blood pumped out of the heart per minute and is the product of stroke volume and heart rate:

Cardiac output (Q) = Stroke volume (SV) × Heart rate (HR)

As such, the response of cardiac output during exercise is easy to predict. You have just discovered that during exercise both heart rate and stroke volume increase linearly with increasing exercise intensity. Consequently, the pattern of cardiac output during exercise is the same and will continue to increase linearly until maximum exercise capacity, where it will plateau. This is shown in Figure 4.9.

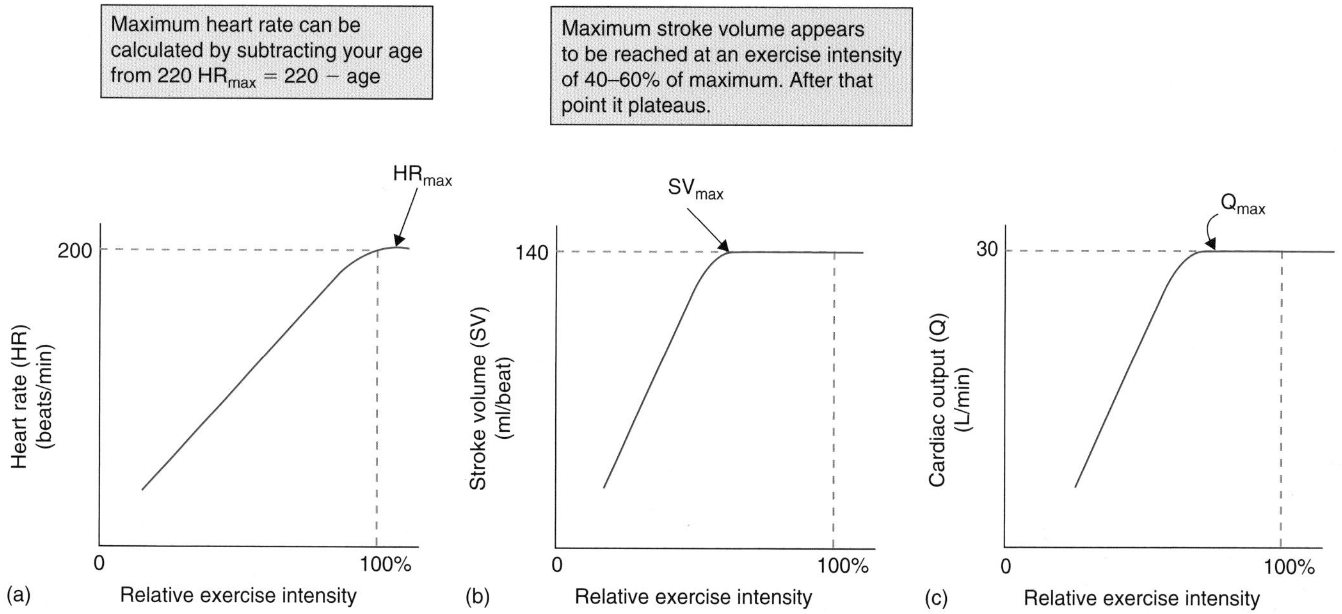


Figure 4.9 Cardiac responses to exercise (a) Heart rate response (b) Stroke volume response (c) Cardiac output response

Table 4.2 Cardiac output values at rest and during exercise for trained and untrained subjects (approximate values)

| | Resting cardiac output | Submaximal exercise | Maximal exercise |
|---|---|---|---|
| **Trained** | 5L/min | 15–20L/min | 30–40L/min |
| **Untrained** | 5L/min | 10–15L/min | 20–30L/min |

## Activity 4

Using the text and Figure 4.10, complete the table below. Note: Don't forget the units!

| Variable | Definition | Approximate resting value | Approximate exercise values |
|---|---|---|---|
| Heart rate | | | |
| Stroke volume | | | |
| Cardiac output | | | |

Cardiac output represents the ability of the heart to circulate blood in the body, delivering oxygen to the working muscles. During maximum exercise, cardiac output may reach values of between four and eight times resting values and is therefore a major factor in determining endurance capacity.

## The pulse

The pulse is a pressure wave which is generated from the heart each time the left ventricle pumps blood into the aorta. The increased pressure causes slight dilation of the arteries as the blood travels through them around the body, and this can be felt at various sites on the body. The most common sites where the pulse can be palpated are as follows:

- radial artery;
- carotid artery;
- femoral artery;
- brachial artery;
- temporal artery.

## Exam-style questions

**1** On the graph opposite, draw a graph to show how the cardiac output of a swimmer completing a 20-minute steady swim, changes during the following stages:

- Immediately prior to the swim
- During the swim
- During recovery from the swim (4 marks)

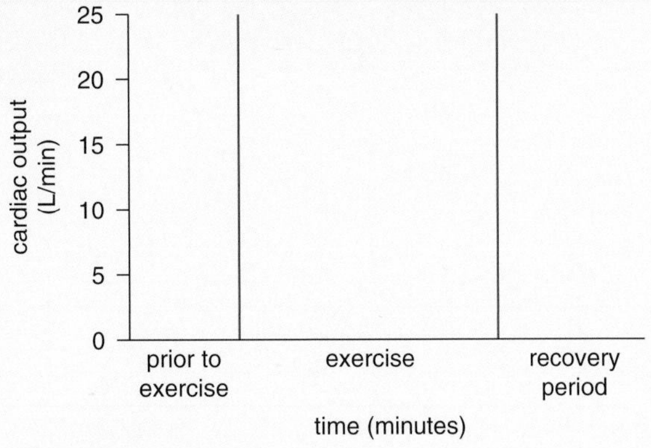


**2** Exercise produces changes in the pattern of heart rate and corresponding changes in the blood flow around the body.

(a) What do you understand by the terms heart rate, stroke volume and cardiac output, and how are they related? (4 marks)

**3** During exercise both heart rate and stroke volume increase.

(a) Explain the processes in the body that allow stroke volume to increase (2 marks)

(b) How does the cardiac control centre regulate heart rate? (4 marks)

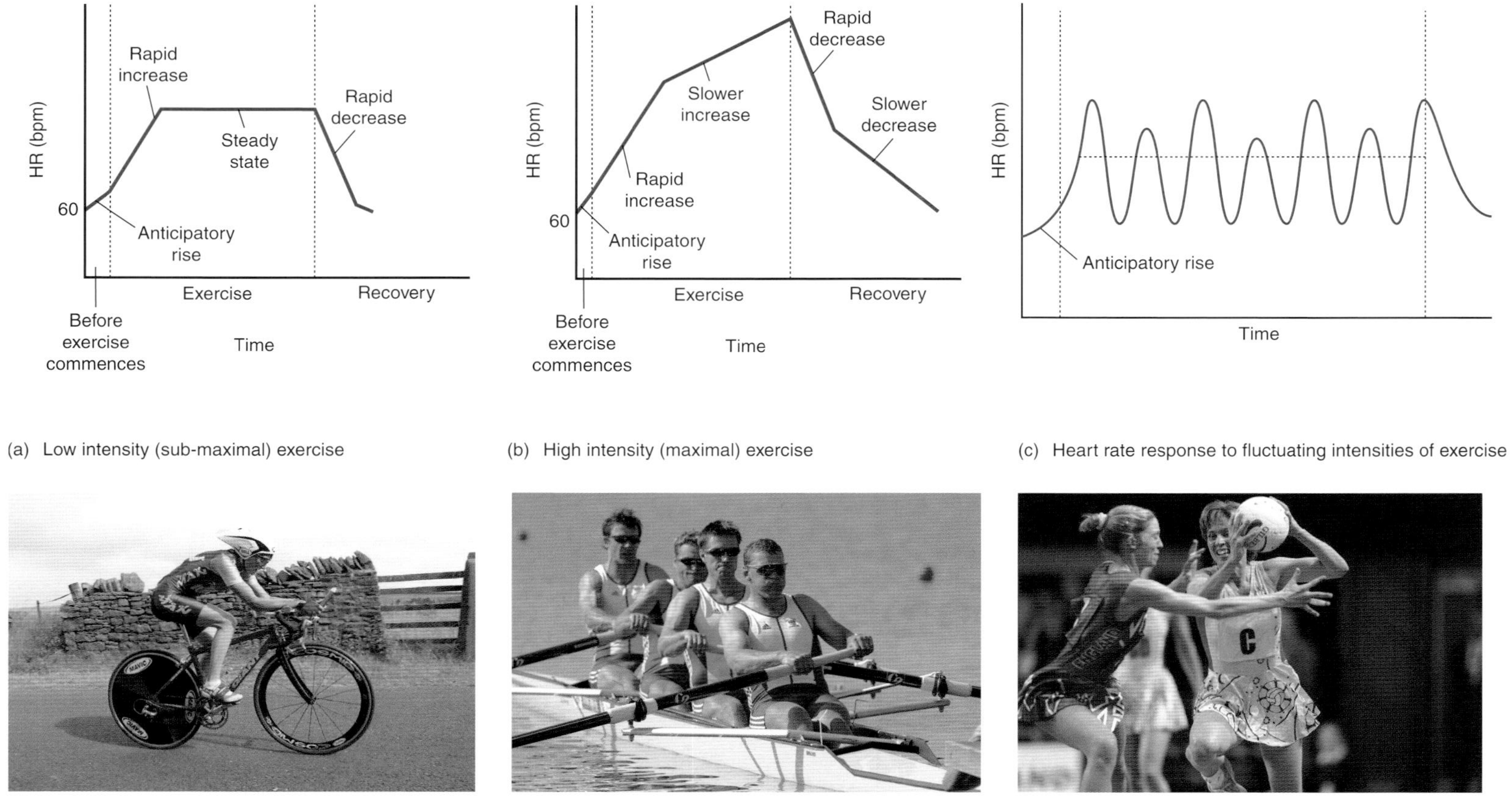


Figure 4.10 Expected heart rate curves for different intensities of exercise

## Activity 5

1 Record your pulse for a 10-second count at each of the following sites:
- carotid artery;
- radial artery;
- brachial artery.

Remember to start counting from zero.

2 Multiply your scores by six to achieve your heart rate score in beats per minute.
3 Account for any differences in your heart rate scores at the different sites.
4 Why should you never use your thumb to measure your pulse?

## Activity 6

You are going to carry out an investigation to examine heart rate response to varying intensities of exercise. You will need a stopwatch, a gymnastics bench and a metronome.

1 Record resting heart rate for a 10-second count at the beginning of the class.
2 Record heart rate for a 10-second count at the carotid artery immediately prior to exercise.
3 Start exercising by stepping on and off the bench at a low intensity, keeping time with the metronome.
4 Record your pulse after one, two and three minutes of exercise. After the third minute of exercise, stop the test. Continue to record your pulse each minute during recovery.
5 Once your heart rate has returned to its resting value (or within a few beats), repeat the test at a medium intensity. Record your results as before.
6 Repeat the exercise for a third time, but at a very high intensity. Once again, record your results.
7 Convert your heart rate scores into beats per minute by multiplying by six.
8 Now use your results to plot a graph for each of the three workloads. Plot each graph using the same axes, placing heart rate along the Y axis and time along the X axis. Don't forget to show your resting heart rate values on the graph.
9 For each of your graphs, explain the heart rate patterns prior to, during and following exercise.

| Time | Exercise intensity | | |
|---|---|---|---|
| | Low | Medium | High |
| Resting HR | | | |
| HR prior to exercise | | | |
| Exercise 1 min | | | |
| Exercise 2 min | | | |
| Exercise 3 min | | | |
| Recovery 1 min | | | |
| Recovery 2 min | | | |
| Recovery 3 min | | | |
| Recovery 4 min | | | |
| Recovery 5 min | | | |
| Recovery 6 min | | | |
| Recovery 7 min | | | |

## Activity 7

Using Figure 4.10, account for the different patterns in heart rate for submaximal and maximal exercise.

## Activity 8

Wearing a heart rate monitor, participate in an invasion game of your choice (e.g. netball, football, basketball) for at least 15 minutes. Don't forget to record your resting heart rate and your heart rate immediately prior to the start.

At a maximum of three-minute intervals, record your heart rate for the duration of the game. Note: The longer you participate in the game, the better!

Copy out and complete the table and graph.

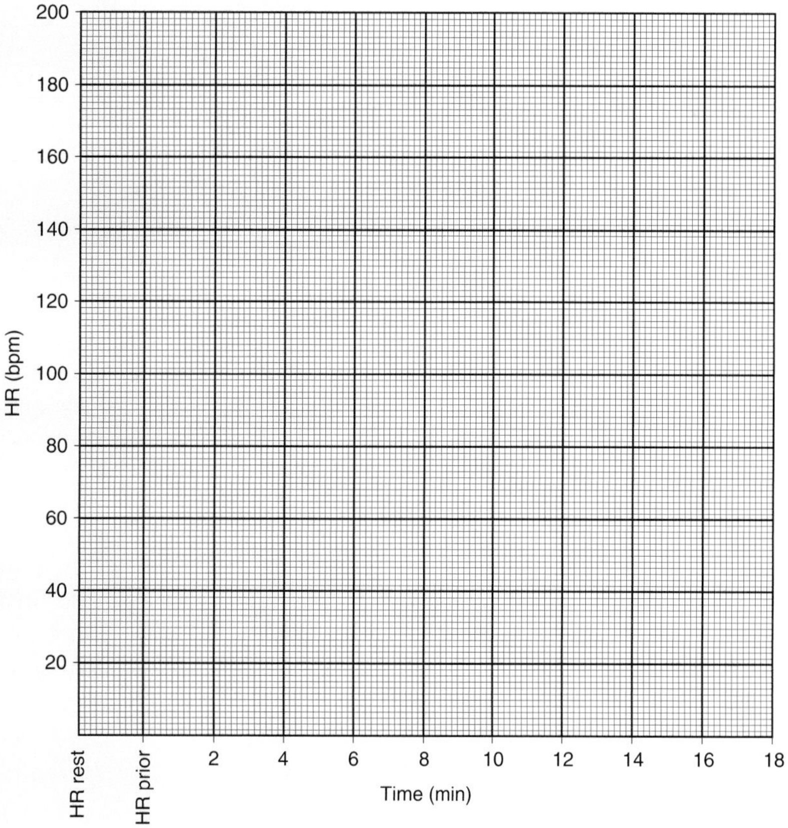


| Time | Heart rate |
|---|---|
| Rest | |
| Prior to exercise | |
| 1 | |
| 2 | |
| 3 | |
| 4 | |
| 5 | |
| 6 | |
| 7 | |
| 8 | |
| 9 | |
| 10 | |
| 11 | |
| 12 | |
| 13 | |
| 14 | |
| 15 | |

Explain the pattern of heart rate illustrated by the graph.

# The control and regulation of the heart

The heart is governed by the autonomic nervous system (ANS), which operates without us having to think about it. In respect to the heart, it is the ANS which determines the rate at which the pacemaker (SA node) sends out impulses. The sympathetic and parasympathetic nervous systems are the two subdivisions of the autonomic nervous system which determine the actions of the cardiac control centre (CCC) in the medulla oblongata of the brain. They are fundamental to the regulation of the heart and work antagonistically as follows:

1 The sympathetic nervous system increases the heart rate by releasing adrenaline and noradrenaline from the adrenal medulla. Adrenaline increases the strength of ventricular contraction, and therefore stroke volume, while noradrenaline (a transmitter substance) aids the spread of the impulse throughout the heart, and therefore increases heart rate.
2 The parasympathetic nervous system, on the other hand, releases acetylcholine, which slows the spread of impulses and therefore reduces heart rate, returning it to the normal resting level.

Essentially, there are three main factors that determine the action of the CCC:

1 Neural factors – Once exercise begins, proprioceptors and mechanoreceptors within the muscles, tendons and joints relay messages to the cardiac centre, informing it that the amount of movement has increased and therefore muscles will require a greater supply of blood. Chemoreceptors located in the aorta and carotid arteries inform the centre of changes to the chemical composition of the blood, in particular reacting to increased levels of carbon dioxide. The cardiac centre increases the heart rate in order to speed up carbon dioxide removal. Baroreceptors, meanwhile, respond to changes in blood pressure as a result of increased activity.
2 Hormonal factors – Once stimulated, the sympathetic nerves cause the release of adrenaline and noradrenaline, which increases the strength of ventricular contractions of the heart and increases heart rate, which together greatly increase cardiac output. In addition, these hormones help to control blood pressure and assist in the redistribution of blood to the working muscles through vasoconstriction and vasodilation of arterioles.
3 Intrinsic factors – When exercise commences there is an increase in body temperature, which helps increase the flow of blood round the body (as blood becomes less viscous) and helps raise heart rate by increasing the speed of nerve impulse transmission.

**Key terms**

**Sympathetic nervous system:** One of the two subdivisions of the autonomic nervous system which is primarily responsible for increasing heart rate, particularly during exercise.
**Parasympathetic nervous system:** The second of the two subdivisions of the autonomic nervous system. Its actions oppose those of the sympathetic nervous system and it is primarily responsible for returning the heart and respiratory rate to normal resting levels following exercise.
**Cardiac control centre:** Located in the medulla oblongata in the brain, the cardiac control centre is primarily responsible for controlling the heart rate.

Table 4.3 The autonomic nervous system and cardiac function

| The sympathetic function | The parasympathetic function |
|---|---|
| Increased heart rate | Decreased heart rate |
| Increased strength of contraction | Decreased strength of contraction |
| Vasodilation of arteries supplying the muscles and the heart | Vasoconstriction of arteries supplying the muscles and the heart |
| Some vasoconstriction of arteries of the abdomen, kidneys and skin | Vasodilation of arteries of the abdomen, kidneys and skin |

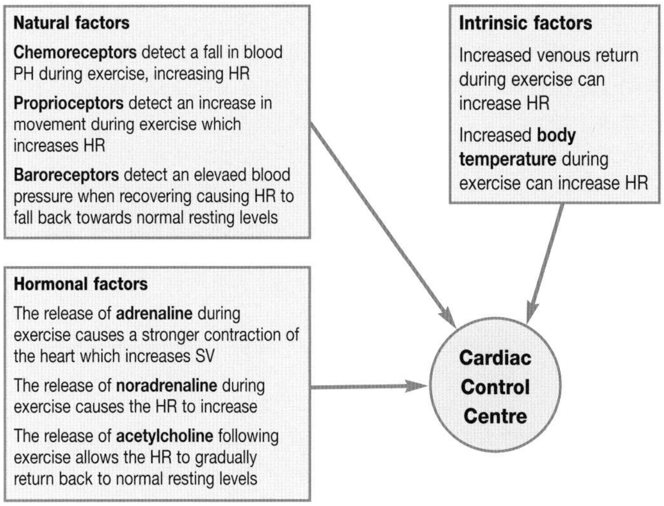
Natural factors
**Chemoreceptors** detect a fall in blood PH during exercise, increasing HR
**Proprioceptors** detect an increase in movement during exercise which increases HR
**Baroreceptors** detect an elevaed blood pressure when recovering causing HR to fall back towards normal resting levels
Intrinsic factors
Increased venous return during exercise can increase HR
Increased **body temperature** during exercise can increase HR
Hormonal factors
The release of **adrenaline** during exercise causes a stronger contraction of the heart which increases SV
The release of **noradrenaline** during exercise causes the HR to increase
The release of **acetylcholine** following exercise allows the HR to gradually return back to normal resting levels
Cardiac Control Centre

Figure 4.11 A summary of the factors that affect the cardiac control centre (CCC)

## Key terms

**Chemoreceptors:** Sensory cells situated in the aorta and the carotid arteries which monitor the level of acidity of the blood. They are particularly sensitive to changes in the carbon dioxide content of the blood and cause the cardiac control centre to adjust heart rate accordingly.

**Mechanoreceptors:** Sensory cells that provide feedback to the central nervous system about any mechanical movement that takes place.

**Baroreceptors:** Sensory cells situated in the aorta, venae cavae and atria which respond to changes in blood pressure. The cardiac control centre and vasomotor centre will respond to changes in blood pressure by adjusting the heart rate and blood vessel diameter accordingly.

## Activity 9

Place the following stages in the control of heart rate in the correct order:

- Sympathetic nerves release adrenaline/noradrenaline.
- Parasympathetic nerves emit impulses and release acetylcholine.
- Proprioceptors (e.g. muscle spindles) detect changes in motor activity.
- Increases the activity of the SA node and causes an increase in heart rate.
- Chemoreceptors detect changes in carbon dioxide and the pH of the blood.
- Once exercise ceases, baroreceptors detect elevated blood pressure in the aorta and carotid arteries.
- Decreases the activity of the SA node and reduces heart rate slowly, back to resting levels.

## Regulation during exercise

At rest, the parasympathetic system overrides the sympathetic system, and keeps the heart rate down. However, once exercise begins, the sympathetic system increases its activity and the parasympathetic system decreases activity, so heart rate is allowed to rise. Increased metabolic activity causes an increased concentration of carbon dioxide and lactic acid content in the blood, which increases acidity and decreases blood pH. These changes are detected by chemoreceptors sited in the aortic arch and carotid arteries. They inform the sympathetic centre in the upper thoracic area of the spinal cord to increase the heart rate in order to transport the carbon dioxide to the lungs, where it can be expelled. Messages from the sympathetic centre are sent to the SA node via accelerator nerves, which release adrenaline and noradrenaline on stimulation.

Adrenaline and noradrenaline released from the adrenal medulla (situated at the top of the kidneys) generally have the same effect – increasing heart rate and increasing the strength of contraction. They also help to increase metabolic activity, convert glycogen into its usable form, glucose, make glucose and free fatty acids available to the muscle, and redistribute blood to the working muscles.

Other factors which increase heart rate during exercise include:

- increased body temperature – and therefore decreased blood viscosity (the relative 'thickness' of the blood);
- increased venous return (a result of the increased action of the muscle pump).

Both these factors will result in greater cardiac output.

Once exercise ceases, sympathetic stimulation decreases and the parasympathetic system takes over once again. The parasympathetic system responds to information from baroreceptors – the body's inbuilt blood pressure recorders. When blood pressure is too high, messages are sent from the cardiac inhibitory centre to the SA node via the vagus nerve. The parasympathetic nerve then releases acetylcholine, which decreases the heart rate.

This continuous interaction of the sympathetic and parasympathetic systems ensures that the heart works as efficiently as possible, and enables sufficient nutrients to reach the tissue cells to ensure effective muscle action.

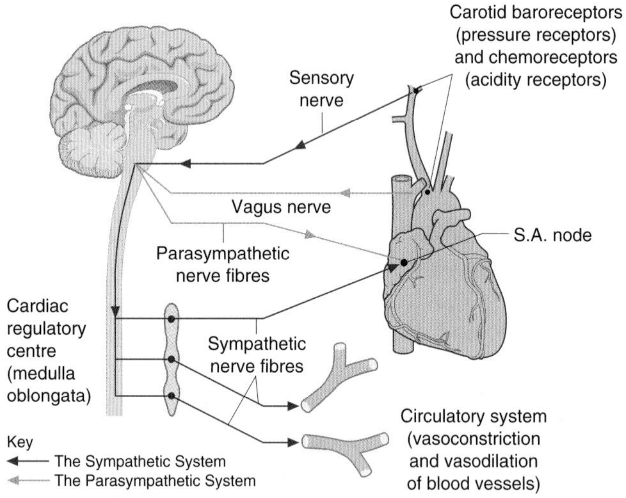


Figure 4.12 The regulation of heart rate

## Athlete's heart

We have examined how the heart responds and adjusts to exercise in a short exercise session. Let us now turn our attention to the effects of long-term training on the heart.

As mentioned above, the heart of an athlete is larger than that of a non-athlete and often displays greater vascularisation. Cardiac hypertrophy is characterised by a larger ventricular wall and a thicker myocardium. Endurance athletes tend to display larger ventricular cavities, while those following high-resistance or strength-training regimes display thicker ventricular walls.

Cardiac hypertrophy is accompanied by a decreased resting heart rate. This can easily be demonstrated by comparing the resting heart rates of trained and untrained people. When the heart rate falls below 60 beats per minute, bradycardia is said to have occurred, and is due to a slowing in the intrinsic rate of the atrial pacemaker (SA node) and an increase in the predominance of the parasympathetic system acting on the pacemaker.

### Key terms

**Cardiac hypertrophy:** The enlargement of the heart due to the effects of training. Endurance athletes tend to display larger ventricular cavities, while those following high-resistance strength training will display thicker ventricular walls.

**Bradycardia:** Literally meaning 'slow heart', bradycardia is the term used to describe the reduction in resting heart rate that accompanies training (usually when resting heart rate falls below 60 beats per minute).

Some endurance athletes have recorded resting heart rates of below 30 beats per minute! Since the resting cardiac output for an athlete is approximately the same as that of a non-athlete, the athlete compensates for the lower resting heart rate by increasing stroke volume. This increased resting stroke volume is greatest among endurance athletes (as great as 200ml/beat), due to the increased size of the ventricular cavity. The increase can also be the result of improved contractility of the myocardium, which is highlighted by the increased ejection fraction reported by athletes. The ejection fraction represents the percentage of blood entering the left ventricle which is actually pumped out per beat. It is calculated by dividing the stroke volume by the volume of blood in the ventricles at the end of the diastolic phase (EDV). On average, this is approximately 60 per cent, but can reach 85 per cent following training (see Figure 4.13).

Training signals an improvement in cardiac output during exercise, brought about by an increase in

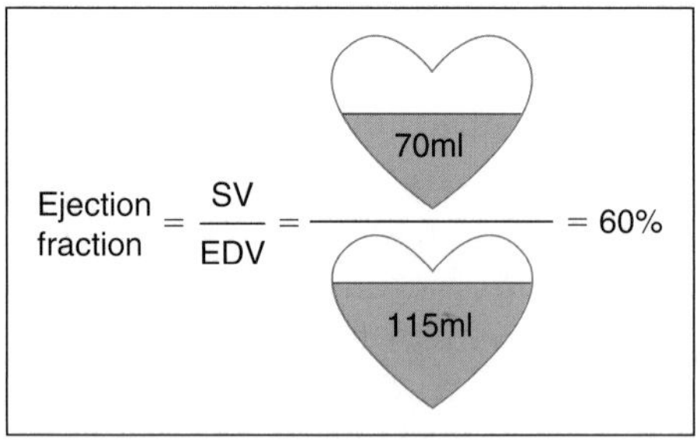


Figure 4.13 Calculation of the ejection fraction

**Key terms**

**Starling's law:** Starling's law states that stroke volume increases in response to an increase in the diastolic filling of the heart (which is dependent on venous return). The increased volume of blood stretches the ventricular wall, causing the cardiac muscle to contract more forcefully.

**Ejection fraction:** The proportion of blood actually pumped out of the left ventricle per contraction.

stroke volume, due to the larger volume of the left ventricle and the hypertrophy (enlargement) of the heart (sometimes referred to as athlete's heart). At rest, cardiac hypertrophy plays an important role, since increased stroke volume (which accompanies hypertrophy) allows the resting heart rate to decrease. This is known as bradycardia. The increased size of the ventricular cavity in trained athletes allows a longer diastolic phase, during which time the heart can fill up with more blood. This stretches cardiac fibres and increases the strength of contraction, with the resultant effect of increasing stroke volume. Consequently, cardiac output does not change at rest following training.

**IN CONTEXT**

**Seven times winner of the Tour de France, Lance Armstrong, has a heart approximately 30 per cent larger than average.**

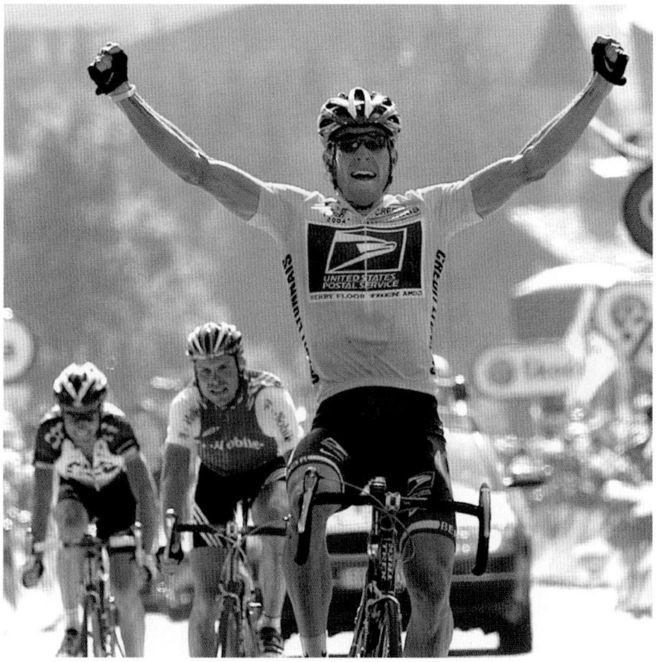

Figure 4.14 Lance Armstrong is reported to have a heart 30 per cent larger than the average

**Exam-style questions**

(a) Describe the physiological changes that occur to the heart following a period of endurance training. (3 marks)

(b) What effect do these physiological changes have on an individual's performance? (2 marks)

# Cardiovascular drift

When we exercise for prolonged periods of time, particularly in warm weather or in hot environments, we can often experience an increase in heart rate, despite working at a constant intensity. This elevation in heart rate is known as cardiovascular drift. The most likely explanation for this upwards drift in heart rate is the reduction in blood volume that arises from the increased sweating response of the body. When the body becomes hot during exercise, blood is shunted to the skin (peripheral circulation) to release heat from the body, while at the same time the sweat glands increase their output to cool the body through evaporation. The outcome of this is that body fluids are lost, which reduces the volume of blood returning to the heart. You will recall from Starlings Law that stroke volume is dependent upon venous return, so if less blood is returning to the heart, stroke volume decreases. In order to maintain the same level of cardiac output the heart rate must increase (since Cardiac output = Stroke volume x Heart rate). To minimise cardiovascular drift it is essential that performers remain hydrated by drinking plenty of fluids before and during the exercise period.

# The vascular system

Having examined how the heart works to pump the blood into the network of blood vessels, we will now take a closer look at how the blood supports the functioning of the body and how the blood vessels ensure that sufficient blood reaches the body's tissues.

## The blood

Blood consists of cells and cell fragments, surrounded by a liquid known as plasma. The average male has a total blood volume of 5–6L, and the average female blood volume is approximately 4–5L.

## Functions of blood

The blood's functions are fundamental to life itself and include:

- transportation of nutrients such as glucose and oxygen;
- protection and fighting disease through interaction with the lymphatic system;
- maintenance of homeostasis, including temperature regulation and maintenance of the acid–base (pH) balance.

The blood is responsible for transporting oxygen to the body's cells and removing metabolites, such as carbon dioxide, from the muscle to the lungs. The blood also transports glucose from the liver to the muscle, and lactic acid from the muscle to the liver, where it can be converted back to glucose. Further functions include the transportation of enzymes, hormones and other chemicals, all of which have a vital role to play in the body, no more so than during exercise.

The blood protects the body by containing cells and chemicals which are central to the immune system. When damage to blood vessels occurs, the blood clots in order to prevent cell loss.

The blood is vital in maintaining the body's state of equilibrium; for example, through hormone and enzyme activity, and the buffering capacity of the blood, the blood's pH should remain relatively stable. In addition, the blood is involved in temperature regulation and can transport heat to the surface of the body where it can be released. All these factors are particularly important during exercise, to ensure optimal performance.

## Blood viscosity

Viscosity refers to the thickness of the blood and its resistance to flow. The more viscous a fluid, the more resistant it is to flow. The greater the volume of red blood cells, the greater the capacity to transport oxygen. However, unless it is accompanied by an increase in plasma, viscosity may also increase, and restrict blood flow. Viscosity may also increase when plasma content decreases, due to dehydration (which may accompany endurance-based exercise).

Training brings about an increase in total blood volume, and therefore an increase in the number of red blood cells. However, the plasma volume increases more than blood cell volume, so the blood viscosity decreases. This facilitates blood flow through the blood vessels, and improves oxygen delivery to the working muscles.

**Key term**

**Blood viscosity:** A term used to describe the relative thickness of the blood. If the blood is very viscous, it has a high amount of blood cells to plasma and consequently does not flow very quickly.

# The transport of blood gases

## The transport of oxygen and the oxyhaemoglobin dissociation curve

We established in Chapter 2 that the majority of oxygen is carried by the red blood cells combined with haemoglobin; this is an iron-based protein which chemically combines with oxygen to form oxyhaemoglobin.

Haemoglobin + Oxygen → Oxyhaemoglobin
$Hb + O_2 \rightarrow HbO_2$

Each molecule of haemoglobin can combine with four molecules of oxygen, which amounts to approximately 1.34ml. The concentration of haemoglobin in the blood is about 15g per 100ml; thus, each 100ml of blood can transport up to 20ml of oxygen (1.34 × 15). However, the amount of oxygen that can combine with haemoglobin is determined by the partial pressure of oxygen ($pO_2$). A high $pO_2$ results in complete haemoglobin saturation; while at a lower $pO_2$, haemoglobin saturation decreases.

Haemoglobin is almost 100 per cent saturated with oxygen, at a $pO_2$ of 100mmHg (which is the $pO_2$ in the alveoli). Therefore, at the lungs, haemoglobin is totally saturated with oxygen, and even if more oxygen were available, it could not be transported. As the $pO_2$ is reduced, haemoglobin saturation decreases accordingly. This is largely due to the increased acidity of the blood (decrease in blood pH), caused by an increase in $CO_2$ content or lactic acid, and the increase in body temperature, which causes a shift to the right in the haemoglobin saturation curve. This is known as the Bohr shift, and explains how oxygen is dissociated from haemoglobin at lower pH values in order to feed the tissues.

During exercise, increased $CO_2$ production causes a greater dissociation of oxygen due to the decrease in muscle pH. A further cause is the increase in body temperature that accompanies exercise; as oxygen unloading becomes more effective, the dissociation curve shifts to the right.

**Key term**

**Bohr shift:** A shift in the oxyhaemoglobin dissociation curve to the right that is caused by increased levels in carbon dioxide and the subsequent increase in blood acidity.

To summarise, endurance performance is reliant on the quick and effective dissociation of oxygen from haemoglobin, which in turn is dependent on four factors:

1. a fall in the $pO_2$ within the muscle;
2. an increase in blood and muscle temperature;
3. an increase in the $pCO_2$ within the muscle;
4. a fall in pH due to the production of lactic acid.

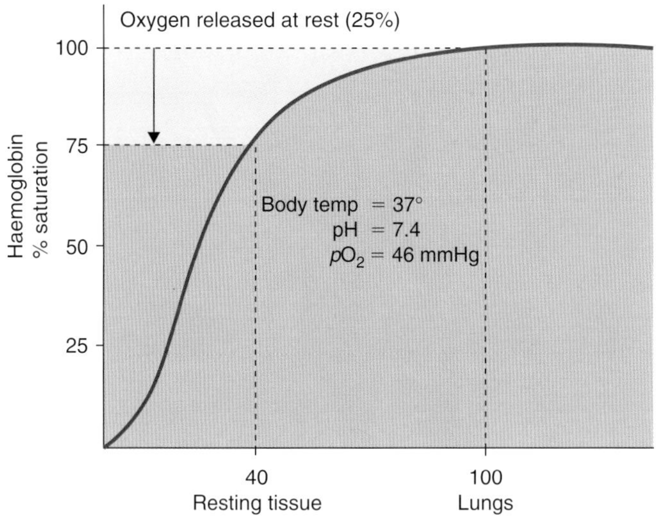


(a) **At rest**

At rest the $pO_2$ in the alveoli is approximately 100 mmHg. At this point the haemoglobin is almost 100% saturated with oxygen. In resting muscles and tissues the $pO_2$ is approximately 40 mmHg. At this point haemoglobin is only 75% saturated with oxygen. This means that 25% of the oxygen picked up at the lungs is released into the muscle to help in energy production

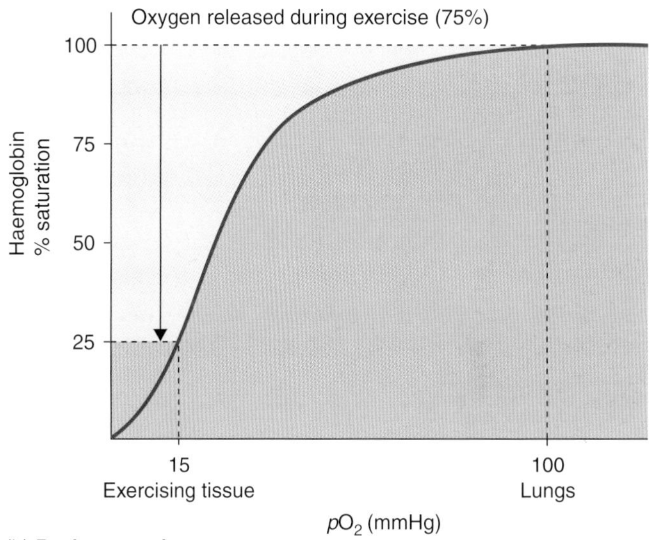


(b) **During exercise**

During exercise the $pO_2$ in the alveoli remains at approximately 100 mmHg with almost 100% haemoglobin saturation. In working muscles the $pO_2$ can be greatly reduced when compared to resting figures. The diagram shows a $pO_2$ in working muscles of 15 mmHg. This represents an oxy-haemoglobin saturation of 25% meaning that 75% of the oxygen picked up at the lungs is released into the muscle to help meet the extra energy demands.

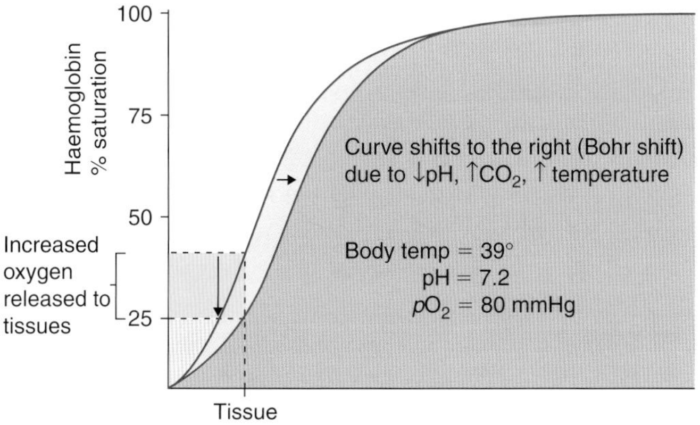


(c) **The Bohr shift**

During exercise there is an increase in the production of carbon dioxide in the muscle cell raising the $pCO_2$. As a result of this and increases in the concentration of lactic acid, blood acidity increases causing a fall in the pH. Energy produced in the muscle cell increases temperature. These factors cause a shift in the curve to the right (known as the Bohr shift) which results in an increased release of oxygen.

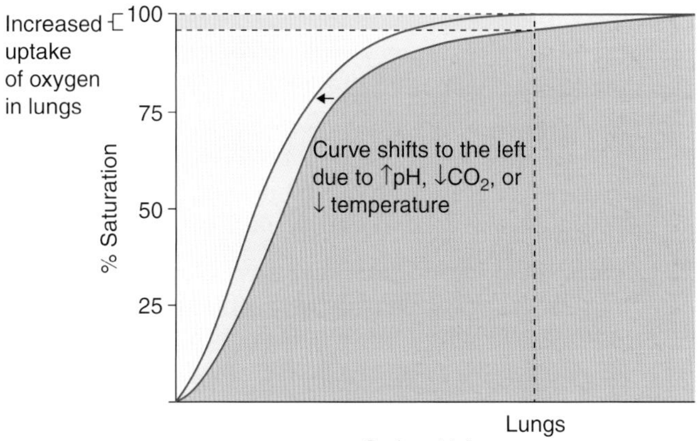


(d) **Following exercise**

Once exercise ceases we see an increase in blood pH, a decrease in $pCO_2$ and a decrease in temperature in the lungs. The curve shifts to the left returning to its resting position. It results in an increased ability of haemoglobin to pick up oxygen at the lungs.

Figure 4.15 The oxygen–haemoglobin dissociation curve

## Activity 10

1 During resting conditions, approximately 5ml of oxygen is transported to the tissues in each 100ml of blood. We know from earlier discussions that cardiac output at rest is approximately 5,000ml/min. Calculate how much oxygen is delivered to the tissues each minute.

2 During exercise, the oxygen transport can be increased by up to three times, due to the greater release of oxygen from haemoglobin. In addition, the rate of oxygen transport can increase fivefold, due to the increase in cardiac output while exercising. Calculate how much oxygen can now be delivered to the tissues when exercising.

## Activity 11

1 Explain how the oxyhaemoglobin disassociation curve can aid our understanding of gaseous exchange. How might increases in blood acidity affect the curve?

2 Outline how $CO_2$ is transported in the body. What is the role of the bicarbonate ion in this process?

### IN CONTEXT

**Paula Radcliffe's record as an endurance performer speaks for itself. The defining factor that determines successful performance in activities such as a marathon run is undoubtedly the availability of oxygen to the runner's muscles. The marathon runner's body has adapted to increase the supply of oxygen to the working muscles. We already know that during exercise, the oxyhaemoglobin curve shifts to the right (the Bohr shift), which facilitates the dissociation of oxygen from haemoglobin. This shift to the right arises due to the following factors:**

1 **A fall in the $pO_2$ inside the muscle cell, due to an increased oxygen uptake by the muscles. This increases the oxygen diffusion gradient.**

2 **An increase in $pCO_2$ inside the muscle cell. Carbon dioxide is produced when the body releases energy from our food fuels. This increases the carbon dioxide diffusion gradient.**

3 **A fall in blood pH (increased acidity), resulting from both carbon dioxide and lactic acid production in the muscle cell.**

4 **An increase in body temperature, which arises from the heat energy produced during the increased muscle contractions that accompany physical activity.**

**Together, these four factors ensure that the muscles of the runner receive the necessary oxygen to complete the marathon, delaying fatigue and increasing the intensity of the performance.**

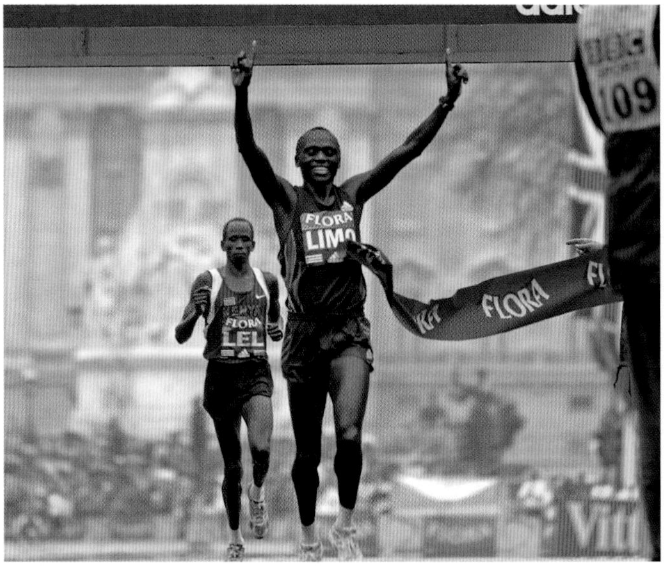


**Figure 4.16** The marathon runner's body has adapted to increase the supply of oxygen to the working muscles

The arterial–venous oxygen difference (a–$\bar{V}O_2$ diff.) is the difference in oxygen content between the arterial blood and venous blood, and can measure how much oxygen is actually being consumed in the muscles and tissues. At rest, only about 25 per cent of oxygen is actually used. This increases dramatically during intense exercise, however, to as much as 85 per cent. Figure 4.16 illustrates the a–$\bar{V}O_2$ diff. at rest and during intense exercise.

### Key terms

**a–$\bar{V}O_2$ diff.:** The arterial–venous oxygen difference is the difference in oxygen content of the blood in the arteries and the veins. It is a measure of the amount of oxygen consumed by the muscles.

**IN CONTEXT**

The overall efficiency of oxygen transport is dependent on haemoglobin content, and many athletes have sought to increase haemoglobin content through the illegal practice of **blood doping**. By removing blood, which is subsequently replaced by the body, the athlete reinfuses it, to increase blood volume and, more importantly, haemoglobin content. Results of research on the practice of blood doping are conflicting, and it should always be remembered that it is illegal under the current Olympic Committee doping rules.

More recently, the preferred cheater's drug has been **EPO** – a synthetic version of **erythropoietin**, a glycoprotein that occurs naturally in the body and stimulates the production of red blood cells. The drug's advantages are that it can increase the oxygen-carrying capacity of the blood and therefore improve endurance performance. But EPO has potentially fatal effects, as well as being illegal for competition (and very expensive). Several top cyclists have died following misuse of the drug. Thankfully, a new test has recently become available to detect the use of this dangerous drug.

## Exam-style questions

**1** With reference to the oxyhaemoglobin dissociation curve, explain how a greater amount of oxygen is released to the working muscles.(2 marks)

**2** During exercise the oxyhaemoglobin dissociation curve shifts to the right. What is the significance of this to an athlete's performance? (3 marks)

## The transport of carbon dioxide

Carbon dioxide produced in the body's tissues is also transported in the blood in various ways:

- approximately 8 per cent is dissolved in the blood plasma;
- up to 20 per cent combines with haemoglobin to form carbaminohaemoglobin;
- up to 70 per cent of carbon dioxide is dissolved in water as carbonic acid.

Removal of carbon dioxide from the body is necessary if effective performance is to be maintained.

## The circulatory system

The blood flows through a continuous network of blood vessels, which form a double circuit. This connects the heart to the lungs, and the heart to all other body tissues.

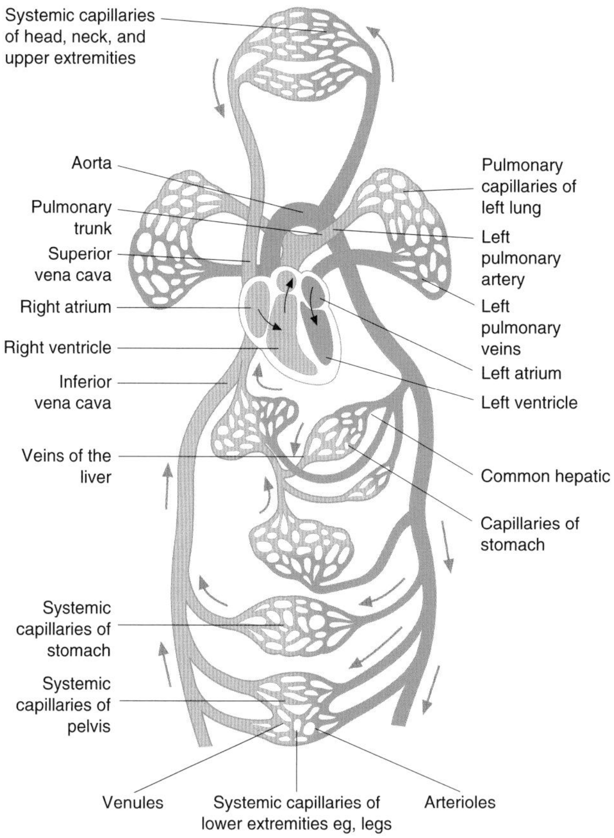


**Figure 4.17** The double-circulatory system

## The double circulatory system

Pulmonary circulation transports blood between the lungs and the heart. The pulmonary artery carries blood low in oxygen concentration from the right ventricle to the lung, where it becomes oxygen-rich and unloads carbon dioxide. The pulmonary vein then transports the freshly oxygenated blood back to the heart and into the left atrium.

The blood returning to the left atrium is pumped through the left side of the heart and into the aorta, where it is distributed to the whole of the body's tissues by a network of arteries. Veins then return the blood, which is now low in oxygen and high in carbon dioxide concentration, to the heart, where it enters the right atrium via the venae cavae. This circuit is known as systemic circulation.

## Blood vessels

The vascular network through which blood flows to all parts of the body comprises arteries, arterioles, capillaries, veins and venules.

## Arteries and arterioles

Arteries are high-pressure vessels which carry blood from the heart to the tissues. The largest artery in the body is the aorta, which is the main artery leaving the heart. The aorta constantly subdivides and gets smaller. The constant subdivision decreases the diameter of the vessel arteries, which now become arterioles. As the network subdivides, blood velocity decreases, which enables the efficient delivery and exchange of gases.

Arteries are composed of three layers of tissue:

1 an outer fibrous layer – the tunica adventitia or tunica externa;
2 a thick middle layer – the tunica media;
3 a thin lining of cells to the inside – the endothelium or tunica intima.

The tunica media comprises smooth muscle and elastic tissue, which enables the arteries and arterioles to alter their diameter. Arteries tend to have more elastic tissue, while arterioles have greater amounts of smooth muscle; this allows the vessels to increase the diameter through vasodilation, or to decrease the diameter through vasoconstriction. It is through vasoconstriction and vasodilation that the vessels can regulate blood pressure and ensure the tissues are receiving sufficient blood – particularly during exercise.

### Key terms

**Vasodilation:** A process by which blood vessels in the body (namely arteries and arterioles) become wider.
**Vasoconstriction:** A process by which blood vessels in the body (namely arteries and arterioles) become narrower.

Arteries and arterioles have three basic functions:

- to act as conduits, carrying and controlling blood flow to the tissues;
- to cushion and smooth out the pulsatile flow of blood from the heart;
- to help control blood pressure.

## Veins and venules

Veins are low-pressure vessels which return blood to the heart. Their structure is similar to that of arteries, although they possess less smooth muscle and elastic tissue. Venules are the smallest veins and transport blood away from the capillary bed into the veins. Veins gradually increase in thickness the nearer to the heart they get, until they reach the two largest veins in the body, the venae cavae, which enter the right atrium of the heart.

The thinner walls of the veins often distend and allow blood to pool in them. This is also allowed to happen as the veins contain pocket valves which close intermittently to prevent backflow of blood. This explains why up to 70 per cent of total blood volume is found in the venous system at any one time, at rest.

## Capillaries

Capillaries are the functional units of the vascular system. Composed of a single layer of endothelial cells, they are just thin enough to allow red blood

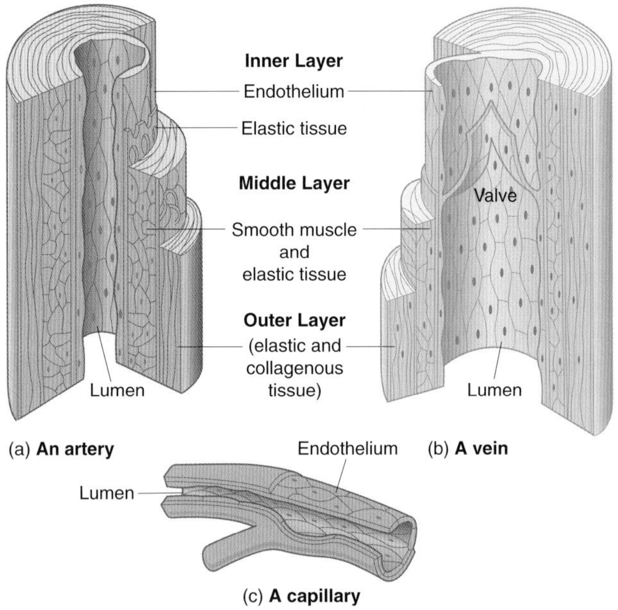


Figure 4.18 The structure of blood vessels

*Source*: Tortora (1991) *Introduction to the Human Body: The Essentials of Anatomy and Physiology*, 2nd edn, HarperCollins

### Activity 12

Copy out the table below and write a short explanation in each box.

| Vessel | Brief outline of structure | Function |
|---|---|---|
| Arteries/ arterioles | | |
| Capillaries | | |
| Veins/venules | | |

cells to squeeze through their wall. The capillary network is very well developed as they are so small; large quantities are able to cover the muscle, which ensures efficient exchange of gases. If the cross-sectional area of all the capillaries in the body were to be added together, the total area would be much greater than that of the aorta.

Distribution of blood through the capillary network is regulated by special structures known as pre-capillary sphincters, the structure of which will be dealt with later in this chapter.

**Key term**

**Pre-capillary sphincters:** A ring-shaped band of muscle tissue located at the opening to the capillary bed which controls and regulates the volume of blood entering it.
**Venous return:** Blood returning to the right side of the heart.

## The venous return mechanism

Venous return is the term used for the blood which returns to the right side of the heart via the veins. As mentioned earlier, up to 70 per cent of the total volume of blood is contained in the veins at rest. This provides a large reservoir of blood which is returned rapidly to the heart when needed. The heart can only pump out as much blood as it receives, so cardiac output is dependent on venous return. A rapid increase in venous return enables a significant increase in cardiac output due to Starling's law.

There are several mechanisms which aid the venous return process:

- The muscle pump – As exercise begins, muscular contractions impinge on and compress the veins, squeezing blood towards the heart.
- Pocket valves inside the veins prevent any backflow of blood that might occur. This is illustrated in Figure 4.19.
- The respiratory pump – During inspiration and expiration, pressure changes occur in the thoracic and abdominal cavities which compress veins and assist blood return to the heart.

These mechanisms are essential at the start of exercise. As exercise commences, the muscles contracting squeeze the vast amount of blood within the veins back towards the heart, enabling stroke volume to increase and optimal delivery of nutrients to the working muscles.

Other factors that aid venous return include:

- smooth muscle within the walls and surrounding the veins which contracts and helps blood on its journey back to the heart;
- gravity, which helps the blood return to the heart from the upper body.

# Blood pressure

Blood pressure is the force exerted by the blood against the walls of the blood vessels. It is necessary to maintain blood flow through the circulatory system and is determined by two main factors:

1. Cardiac output – the volume of blood flowing into the system from the left ventricle.
2. Resistance to flow – the opposition offered by the blood vessels to the blood flow. This is dependent on several factors, including blood viscosity, blood vessel length and blood vessel radius.

Blood pressure = Cardiac output × Resistance

Therefore, blood pressure increases when either cardiac output or resistance increases.

Blood pressure in the arteries also increases and decreases in a pattern which corresponds to the cardiac cycle during ventricular systole. It is highest when blood is pumped into the aorta and lowest during ventricular diastole.

Blood pressure is usually measured at the brachial artery using a sphygmomanometer, and is recorded as millimetres of mercury (mmHg) of systolic pressure over diastolic pressure:

- Systolic pressure is experienced when the heart pumps blood into the system.
- Diastolic pressure is recorded when the heart is relaxing and filling with blood.

The typical reading for a subject at rest is:

$$\frac{120 \text{ mmHg}}{80 \text{ mmHg}} = \frac{\text{Systolic}}{\text{Diastolic}}$$

**Key terms**

**Blood pressure:** The force exerted by the blood against the walls of the blood vessels.
**Systolic pressure:** The peak pressure in the arteries which occurs when the heart is contracting and emptying blood into the arterial system.
**Diastolic pressure:** The lowest pressure in the arteries which occurs when the heart is relaxing and filling with blood.

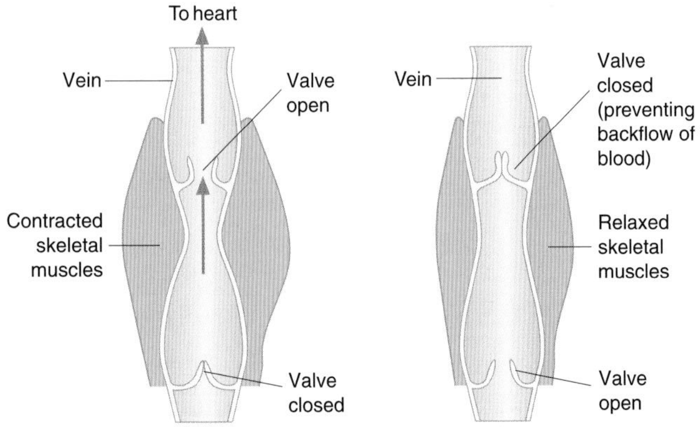


**Figure 4.19** The muscle pump and venous return. The massaging action of the muscles when we exercise squeezes blood back towards the heart, increasing venous return and therefore cardiac output

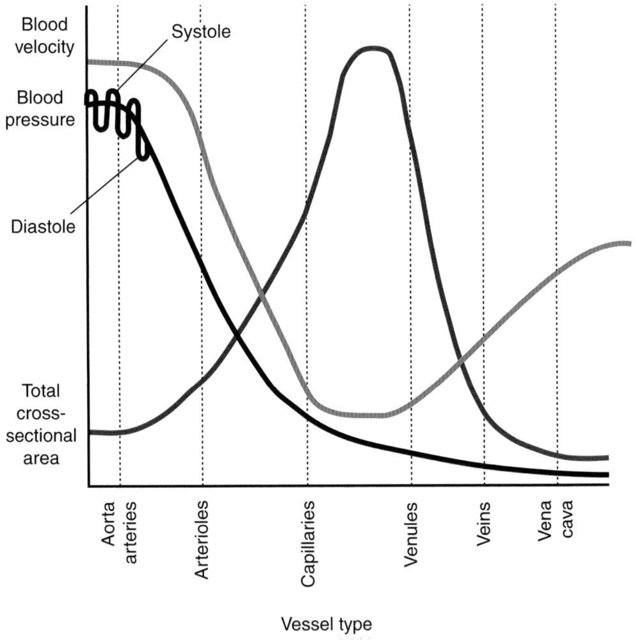


**Figure 4.20** The relationship between blood vessel type, total cross-sectional area, blood velocity and blood pressure

## Activity 13

You are going to investigate blood pressure, using a digital blood pressure meter, or sphygmomanometer.

1. Under the guidance of your teacher, wrap the cuff round the brachial artery.
2. Pump air into the cuff, up to approximately 190mmHg.
3. Slowly release the air inside the cuff by pressing the attachment on the bulb. The systolic pressure can now be read and recorded.
4. Continue to release air from the cuff until the diastolic pressure is displayed on the screen. Record your diastolic pressure.
5. Discover your blood pressure by placing the systolic reading over the diastolic reading:

   $$\frac{\text{Systolic}}{\text{Diastolic}}$$

6. Follow the above procedure after completing two minutes of intense exercise.
7. Account for any differences in your readings.

## Exam-style questions

**1** An increase in venous return leads to a corresponding increase in cardiac output. Explain this relationship. (3 marks)

**2** During exercise blood flow is maintained by the venous return mechanism. Describe three mechanisms involved in venous return. (3 marks)

**3** Explain the importance of the skeletal muscle pump when performing a cool down. (3 marks)

**4** Endurance training will cause changes to the structure and functioning of the body which helps to enhance performance. Describe these changes with reference to the vascular system. (4 marks)

**5** Identify three factors that affect cardiac output during the first few moments of exercise and explain what they do. (6 marks)

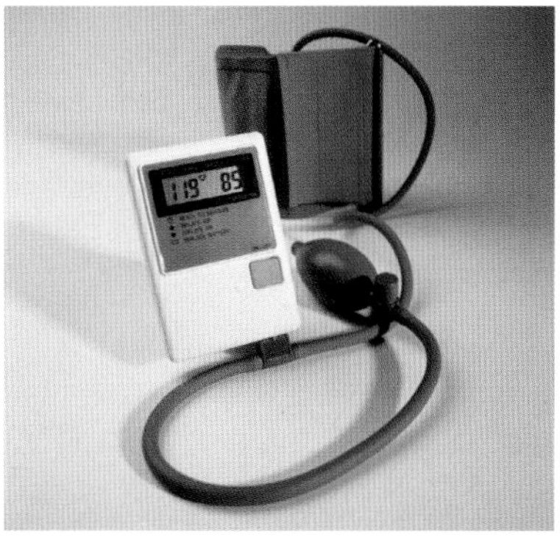


Figure 4.21 The ideal blood pressure reading is 120mmHg/80mmHg

During exercise, blood pressure change is dependent on the type and intensity of the exercise being performed. During steady aerobic exercise involving large muscle groups, the systolic pressure increases as a result of increased cardiac output, while diastolic pressure remains constant or, in well-trained athletes, may even drop, as blood feeds into the working muscles due to increased arteriole dilation. The increased systolic pressure associated with exercise is largely the result of increased cardiac output due to a greater intensity. This ensures that adequate blood is supplied to the working muscle quickly. During high-intensity isometric and anaerobic exercise, both systolic and diastolic pressure rise significantly due to increased resistance of the blood vessels. This is a result of muscles squeezing the veins, increasing peripheral resistance, and an increase in intra-thoracic pressure due to the contraction of the abdominals. When weightlifting, for example, competitors often hold their breath during exertion, which causes a significant increase in both systolic and diastolic pressure.

It is essential that blood pressure is regulated and, where possible, at rest maintained within a normal range. High blood pressure can cause serious complications to the heart, brain and kidneys, whereas low pressure can result in insufficient oxygen and other nutrients reaching the muscle cells.

Blood pressure that is constantly above the 'normal' range is referred to as hypertension and usually results from a hardening of the arteries, which puts excess strain on the cardio-vascular system.

The vasomotor control centre outlined in the following section is responsible for regulating blood pressure.

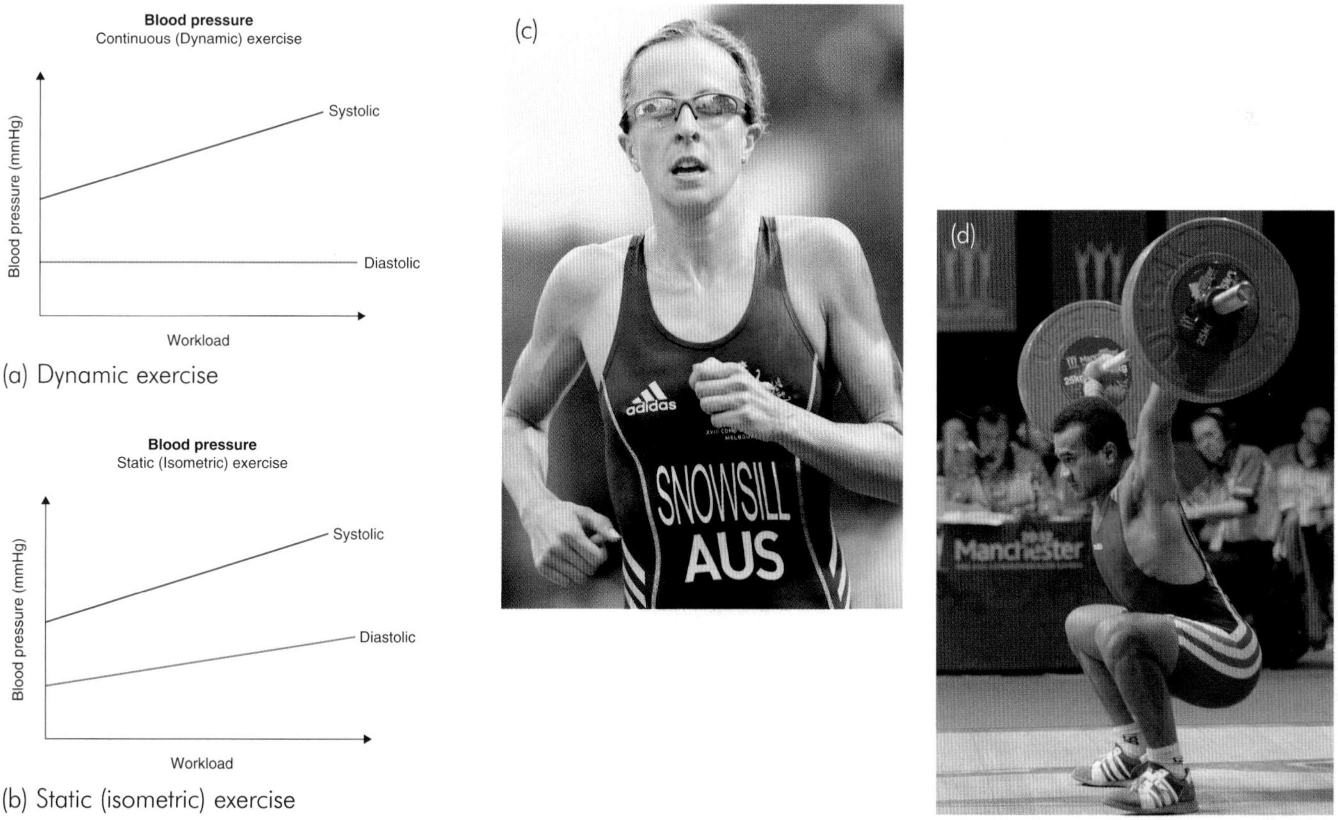


Figure 4.22 The effects of exercise on both systolic and diastolic blood pressure
(a) Dynamic exercise (e.g. a marathon runner), (b) Static (isometric) exercise (e.g. a weight-lifter)

**IN CONTEXT**

**The systolic blood pressure of a powerlifter such as Mariusz Pudzianowski, a former World's Strongest Man, may reach levels of 200mmHg or more when competing.**

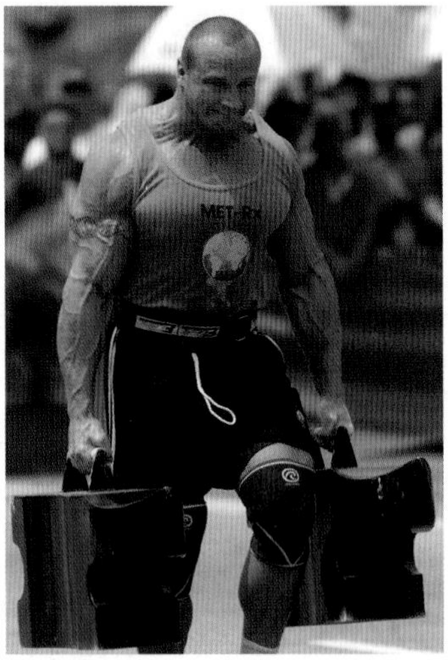


**Figure 4.23** The systolic and diastolic blood pressure of former World's Strongest Man Mariusz Pudzianowski will increase dramatically during exercise

### Activity 14

Explain the importance of blood pressure with regard to sporting activity.

**Key term**

**Hypertension:** Abnormally high blood pressure, which is characterised in adults by systolic readings above 140mmHg or diastolic readings above 90mmHg.

## The re-distribution of blood from rest to exercise

Blood flow changes dramatically once exercise commences. At rest, only 15–20 per cent of cardiac output is directed to skeletal muscle; the majority goes to the liver (27 per cent) and kidneys (22 per cent). During exercise, however, blood is redirected to areas where it is needed most. For example, during exhaustive exercise, the working muscles may receive over 80 per cent of cardiac output. This increased blood flow to the muscle results from a restriction of blood flow to the kidneys, liver and stomach. This process is known as the vascular shunt mechanism. Figure 4.24 illustrates the distribution of cardiac output at rest and during exercise.

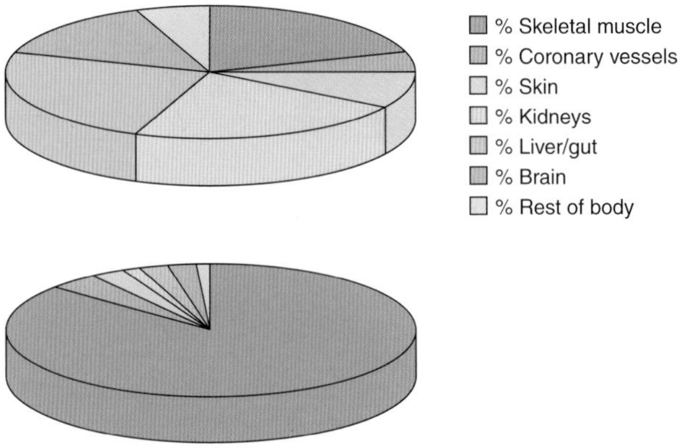


**Figure 4.24** (a) distribution of cardiac output at rest (b) distribution of cardiac output during exercise

### Activity 15

If you have access to a programme such as Microsoft Excel®, use the data in Table 4.4 to construct a pie chart that shows the relative distribution of blood at rest and during maximal effort. (If you do not have access to such a programme, simply draw a pie chart.) Explain the changes shown in your pie chart.

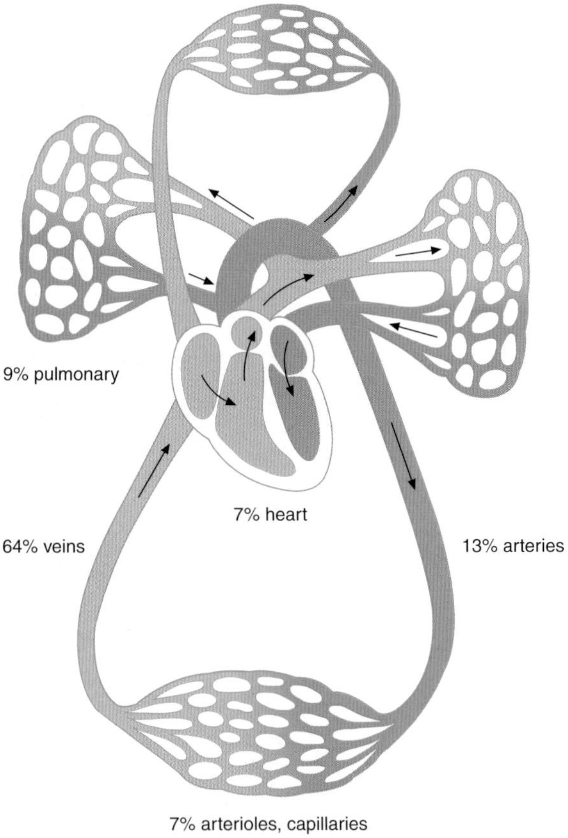


**Figure 4.25** The distribution of blood in the body at rest

**Table 4.4** Blood flow changes during exercise in $cm^3$/min

| Organ | At rest ($cm^3$) | % Blood flow | Maximum effort ($cm^3$) | % Blood flow |
|---|---|---|---|---|
| Skeletal muscle | 1,000 | 20 | 26,000 | 88 |
| Coronary vessels | 250 | 5 | 1,200 | 4 |
| Skin | 500 | 10 | 750 | 2.5 |
| Kidneys | 1,000 | 20 | 300 | 1 |
| Liver/gut | 1,250 | 25 | 375 | 1.25 |
| Brain | 750 | 15 | 750 | 2.5 |
| Whole body | 5,000 | 100 | 30,000 | 100 |

*Source:* Clegg, *Exercise Physiology*, Feltham Press, 1995

**Key term**

**Vascular shunt mechanism:** The redistribution of blood in the body during exercise so that the working muscles receive an increased proportion. Through vasodilation and vasoconstriction of arteries and arterioles, the volume of blood reaching the working muscles can increase fourfold, from approximately 20 per cent to 88 per cent.

## Vasomotor control

The redistribution of blood is determined primarily by the vasoconstriction and vasodilation of arterioles. It reacts to chemical changes of the local tissues. For example, vasodilation will occur when arterioles sense a decrease in oxygen conc entration or an increase in acidity due to higher $CO_2$ and lactic acid concentrations. When embarking on a distance run, the increased metabolic activity increases the amount of carbon dioxide and lactic acid in the blood. This is detected by chemoreceptors, and sympathetic nerves stimulate the blood vessel size to change shape. Vasodilation will then allow greater blood flow, bringing the much needed oxygen and flushing away the harmful waste products of metabolism.

Sympathetic nerves also play a major role in redistributing blood from one area of the body to another. The smooth muscle layer (tunica media) of the blood vessels is controlled by the sympathetic nervous system, and remains in a state of slight contraction, known as vasomotor tone. By increasing sympathetic stimulation, vasoconstriction occurs and blood flow is restricted and redistributed to areas of greater need. When stimulation by sympathetic nerves decreases, vasodilation is allowed, which will increase blood flow to that body part.

Further structures which aid blood redistribution are pre-capillary sphincters. Pre-capillary sphincters are ring-shaped muscles which lie at the opening of capillaries and control blood flow into the capillary bed. When the sphincter contracts, it restricts blood flow through the capillary and deprives tissues of oxygen; conversely, when it relaxes, it increases blood flow to the capillary bed. These are illustrated in Figure 4.26.

**IN CONTEXT**

**For a triathlete such as world champion Tim Don, the vascular shunt mechanism will be in operation and will change according to the specific needs of the working muscles. To start with, the swim will require much blood to be redistributed to the shoulders (deltoids) and quadriceps group of the legs, reducing blood flow to the vital organs. During the cycle and run sections of the triathlon, a much greater proportion of the blood will be distributed to the quadriceps femoris and biceps femoris muscles of the leg.**

### Exam-style questions

**1** With reference to an activity of your choice, explain how and why blood redistribution occurs during exercise. (4 marks)

**2** (a) Using Figure 4.4 explain why the volume of blood flow to the brain remains the same during rest and during maximum effort. (2 marks)

(b) Explain why the percentage of total blood flow to the brain actually decreases (1 mark)

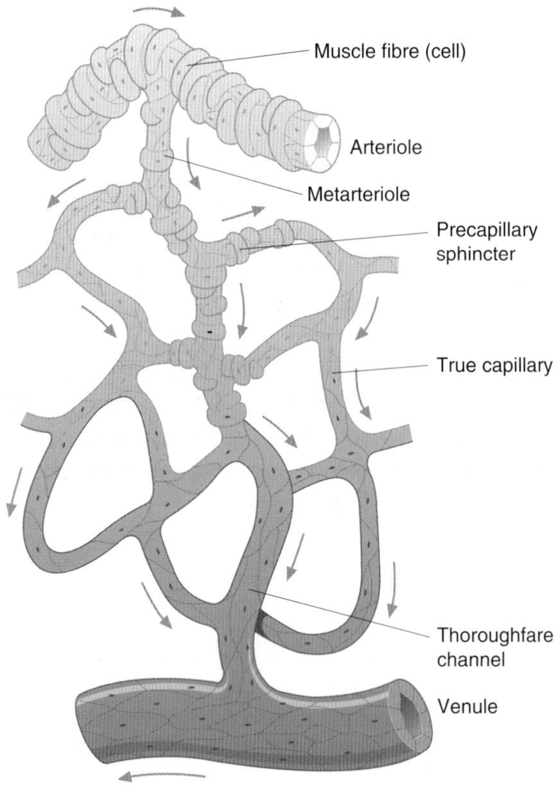


Figure 4.26 A pre-capillary sphincter

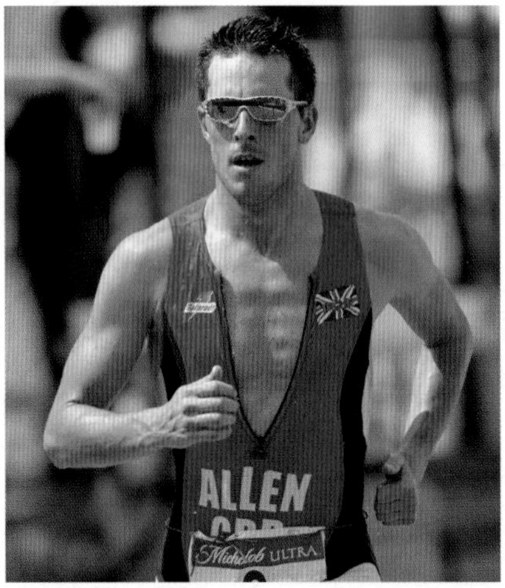


Figure 4.27 Redistribution of blood is vital for effective performance in the triathlon

## Activity 16

Copy the outline of the graph here. On your graph, draw two lines: one to show what happens to blood flow to skeletal muscle during exercise, and the other to illustrate blood flow to all other organs of the body while exercising. Make sure you label each of the lines and give a brief explanation for each one.

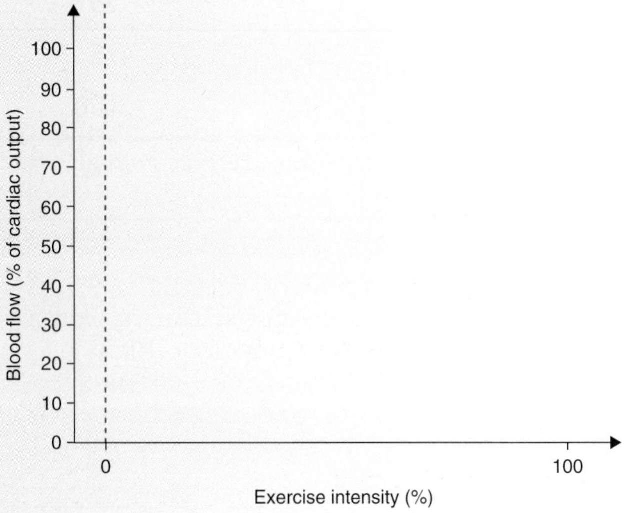


## Activity 17

1 Name the major blood vessels in the body, beginning with those affecting the heart. In each case, state how the structure is suited to the function.
2 Explain how vasoconstriction and vasodilation function in the body, and how they can affect the athlete while exercising.
3 What are the major differences between the heart of a trained athlete and that of an untrained person?
4 Discuss how the vasomotor centre operates.

## Exam-style questions

**1** During exercise the arterio-venous oxygen difference (a-$\bar{V}O_2$ diff) increases. What do you understand by this term and what is the result of this increase? (2 marks)

**2** Figure 4.27 shows a tri-athlete competing in an event.

(a) Explain how the body ensures a constant supply of blood reaches the working muscles (4 marks)

(b) During the event explain how the cardiac control centre regulates heart rate (3 marks)

(c) At the end of the triathlon, the athlete will perform a cool down. Describe the mechanisms that are used to return blood to the heart (3 marks)

## Activity 18

Copy and complete the table below showing the responses of the cardiovascular system to exercise, giving a brief explanation for each. The heart rate response has been completed as an example.

| Factor | Increase/decrease | Explanation |
|---|---|---|
| Heart rate | Increase | During submaximal exercise, HR increases rapidly at first and then plateaus into a steady state, where oxygen demand is being met by supply. During maximal exercise, HR increases proportionally with exercise intensity until a maximum level is reached. This will also be the point of $\bar{V}O_2$ max. The release of hormones such as adrenaline and noradrenaline causes the increase in heart rate. |
| Stroke volume | | |
| Cardiac output | | |
| Blood pressure | | |
| Blood flow to working muscles | | |
| a–$\bar{V}O_2$ diff. | | |
| Blood acidity | | |
| Parasympathetic activity | | |
| Sympathetic activity | | |

## Exam-style questions

**1** A cyclist completes a 60-minute sub-maximal training ride.

On the graph opposite, sketch the graph that represents the following stages of the cycle ride:

- Immediately prior to the bike ride
- During the first 10 minutes
- Between 10 minutes and 60 minutes
- During a 10-minute recovery period (5 marks)

**2** Outline the process of cardiac control that accounts for this pattern of heart rate. (6 marks)

**3** Give three long term adaptive physiological responses of the heart and three physiological responses of the vascular system following a period of endurance training. (6 marks)

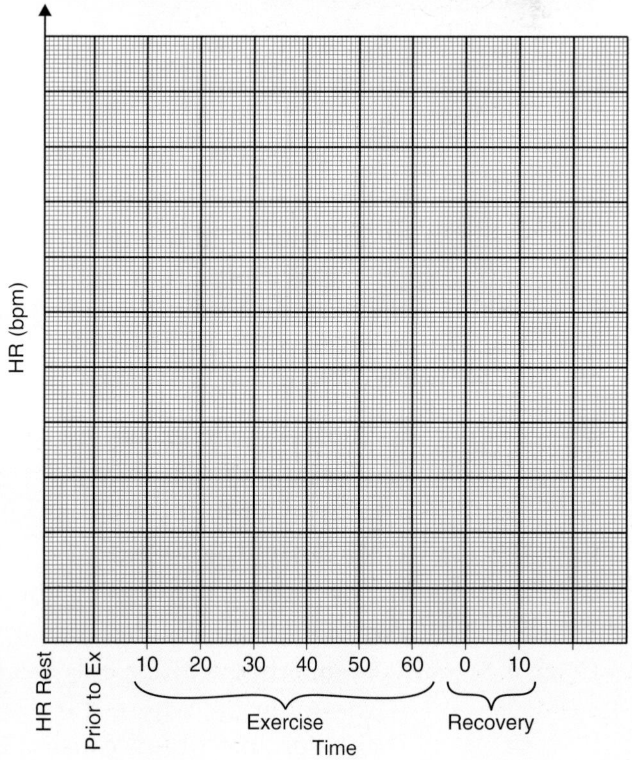

## The impact of training on the vascular system

Earlier in the chapter we established how the heart adapts in response to training specifically in relation its enlargement (hypertrophy) and the reduction in resting heart rate (bradycardia). This section now considers the physiological changes that happen to the vascular system, in particular the adaption to the blood and blood vessels following a period of endurance training.

### Adaptive responses of the blood

#### Increased blood volume

Blood volume increases following a period of endurance training as a result of an increased blood plasma volume. This has the important function of decreasing the viscosity of the blood which enables the blood to flow around the body more easily, thus enhancing oxygen delivery to the muscles and tissues.

#### Increased red blood cells

The amount of red blood cells (and therefore haemoglobin content) increases following a period of endurance training, which again facilitates the transport of oxygen around the body.

### Adaptive responses of the blood vessels

#### Capillarisation

Endurance training promotes the formation of new capillaries surrounding the alveoli and body's tissues, including the muscles which allow more effective gaseous exchange, thus enabling more oxygen to reach the muscle cells.

#### Enhanced redistribution of blood

Improvements in the vasculature efficiency (especially the arteries) to vasoconstrict and vasodilate enhances the redistribution of blood by shunting the supply to the active muscles and tissues so that there is a greater supply of oxygen for energy production in these working muscles.

#### Decreased resting blood pressure

Exercise maintains blood pressure within a 'healthy' range due to the enhanced elasticity of the arteries and the production of high density lipoproteins within the blood which prevent the laying down of fatty deposits and the consequential advancement of atherosclerosis.

### What you need to know

* The structure of the heart is specially adapted to its function.
* Valves within the heart ensure a unidirectional flow of blood.
* The sounds of the heart are a result of these valves snapping shut. The 'lub' sound results from the closing of the atrioventricular valves, while the 'dub' results from the closure of the semilunar valves.
* Typically, the heart is composed of three layers: an outer pericardium, a thick muscular layer called the myocardium, and a smooth inner endocardium.
* Coronary arteries ensure that the heart receives an adequate supply of blood.
* The cardiac cycle explains the passage of blood through the heart. It consists of four stages: atrial diastole, atrial systole, ventricular diastole and ventricular systole.
* The heart is myogenic – it creates its own impulses.
* The impulse is emitted from the SA node and the surrounding fibres are innervated, causing the atria to contract. The impulse eventually arrives at the AV node, where it is dispersed down the bundle of His and throughout the Purkinje fibres, causing the ventricles to contract.

* The heart rate is governed by the parasympathetic and sympathetic nervous systems. The sympathetic nervous system increases heart rate by releasing adrenaline and noradrenaline, while the parasympathetic nervous system slows the heart down through the action of another hormone, acetylcholine.
* Increases in heart rate during exercise are largely the result of increased metabolic activity increasing the concentration of carbon dioxide.
* Cardiac output is the volume of blood pumped out of one ventricle in one minute. Stroke volume is the volume of blood pumped out of one ventricle in one beat. Heart rate is the number of times the heart beats per minute.
* Cardiac hypertrophy is the enlargement of the heart, often resulting from endurance training.
* Bradycardia is the reduction in resting heart rate (usually below 60 beats per minute) which accompanies cardiac hypertrophy.
* The vascular system encompasses the blood and blood vessels.
* The blood's main functions are the transportation of oxygen and the maintenance of homeostasis.
* Oxygen is transported round the body by combining with haemoglobin to form oxyhaemoglobin.
* During exercise, oxygen dissociates more easily from haemoglobin due to the increase in body temperature, a reduced $pO_2$, an increased $pCO_2$ and a lower blood pH (increased acidity). This is illustrated by a shift to the right in the oxyhaemoglobin dissociation curve, and is known as the Bohr shift.
* Major blood vessels consist of arteries, arterioles, capillaries, venules and veins.
* The continuous network of blood vessels in the body is known as the circulatory system, which is composed of the pulmonary and systemic circuits.
* Blood returning to the heart via the veins is known as venous return. It is aided by the muscle and respiratory pumps.
* Blood pressure is the force exerted by the blood on the inner walls of the blood vessels. It is a product of cardiac output and resistance of the vessel walls.
* Blood flow is controlled by the vasomotor centre, which causes blood vessels to vasodilate and vasoconstrict, and determines the amount of blood reaching various parts of the body.
* The vascular shunt mechanism aids in the redistribution of blood during exercise.
* Oxygen is transported in the blood by combining with haemoglobin.
* Smoking can impair the transport of oxygen since haemoglobin has a much higher affinity for carbon monoxide (found in cigarette smoke) than for oxygen.
* The majority (70 per cent) of carbon dioxide is transported as carbonic acid (dissolved in water); 20 per cent is transported by combining with haemoglobin, and 8 per cent is dissolved in blood plasma.

## Review Questions

1 Describe the path that blood takes through the heart, from the point at which it enters via the venae cavae, to where it exits via the aorta.

2 When using a stethoscope, is it possible to hear the heart beating? What creates the heartbeat, and when do these sounds occur during the cardiac cycle?

3 Describe the action of the sympathetic and parasympathetic nervous systems on the heart, before, during and following exercise.

4 Outline the major functions of the blood. Explain the importance of blood when exercising.

5 Sketch and label a graph showing the heart rate pattern expected from an athlete completing a 400m run in a personal best time of 45 seconds, followed by a 15-minute recovery period. Account for these changes.

6 Outline the major factors which affect cardiac output during exercise.

7 How are oxygen and carbon dixoide transported in the body?

8 During exercise, the return of blood to the heart is paramount. Explain how the body achieves this and relate it to Starling's law.

9 How is the redistribution of blood during exercise accomplished?

10 Explain what you would expect to happen to blood pressure in the following instances:

   1 an athlete undertaking a steady swim;
   2 an athlete completing a 100m sprint;
   3 a weightlifter performing a maximal lift;
   4 an athlete completing the cycling stage of a triathlon.

11 Endurance training results in significant benefits to the heart and vascular system. What are these benefits and how do they contribute to a 'healthier lifestyle'?

# CHAPTER 5

# An analysis of human movement in sporting activity

## Learning outcomes

**By the end of this chapter you should be able to:**

- name the major bones and muscles of the body;
- describe the structure of a synovial joint and explain the function of its features;
- describe the movement patterns that can occur at synovial joints in relation to planes and axes using examples from a range of sporting activities;
- describe the different types of muscle contraction, using examples from a range of sporting activities;
- complete a movement analysis at the shoulder and elbow during:
  - a push up
  - overarm throwing
  - forehand racket strokes
- complete a movement analysis at the hip, knee and ankle during:
  - running
  - jumping
  - kicking
  - performing squats
- identify the 3 classes of lever system in the human body giving examples from sporting activity when each operates
- explain the relative efficiency of lever systems with reference to mechanical advantage and disadvantage.
- critically evaluate the impact of different types of physical activity on the skeletal and muscular systems.

## CHAPTER INTRODUCTION

In order for humans to move and perform sporting activity, the interaction of the skeletal and muscular systems is necessary.

Muscles contract, moving bones, which pivot and rotate about the joints of the body. In doing so, a series of lever systems operate that enable a force to be transferred through the body, causing the body, or an object, to move in a desired direction. There now follows a brief discussion of each of the following components:

- bones;
- joints;
- muscles.

First, we will consider each of the components individually. Towards the end of the chapter we will look at them collectively and will see how they interact to enable the body to perform such a wide range of movements.

# The skeleton

## The skeletal system

The 206 bones that make up the human skeleton are specifically designed to provide several basic functions which are essential for participation in physical activity. In conjunction with other components of the skeletal system (including the ligaments and joints), the skeleton can perform certain functions, as explored below.

## Functions

### Support

The skeleton provides a rigid framework to the body, giving it shape and providing suitable sites for the attachment of skeletal muscle.

### Protection

The skeleton provides protection for the internal organs. For example, the vertebral column

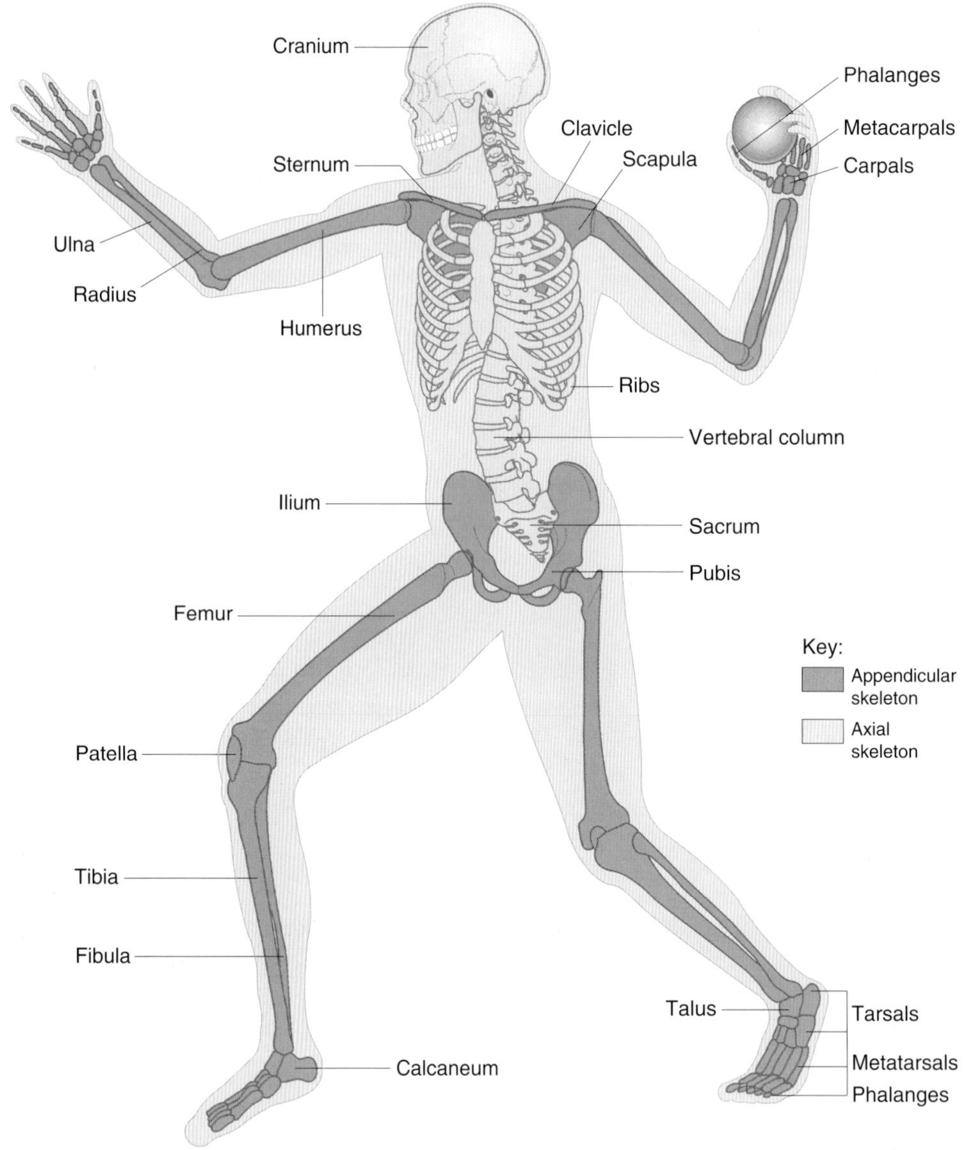


**Figure 5.1** Bones of the axial and appendicular skeleton
*Source*: Davis, Kimmet and Auty (1986) *Physical Education, Theory and Practice*, Macmillan

protects the spinal cord; the cranium protects the brain; and the ribcage principally protects the heart and lungs.

### Movement

The bones of the skeleton provide a large surface area for the attachment of muscles – the engines of movement. The long bones, in particular, provide a system of levers against which the muscles can pull.

### Blood production

Within the bones, bone marrow produces both red and white blood cells. Red blood cells are generally produced at the end of long bones such as the humerus (arm) and the femur (thigh), and in some flat bones such as the pelvis and the sternum (breastbone). White blood cells are usually produced in the shafts of long bones.

### Mineral storage

The bones of the skeleton have storage capabilities for vital minerals such as calcium and phosphorus, which can be distributed to other parts of the body when required.

## The structure of the skeleton

The bones of the skeleton can be divided into two distinct categories: the axial and the appendicular skeleton:

- The axial skeleton provides the main area of support for the body, and includes the cranium (skull), the vertebral column (spine) and the ribcage.
- The appendicular skeleton consists of the appendages, or the bones of the limbs, together with the girdles that join on to the axial skeleton.

Take a moment to study the bones of the axial and appendicular skeleton in Figure 5.1.

**Key terms**

**Axial skeleton:** The main supporting frame of the skeleton, consisting of the skull, vertebral column and ribcage.
**Appendicular skeleton:** Bones of the skeleton that make up the limbs and their associated girdles (hip and shoulder).

### Activity 1

Using sticky labels, label the bones on a partner's body.

### Activity 2

List the bones in the axial and appendicular skeletons in Figure 5.1.

**Key term**

**Articular cartilage:** A smooth tissue that covers the ends of bones which helps to prevent friction.

**IN CONTEXT**

**Ligaments are plastic rather than elastic. This means that once they have been stretched, they remain the same length and do not return to their original length. Consequently, if damage occurs to them, such as a dislocation at the shoulder, it can lead to joint instability.**

**Key term**

**Ligaments:** A band of strong fibrous tissue that attaches one bone to another.

## Joints and articulations

So far we have seen that some bones of the skeleton act as levers, which move when muscles contract and pull on them. Where two or more bones meet, an articulation or joint exists. However, movement does not always occur at these sites, and joints are typically classified according to the degree of movement permitted.

## Classification of joints

### Fixed or fibrous joints

These are very stable and allow no observable movement. Bones are often joined by strong fibres called sutures, such as the sutures of the cranium (skull). See Figure 5.3.

**Long bones**

Long bones are cylindrical in shape and are found in the limbs of the body. Examples of long bones include:

- femur
- tibia
- humerus
- phalanges (although not great in length, these possess the cylindrical shape and so also fall into this category).

The primary function of long bones is to act as levers, and they are therefore essential in movement. When running for example, the psoas, iliacus, and rectus femoris muscles pull on the femur to cause flexion of the hip, effectively lifting the leg off the ground. The rest of the quadricep group (the vasti muscles as well as the rectus femoris) then pull on the tibia causing extension to take place at the knee joint, enabling the lower leg to 'snap' through. This is the first stage of a running action. Their other vital function is the production of blood cells which occurs deep inside the bone.

**Flat bones**

Flat bones offer protection to the internal organs of the body. Examples include:

- the sternum
- the bones of the cranium
- the bones of the pelvis
- upon close inspection, it can be seen that the ribs are also flat.

Flat bones also provide suitable sites for muscle attachment, with the origins of muscles often attaching to them. In this way the muscle contracting has a firm, immovable base against which to pull, and can therefore carry out its function effectively. For example, a major function of the quadricep muscle group is to pull on the tibia, causing extension at the knee. In order to raise the tibia, the muscle must have a stable base against which it can pull, in this case, the ilium. The bone can now act as a lever and cause movement to occur as outlined earlier. The pelvis, sternum and cranium also produce blood cells.

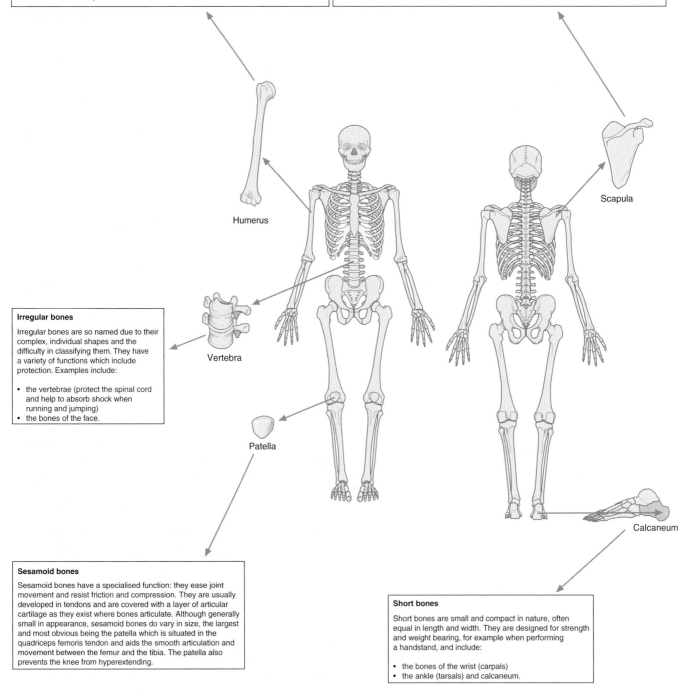

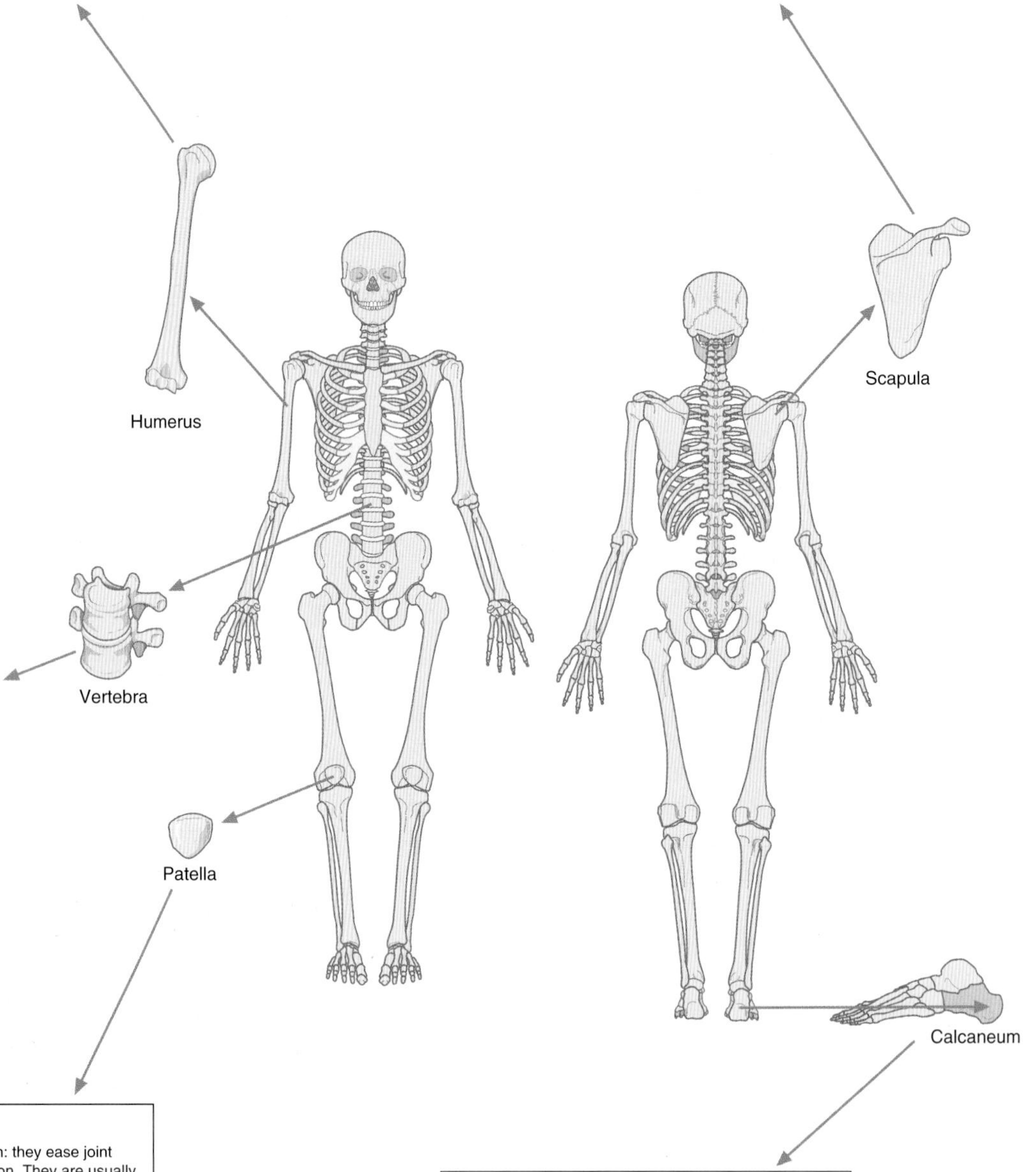


**Irregular bones**

Irregular bones are so named due to their complex, individual shapes and the difficulty in classifying them. They have a variety of functions which include protection. Examples include:

- the vertebrae (protect the spinal cord and help to absorb shock when running and jumping)
- the bones of the face.

**Sesamoid bones**

Sesamoid bones have a specialised function: they ease joint movement and resist friction and compression. They are usually developed in tendons and are covered with a layer of articular cartilage as they exist where bones articulate. Although generally small in appearance, sesamoid bones do vary in size, the largest and most obvious being the patella which is situated in the quadriceps femoris tendon and aids the smooth articulation and movement between the femur and the tibia. The patella also prevents the knee from hyperextending.

**Short bones**

Short bones are small and compact in nature, often equal in length and width. They are designed for strength and weight bearing, for example when performing a handstand, and include:

- the bones of the wrist (carpals)
- the ankle (tarsals) and calcaneum.

**Figure 5.2** Bones are designed to carry out a variety of specific functions and fall into one of five categories, largely according to their shape

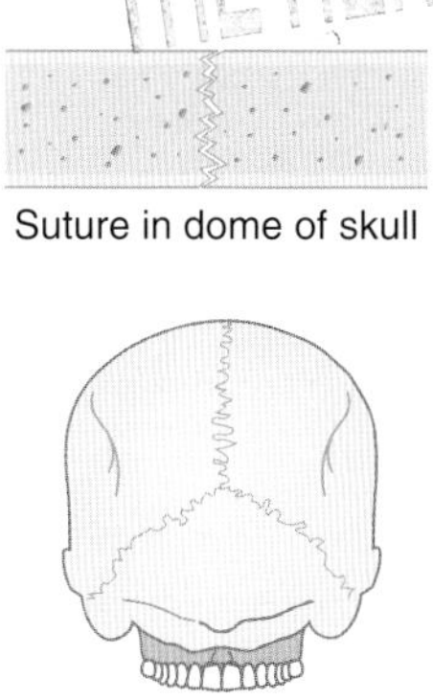


Figure 5.3 A fixed joint

## Cartilaginous or slightly movable joints

These are joined by a tough, fibrous cartilage which provides stability and possesses shock-absorption properties. However, a small amount of movement usually exists. For example, between the lumbar bones, intervertebral discs of cartilage occur, allowing some movement, as shown in Figure 5.4.

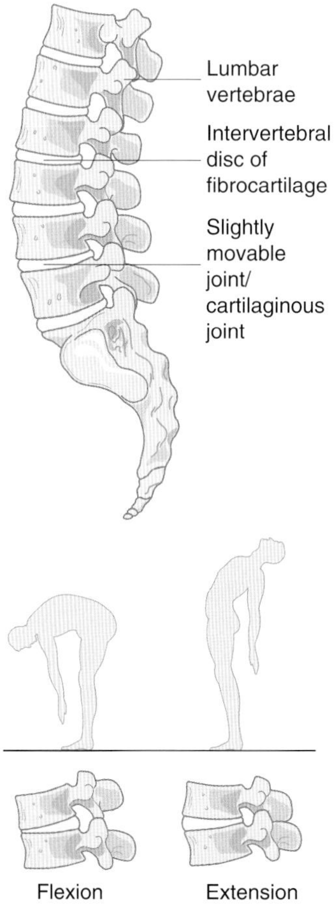


Figure 5.4 A cartilaginous joint

## Synovial or freely movable joints

These are the most common type of joint in the body, and the most important in terms of physical activity, since they allow a wide range of movement.

The joint is enclosed in a fibrous joint capsule, which is lined with a synovial membrane. Lubrication is provided by synovial fluid, which is secreted into the joint by the synovial membrane. In addition, where the bones come into contact with each other, they are lined with smooth yet hard-wearing hyaline or articular cartilage.

Synovial joint stability is provided by the strength of the muscles crossing the joint, which are supported by ligaments that may be inside or outside the capsule. Ligaments are very elastic and lose effectiveness to some degree when torn or stretched.

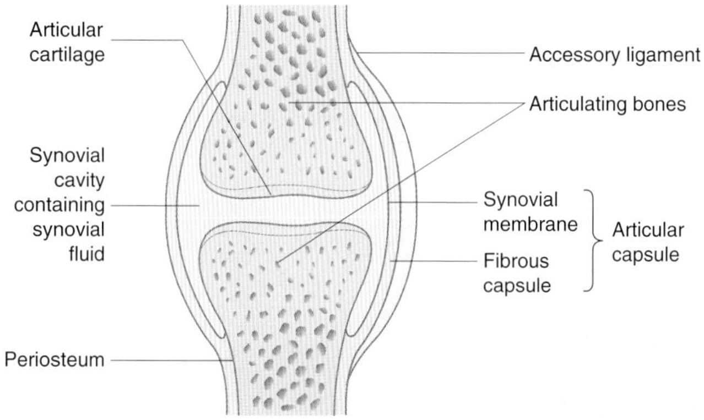


Figure 5.5 A typical synovial joint

Some synovial joints possess sacs of synovial fluid known as bursae, which are sited in areas of increased pressure or stress and help to reduce friction as tissues and structures move past each other. Pads of fat help to absorb shock and improve the 'fit' of the articulating bones. This is particularly true in the knee joint, to help the articulation of the femur and tibia.

**Key term**

**Synovial fluid:** A protein-enriched fluid which lubricates and nourishes the articular cartilage. It helps to reduce friction between the articulating bones.

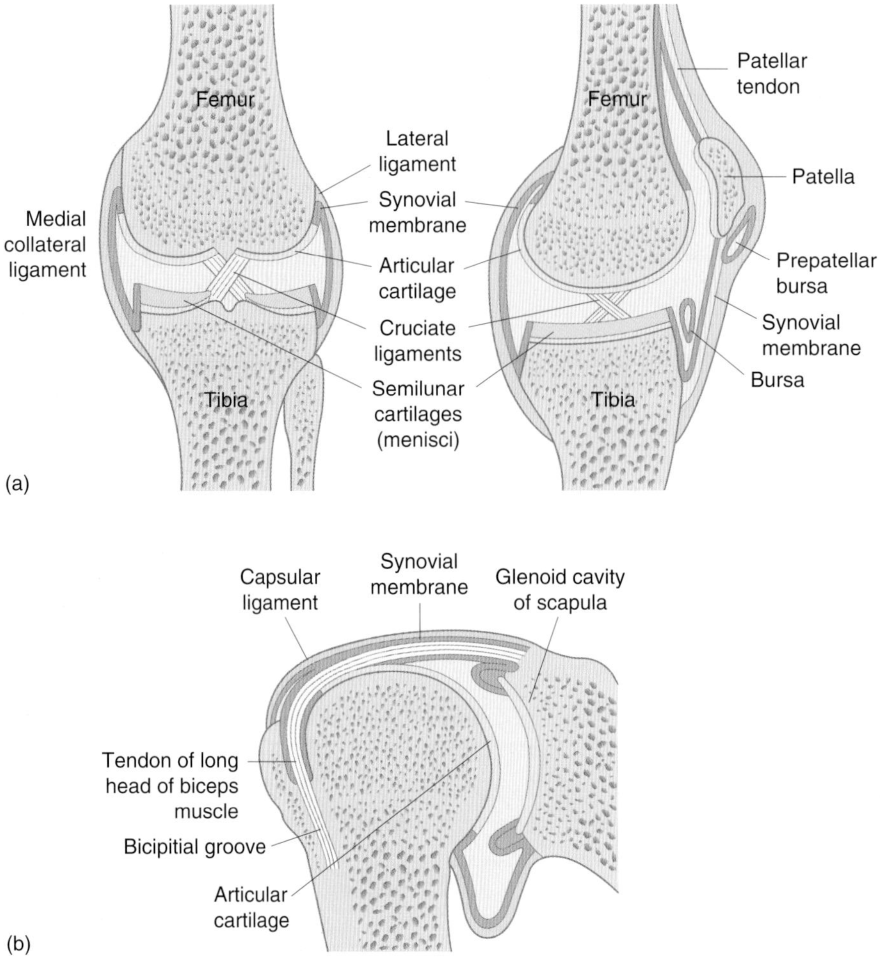


**Figure 5.6** a) The knee joint b) The shoulder joint

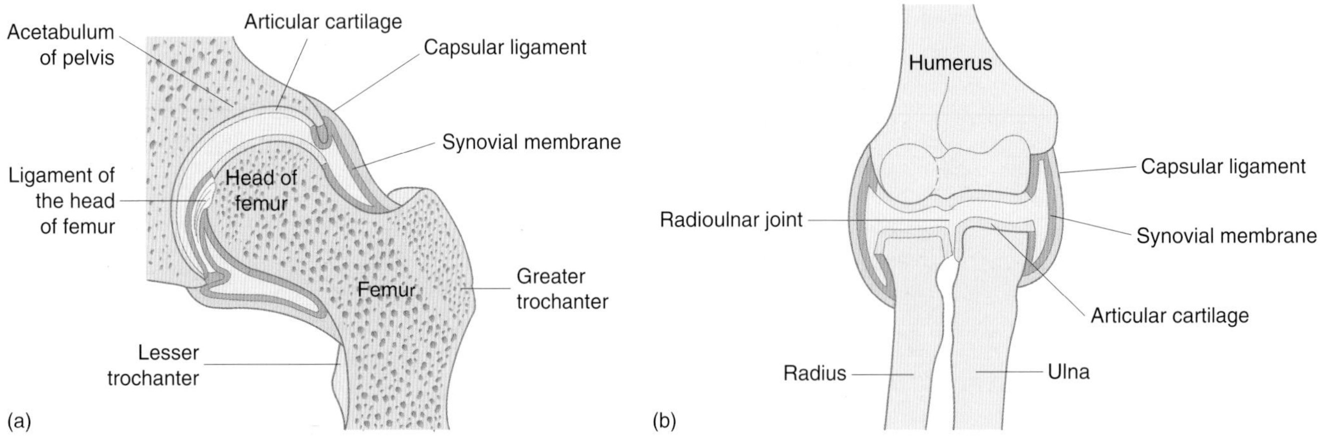


**Figure 5.7** a) The hip joint b) The elbow joint

## Activity 3

Copy and complete the table below.

| Joint feature | Definition | Function |
|---|---|---|
| Joint capsule | | |
| | Glassy smooth tissue that covers the ends of bones in a joint | |
| | | Reduce friction between the articulating bones<br>Nourish articular cartilage |
| | Small sacs of synovial fluid located in the joint at sites of friction | |
| Synovial membrane | | |
| | | Attaches one bone to another |

## Activity 4

Explain how the knee joint is structured and how this suits its function in relation to sporting activity.

### Types of synovial joint

Synovial joints can be further subdivided:

1 A hinge joint is a uniaxial joint, which only allows movement in one plane. For example, the knee joint only allows movement back and forth. Strong ligaments exist in order to prevent any sideways movement.
2 A pivot joint, which is also uniaxial, only allows rotation. For example, in the cervical vertebrae, the axis rotates on the atlas.
3 An ellipsoid joint is biaxial, allowing movement in two planes. For example, the radiocarpal joint of the wrist allows movement back and forth as well as side to side.
4 A gliding joint is formed where flat surfaces glide past one another. Although mainly biaxial, they may permit movement in all directions. For example, in the wrist, the small carpal bones move against each other.
5 A saddle joint is biaxial and generally occurs where concave and convex surfaces meet. For example, the carpo-metacarpal joint of the thumb.
6 The ball-and-socket joint allows the widest range of movement; occurs where a rounded head of a bone fits into a cup-shaped cavity. For example, in the hip and shoulder.

## Activity 5

Try to explain, where possible, how each type of synovial joint shown in Figure 5.8 has a role to play in sporting activity.

### EXAMINER'S TIP

Synovial joints are classified according to the range and type of movement they allow. You must be able to relate the type of synovial joint to its structure. For example, hinge joints only allow movement in one plane due to the large number of ligaments crossing the joint and restricting movement. The ball-and-socket joint of the shoulder, however, enjoys a wide range of movement, due to its shallow socket and relatively few ligaments.

### Movement patterns occurring at synovial joints

The movements that occur at joints can be classified according to the action occurring between the articulating bones. These are called movement patterns. A movement of a limb or body part will always have a starting point (point A) and a finishing point (point B). By analysing the position

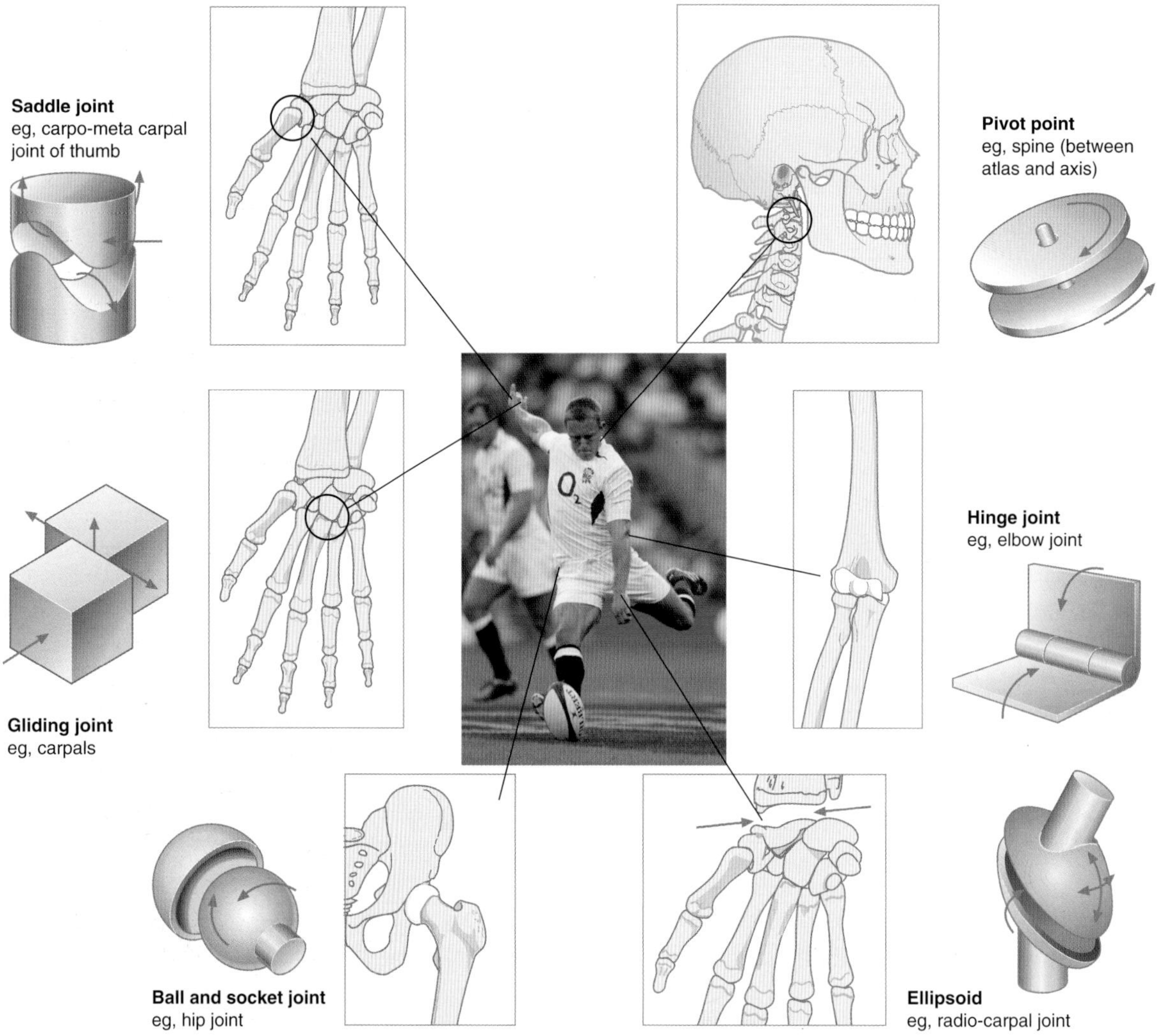


**Figure 5.8** Types of synovial joint

of the finishing point relative to the starting point, we can form a classification of movement. A knowledge of body planes can also aid our understanding and classification of joint actions.

## Planes and axes of the body

In order to explain the body's movements, it is often useful to view the body as having a series of imaginary lines running through it. These are known as the planes of movement or the planes section. The imaginary lines divide the body up in three ways (see Figure 5.9). Firstly, the median or sagittal plane splits the body vertically into the left and right sides, the horizontal or transverse plane divides the body into superior and inferior sections and runs horizontally, while the frontal or coronal plane runs vertically and divides the body into anterior and posterior sections.

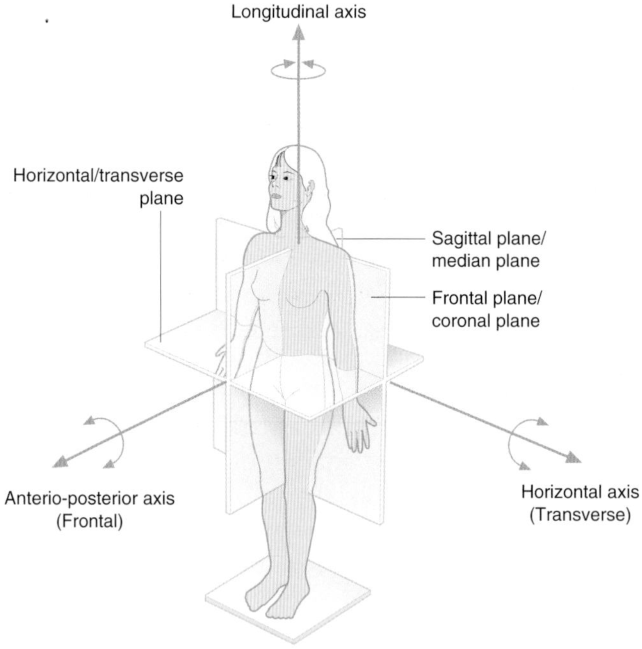


**Figure 5.9** Body planes and axes

Table 5.1 Body planes and movement patterns possible

| Plane | Movement pattern |
|---|---|
| Frontal plane | Abduction<br>Adduction<br>Inversion<br>Eversion<br>Lateral flexion<br>Elevation<br>Depression<br>Protraction<br>Retraction |
| Sagittal/median plane | Flexion<br>Extension<br>Dorsiflexion<br>Plantarflexion |
| Horizontal plane | Medial rotation } rotation<br>Lateral rotation<br>Horizontal abduction<br>Horizontal adduction<br>Pronation<br>Supination |

The body or body parts can move in these planes and a knowledge of them will certainly be of benefit to the coach and athlete. In gymnastics, for example, movement in all planes may occur in the performance of full twisting somersaults. What other sporting situations can you think of where a knowledge of planes of movement may be of use? In addition, the body (or body parts) can rotate around one of three axes in the body. When performing a front somersault, for example, the body rotates about the horizontal axis. A full twisting jump involves the body rotating about the longitudinal axis. Finally, when performing a cartwheel the body rotates about the anterior-posterior or frontal axis. Table A summarises the movement patterns which occur in each of the body's planes.

Major movement patterns that play a significant role in sporting activity are outlined in Table 5.2.

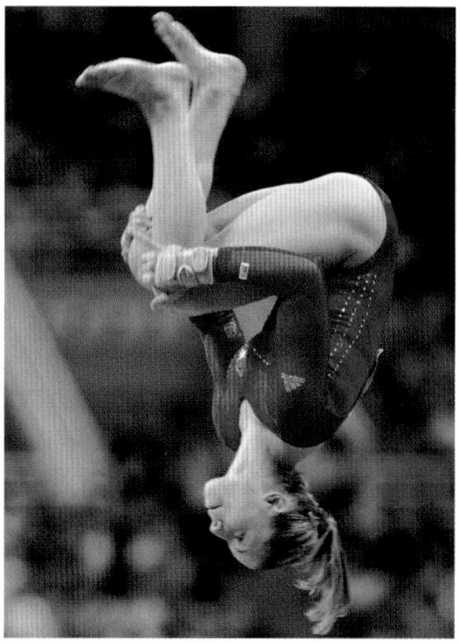

Figure 5.10 A gymnast performing a front somersault in the median plane about the horizontal axis

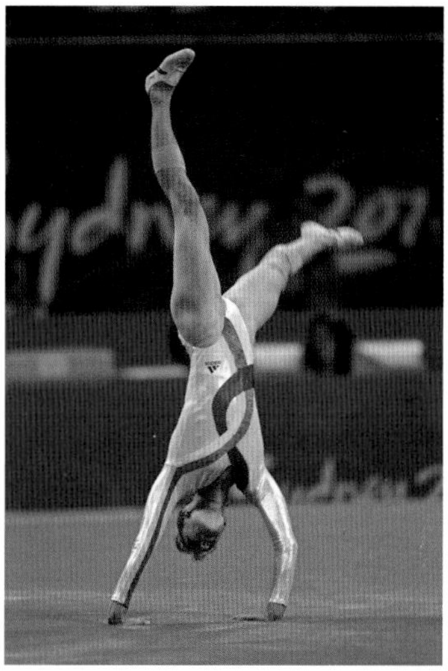

Figure 5.11 A gymnast performing a cartwheel in the frontal plane about the anterio–posterior axis

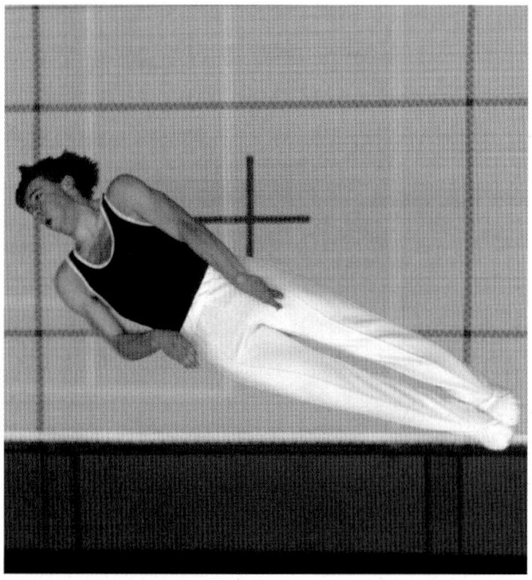

Figure 5.12 A trampolinist performing a full-twisting somersault jump in the horizontal plane about the longitudinal axis

Table 5.2 Movement patterns

| Joint action | Diagram |
| --- | --- |
| **Flexion**<br>Flexion occurs when the angle between the articulating bones is decreased. For example: by raising the lower arm up to touch the shoulder, the angle between the radius and the humerus at the elbow has decreased. Flexion of the elbow has thus occurred. Flexion occurs in the **median plane** about the **horizontal axis.** A muscle that causes flexion is known as a 'flexor'. In the instance at the elbow, the **bicep brachii** is the flexor muscle. | 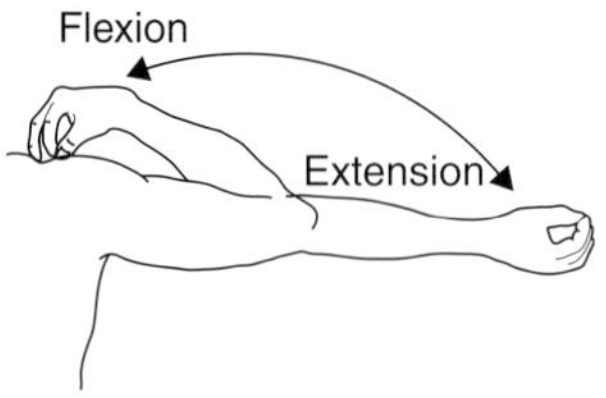 |
| **Extension**<br>Extension of a joint occurs when the angle of the articulating bones is increased. For example: when standing up from a seated position, the angle between the femur and tibia increases, thus causing extension at the knee joint. Extreme extension, usually at an angle of greater than 180° is known as hyper extension. Extension occurs in the median plane about the horizontal axis. A muscle that causes extension is known as an 'extensor'. In the example of the knee joint, the quadricep femoris group is the extensor. | 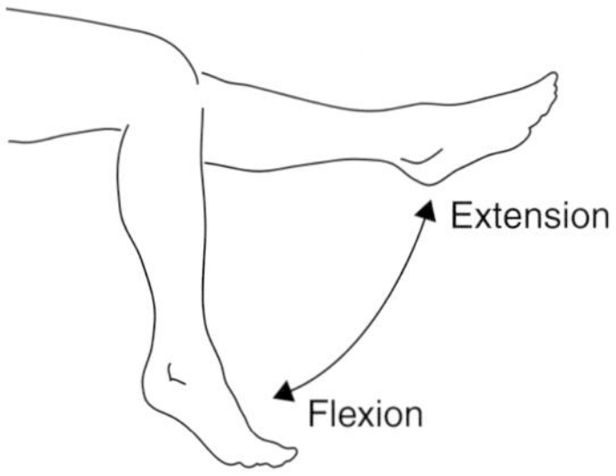 |
| **Abduction**<br>This is movement of a body part away from the midline of the body or other body part. For example:<br>• if arms are placed by the sides of the body and then raised laterally, abduction has occurred at the shoulder joint<br>• if fingers are spread out, movement has occurred away from the midline of the hand, and abduction has occurred.<br>Abduction occurs in the **frontal plane** about an **anterio-posterior axis**. However, horizontal abduction takes place in the **horizontal or transverse plane**. | 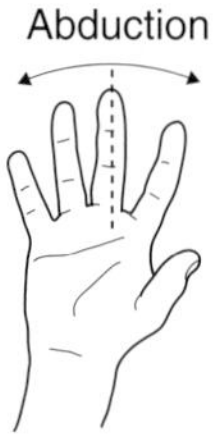 |
| **Adduction**<br>Adduction is the opposite of abduction and concerns movement towards the midline of the body or body part. For example, by lowering the arm back to the sides of the body, movement towards the midline has occurred and is termed adduction. Adduction occurs in the **frontal plane** about an **anterio-posterior axis**. However, horizontal adduction takes place in the **horizontal or transverse plane**. | 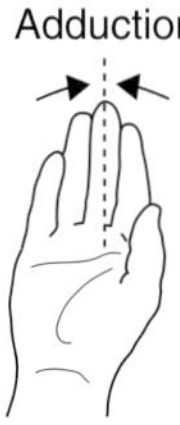 |
| **Circumduction**<br>Circumduction occurs where a circle can be described by the body part and is simply a combination of flexion, extension, abduction and adduction. True circumduction can only really occur at ball and socket joints of the shoulder and hip.<br>As circumduction is a combination of flexion, extension, abduction and adduction it occurs in the **median and frontal planes**. | 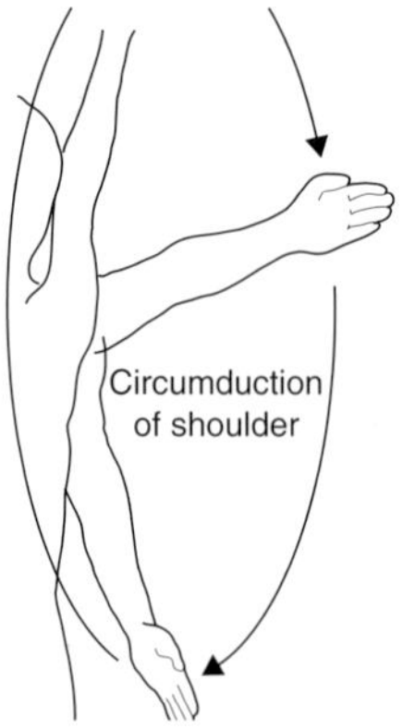 |

Table 5.2 *continued*

| Joint action | Diagram |
| --- | --- |
| **Pronation**<br>Pronation occurs at the elbow and involves internal rotation between the radius and humerus. It typically occurs where the palm of the hand is moved from facing upwards to facing downwards. Pronation occurs in the **horizontal plane** about a **longitudinal axis**.<br><br>**Supination**<br>Supination is the opposite of pronation and again takes place at the elbow. This time the movement is lateral rotation between the radius and humerus and generally occurs when the palm of the hand is turned so that it faces upwards. Supination occurs in the **horizontal plane** about a **longitudinal axis**. | 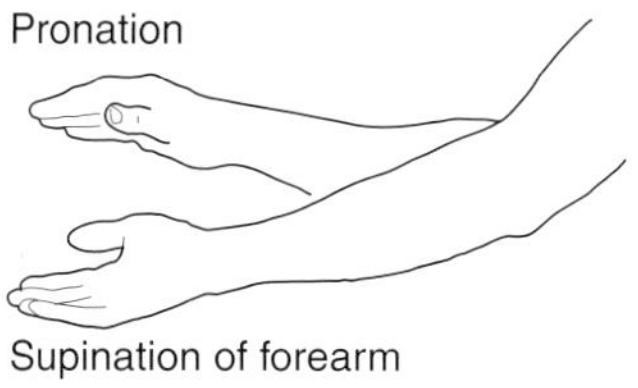 |
| **Horizontal abduction/adduction**<br>Horizontal abduction involves movement of the arm across the body in the **horizontal plane**. To explain this further attempt the following exercise:<br>1. Stand with your arms by your side.<br>2. Raise your right arm up in front of you, until it reaches 'shoulder height'.<br>3. Move your arm (from the shoulder) out to the right. This is horizontal abduction.<br>4. Now move your arm across your body towards your midline – this is horizontal adduction of the shoulder.<br><br>Sometimes horizontal abduction is known as **horizontal extension** and horizontal adduction is known as **horizontal flexion**. | 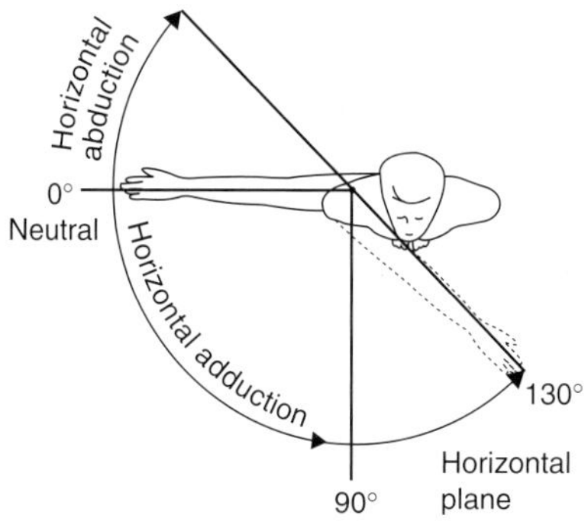 |
| **Rotation**<br>Rotation of a joint occurs where the bone turns about its axis within the joint. Rotation towards the body is termed **internal** or **medial** rotation, while rotation away from the body is called **external** or **lateral** rotation. Rotation occurs in the **horizontal plane** about a **longitudinal axis**.<br>To explain this further attempt the following exercise:<br>1. Grip a ruler at the bottom with your right hand.<br>2. Now raise your arm up in front of your body and move the ruler in an anticlockwise movement. Medial rotation has occurred at the shoulder joint.<br>3. Now move the ruler clockwise so that it ends up pointing to the side. This is lateral rotation and has once again occurred at the shoulder. | 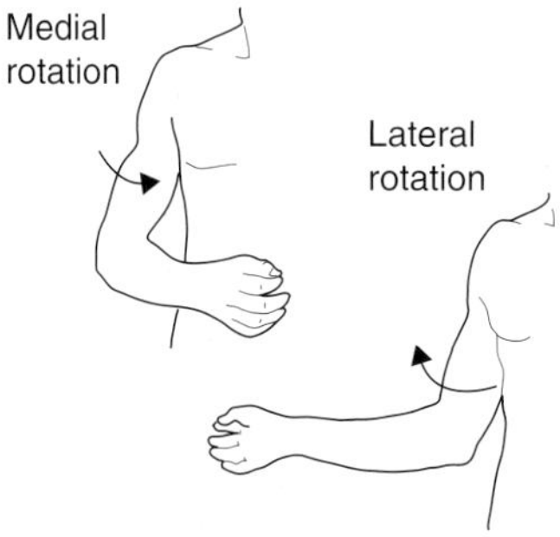 |
| **Plantarflexion**<br>Plantarflexion occurs at the ankle joint and is typified by the pointing of the toes. Plantarflexion occurs in the **median plane** about **a horizontal axis**. | 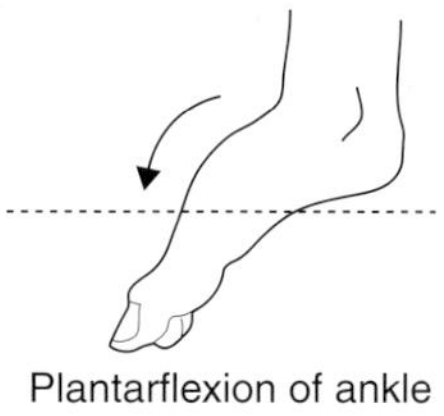 |

Table 5.2 *continued*

| Joint action | Diagram |
|---|---|
| **Dorsiflexion**<br>This also occurs at the ankle and occurs when the foot is raised upwards towards the tibia. Dorsiflexion occurs in the **median plane** about a **horizontal axis**. | 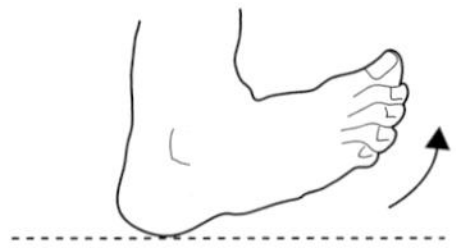<br>Dorsiflexion of ankle |
| **Inversion**<br>This occurs when the sole of the foot is turned inwards towards the midline of the body. Inversion occurs in the **frontal plane**.<br>**Eversion**<br>Eversion occurs when the sole of the foot is turned laterally outwards. Eversion occurs in the **frontal plane**. | 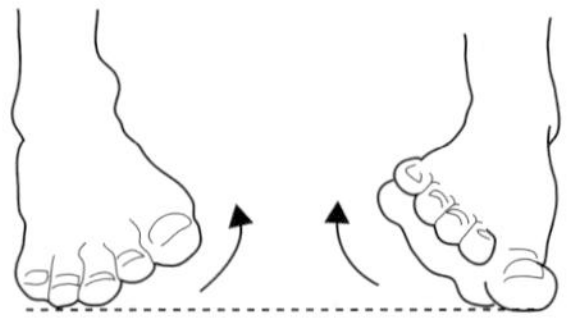<br>Inversion Eversion |

## Activity 6

Using an articulated skeleton, or a partner, examine the joints listed below. Describe the type of joint and the movements possible:

- Radio-ulnar joint
- Knee joint
- Elbow joint
- Hip joint
- Shoulder joint
- Skull and cervical vertebrae
- Ribs and thoracic vertebrae
- Lumbar region

## Activity 7

What movement patterns occur at:

- the shoulder and elbow during the performance of a tennis serve?
- the hip and knee during a squat thrust?
- the hip, knee and ankle during the recovery and kick phase in breaststroke?

**Key term**

**Movement patterns:** Terms used to describe the actions taking place at joints. They include flexion, extension, abduction, adduction, rotation and circumduction.

**IN CONTEXT**

**Look at the javelin thrower in Figure 5.13. The humerus articulates with the scapula at the shoulder joint and moves from the preparation phase shown (starting point), through to the release point (finishing point). In doing so, the action of horizontal flexion/adduction occurs.**

## EXAMINER'S TIP

Candidates often get confused between rotation and circumduction. To distinguish between the two, try the following:

- Grip a ruler at the bottom with your right hand.
- Now raise your arm in front of your body and move the ruler anticlockwise. Medial rotation has just occurred at your shoulder.
- Now move the ruler clockwise so that it ends up pointing to the side. This is lateral rotation.

Circumduction occurs when you describe a circle with your hand, using your whole arm.

## EXAMINER'S TIP

When answering a question on movement patterns, make sure you state the following:

- the name of the joint;
- the type of joint;
- the articulating bones;
- the movement produced.
- the planes in which the movement occurs
- the axes about which the movement occurs

It is often a good idea in your exam to draw up a table to show this information.

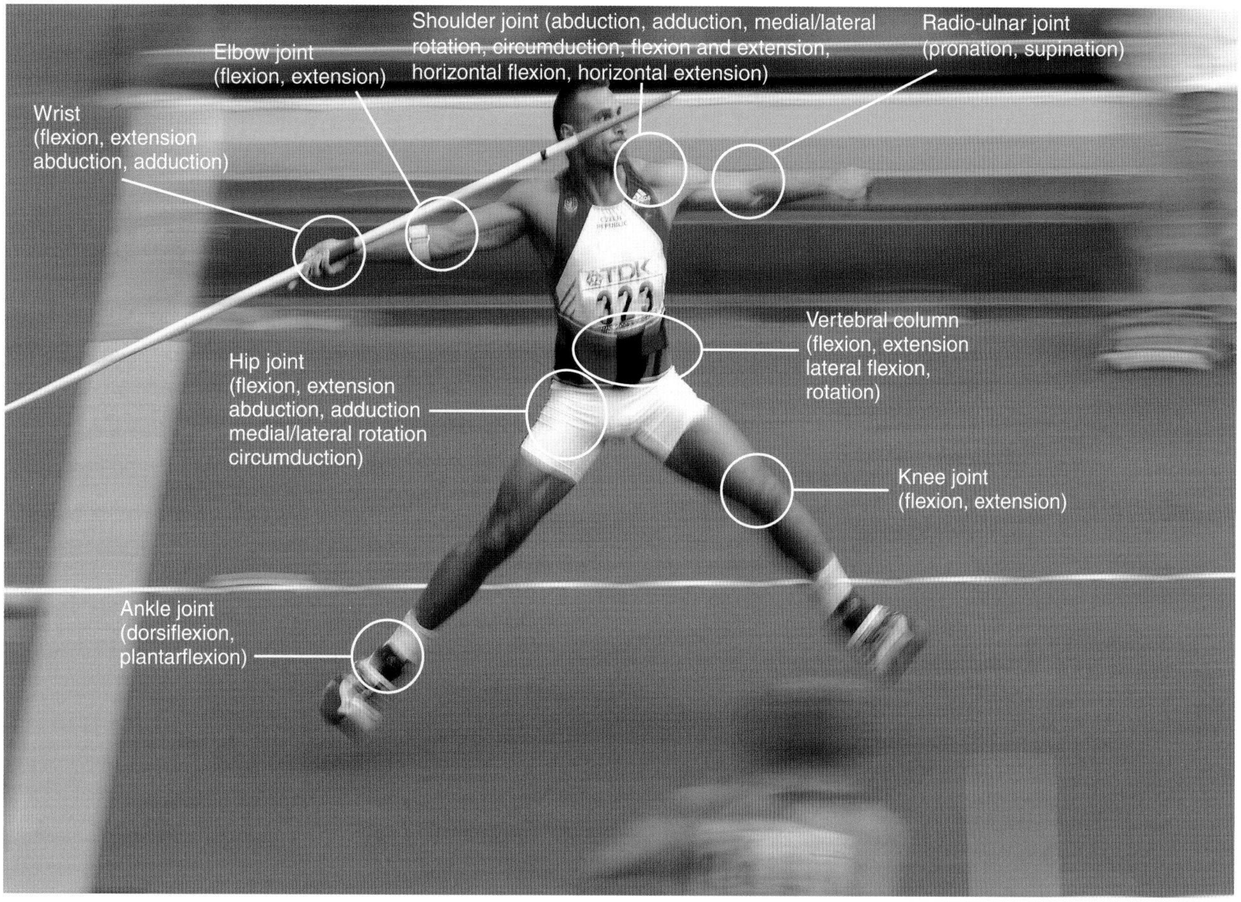


Figure 5.13 Joints and their associated movement patterns

## Activity 8

Participate in the circuit training session outlined in Figure 5.14. For each activity, state what movement patterns are occurring at the stated joints.

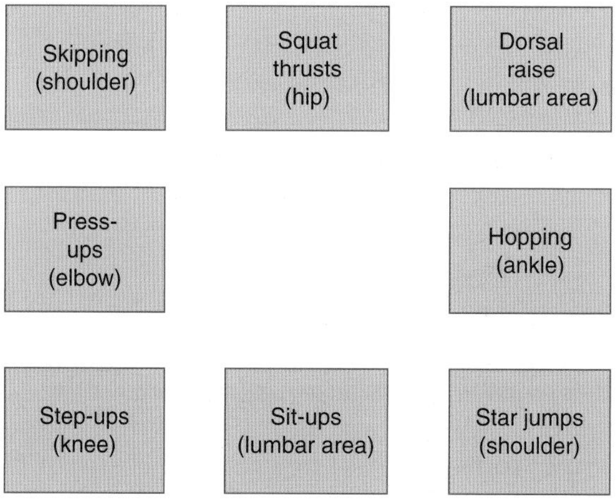


Figure 5.14 A circuit of exercises

# The muscular system

No study of human movement or exercise is complete without a study of the muscular system. The muscles interact with the skeleton to provide movement.

Skeletal muscle is responsible for the body's mechanical movement, and is central to our study of movement analysis. We are now going to examine its properties and functions.

## Properties of skeletal muscle

Skeletal muscle possesses three essential properties:

1 Extensibility: this is the ability of muscle tissue to lengthen when contracting and provide the effort required to move the lever system (bones), producing coordinated movement.
2 Elasticity: this is the ability of muscle tissue to return to its normal resting length once it has been stretched. This can be compared to an elastic band that will always resume its resting

shape, even after stretching. This enables the muscle to prepare for a series of repeated contractions, which is normally required during the performance of exercise.

3 Contractility: this refers to the capacity of a muscle to contract or shorten forcibly when stimulated by nerves and hormones (excitability).

All these properties are essential for all body actions, including locomotion, posture and facial expressions.

## Functions of skeletal muscle

Skeletal muscle has several important functions within the body:

1 Movement: skeletal muscles attach to bones, against which they pull to enable movement. For example, when running, the hip flexor muscles pull on the femur to lift the leg off the ground, while the quadriceps muscles contract to pull on the tibia to straighten the leg at the knee joint.

2 Support and posture: the muscles are seldom fully relaxed and are often in a constant state of slight contraction. In order to adopt an upright position, many muscles within the legs and torso are contracting statically to ensure that the body is balanced. This is also known as muscle tone.

3 Heat production: the contraction of skeletal muscle involves the production of energy. In breaking down glycogen to provide this energy, heat is released. This accounts for why the body becomes hot when exercising. When the body is cold, the muscle often goes through a series of involuntary contractions (commonly known as shivering) in order to release heat and keep the body warm.

## Connective tissue

Connective tissue is responsible for holding all the individual muscle fibres together. It surrounds individual muscle fibres and encases the whole muscle, forming tendons, which attach the muscles to bones and transmit the 'pull' of the muscle to the bones, to cause movement and harness the power of muscle contractions. Tendons vary in length and are composed of parallel fibres of collagen.

The points of attachment for each muscle are termed the origin and the insertion.

- The origin is the end of the muscle attached to a stable bone against which the muscle can pull. *This is usually the nearest flat bone.*
- The insertion is the muscle attachment on the bone that the muscle puts into action.

For example, the biceps brachii has its origin on the scapula. This gives a firm base against which the biceps brachii can pull in order to raise the lower arm. (The biceps is a flexor muscle, and its job is to allow flexion at the elbow.) Since the biceps brachii raises the lower arm, it must be attached to that body part via the insertion. In fact, the biceps brachii has its insertion on the radius.

The muscle belly is the thick portion of muscle tissue sited between the origin and the insertion. It is not unusual for a muscle to have two or more origins, while maintaining a common insertion: the term 'biceps' can be broken down to mean two ('bi') heads ('ceps'). The biceps brachii has two origins, or heads, which pull on one insertion in the radius and put the lower arm into action.

**Key terms**

**Tendon:** A connective tissue that attaches skeletal muscle to a bone. Tendons have a great capacity to withstand stress as they must transmit large muscular forces to put a bone into action.

**Origin:** The tendon or point of attachment of a muscle onto a stationary bone against which the muscle can pull. Usually on the nearest flat bone to the working muscle.

**Insertion:** The tendon or point of attachment of a muscle onto the bone that the muscle puts into action.

**EXAMINER'S TIP**

The origin of a muscle is usually attached to the nearest flat bone, while the insertion is on the bone that the muscle puts into action.

## Antagonistic muscle action

Muscles never work alone. In order for a coordinated movement to be produced, the muscles must work as a group or team, with several muscles working at any one time. Taking the simple movement of flexion of the arm at the elbow, the muscle responsible for flexion (bending of the arm) is the biceps brachii, and the muscle which produces the desired joint movement is called the agonist, or prime mover. However, in order for the biceps muscle to shorten when contracting, the triceps muscle must lengthen. The triceps, in this instance, is known as the antagonist, since its action is opposite to that of the agonist. The two muscles must work together, however, to produce the required movement.

Fixator muscles, or stabilisers, also work in this movement. Their role is to stabilise the origin so that the agonist can achieve maximum and effective contraction. In this case, the trapezius contracts to stabilise the scapula, to create a rigid platform. Neutralisers or synergist muscles in this movement prevent any undesired movements which may occur, particularly at the shoulder, where the biceps works over two joints.

It can thus be seen that for this apparently simple movement of elbow flexion, integrated and synergistic (harmonious) muscle actions are required to enable the necessary smooth movement.

Furthermore, the roles of each muscle are constantly changed for changing actions. For example, in the action of elbow extension, the roles of the biceps and triceps are reversed, so that the triceps becomes the prime mover or agonist (since the triceps is an extensor and thus produces this movement pattern), while the biceps becomes the antagonist, to enable the smooth and effective contraction of the triceps.

Below is a list of commonly used antagonistic pairings.

## Antagonistic pairings

- pectorals/latissimus dorsi;
- anterior deltoids/posterior deltoids;
- trapezius/deltoids;
- rectus abdominis/erector spinalis;
- quadriceps group/hamstring group;
- tibialis anterior/gastrocnemius and soleus;
- biceps brachii/triceps brachii;
- wrist flexors/wrist extensors.

### Activity 9

Explain the antagonistic muscle action occurring in the leg during a kicking action in swimming front crawl.

**IN CONTEXT**

**When a gymnast such as Beth Tweddle takes off when performing a somersault, her quadriceps muscles are the agonists and will undergo concentric contraction as they shorten. On landing, her quadriceps undergo eccentric contraction as they lengthen while contracting and cushion the landing – they remain the agonists. To maintain the tucked position throughout the somersault, her hip flexors (iliopsoas) work isometrically – they do not change length but they are still contracting.**

**Key terms**

**Agonist/prime mover:** A muscle that contracts and is directly responsible for the movement that results at a joint.
**Antagonist:** A muscle that has an action opposite to that of an agonist and helps in the production of a coordinated movement.
**Fixator:** A muscle that stabilises the origin of the agonist so that an effective contraction can take place.

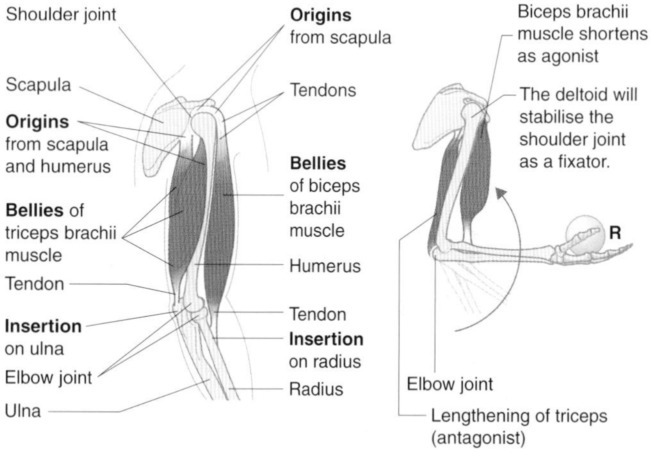


Figure 5.15 Antagonistic muscle action at the elbow joint

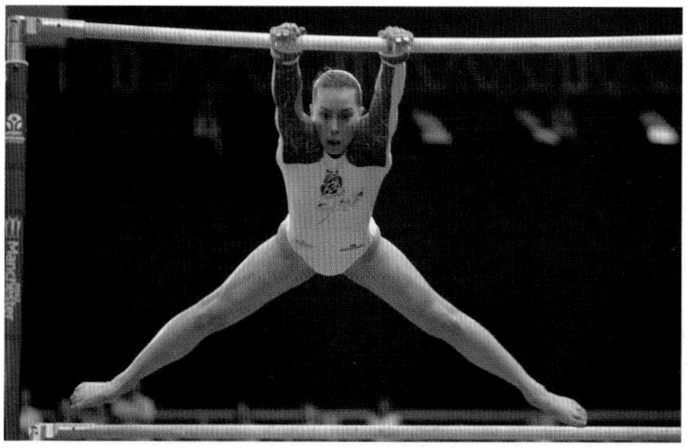

Figure 5.16 The muscles of a gymnast will work antagonistically to produce effective and coordinated movements

## Exam-style questions

1 The putting action of the arm in shot putt involves a series of coordinated movements at the shoulder, elbow and wrist.

(a) Name the main muscle involved at each joint. (3 marks)

(b) Explain the antagonistic muscle action taking place at the elbow joint during the execution stage of the putt. (3 marks)

2 (a) Identify the type of movement pattern occurring at the shoulder wrist and ankle joints of a swimmer as they dive into the swimming pool. (3 marks)

(b) During a 100m race the swimmer will perform a tumble turn. State the plane and the axis about which this action takes place. (2 marks)

3 Explain the roles and types of muscular contraction taking place in the biceps brachii, triceps brachii and deltoid muscles when a weight-trainer performs a bicep curl with a weighted barbell. (6 marks)

4 An athlete is performing a sprint start. The table here illustrates a movement analysis of the leg action during the drive phase.

| Joint | Joint type | Articulating bones | Movement produced | Agonist | Plane | Axis |
|---|---|---|---|---|---|---|
| Knee | A | Femur and tibia | C | D | F | Transverse / Horizontal |
| Hip | Ball and socket | B | Extension | E | Sagittal/ median | H |
| Ankle | Hinge | C | Plantarflexion | Gastrocnemius | G | I |

(i) Provide the missing information for letters A-I (9 marks)

(ii) Identify the muscle function and the type of muscle contraction being performed at D and E. (2 marks)

## Types of muscular contraction

In order to produce the vast range of movements of which it is capable, the body's muscles either shorten, lengthen or remain the same length while contracting. Indeed, muscle contractions are classified depending on the muscle action which predominates. See Table 5.3.

Isotonic contractions refer to those instances when the muscle is moving while contracting. This can be divided further, into concentric and eccentric muscle actions:

- Concentric contractions involve the muscle shortening while contracting, as happens in the biceps brachii during the upward phase of a biceps curl, or in the triceps during the upward phase of a push-up.
- Eccentric contractions, on the other hand, involve the muscle lengthening while contracting (remember that a muscle is not always relaxing while lengthening!). This can be seen in the biceps during the downward phase of the biceps curl, or in the triceps during the downward phase of the press-up. The eccentric contraction of the biceps during the downward phase is used to counteract the force of gravity. This is because gravity acts on the mass of the forearm, causing extension at the elbow. If the biceps does not contract to control the rate of motion caused by gravity, the movement will be very quick, resulting in injury.

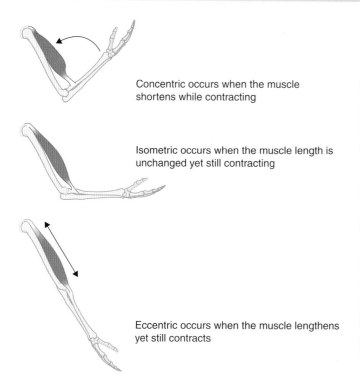

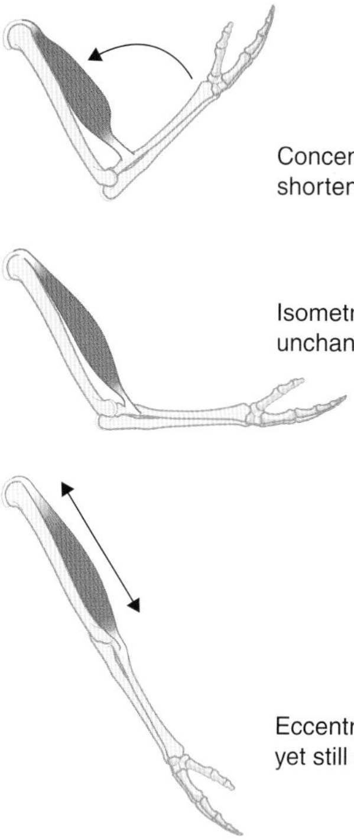
Concentric occurs when the muscle shortens while contracting
Isometric occurs when the muscle length is unchanged yet still contracting
Eccentric occurs when the muscle lengthens yet still contracts

Figure 5.17 Types of muscle contraction at the biceps brachii

## Key terms

**Isotonic concentric contraction:** The shortening of a muscle while contracting. For example, during the upward phase of a biceps curl, the biceps contracts concentrically.

**Isotonic eccentric contraction:** The lengthening of a muscle while contracting. For example, during the downward phase of a biceps curl, the biceps contracts eccentrically.

**Isometric contraction:** Where a muscle contracts, yet there is no visible shortening or lengthening. Also known as a static contraction. For example, when holding a barbell with the elbows flexed at 90°, the biceps contracts isometrically.

**Plyometrics:** A type of training designed to improve power, elastic strength and speed. It involves pre-loading the muscle with an eccentric contraction before performing a powerful concentric contraction. Activities commonly include bounding, hopping and a variety of medicine ball exercises.

Plyometrics is a type of strength training based on a muscle contracting eccentrically.

Sometimes, however, a muscle can contract without actively lengthening or shortening. In this instance, the muscle is going through isometric contraction – the muscle remains the same length while contracting. In fact, the majority of muscles will contract isometrically in order for us to maintain posture. These static contractions also occur while holding a weight in a stationary position, or when performing a handstand.

Normally, when a muscle contracts, the angular velocity of the muscle shortening or lengthening varies throughout the contraction. However, specialist hydraulic machines have been devised so that it is possible to maintain constant the speed at which the muscle lengthens or shortens, but not necessarily maintain the resistance applied. The speed of the movement cannot be increased. Any attempt to increase the velocity results in equal reaction force from the machine. In this way, isokinetic exercise, as it is called, is excellent for strength training.

Figure 5.18 shows the location of the major muscles in the body, while Table 5.4 shows the movements each muscle produces and gives an idea of some simple strengthening exercises. Take a moment to study both of these.

## IN CONTEXT

**When a muscle contracts eccentrically it is often acting as a brake to counteract the effect of gravity. So a triple jumper's quadriceps muscles must contract eccentrically on landing during the hop-and-step phase to stop the leg from buckling and the jumper collapsing to the floor.**

Table 5.3 Types of muscle contraction

| | Isotonic Concentric | Eccentric | Isometric Static |
|---|---|---|---|
| Muscle action | Muscle shortens | Muscle lengthens while contracting | Muscle remains the same length while contracting |
| Example | Biceps: when raising a weight | Biceps: when lowering a weight | Biceps: holding a weight in a static position |

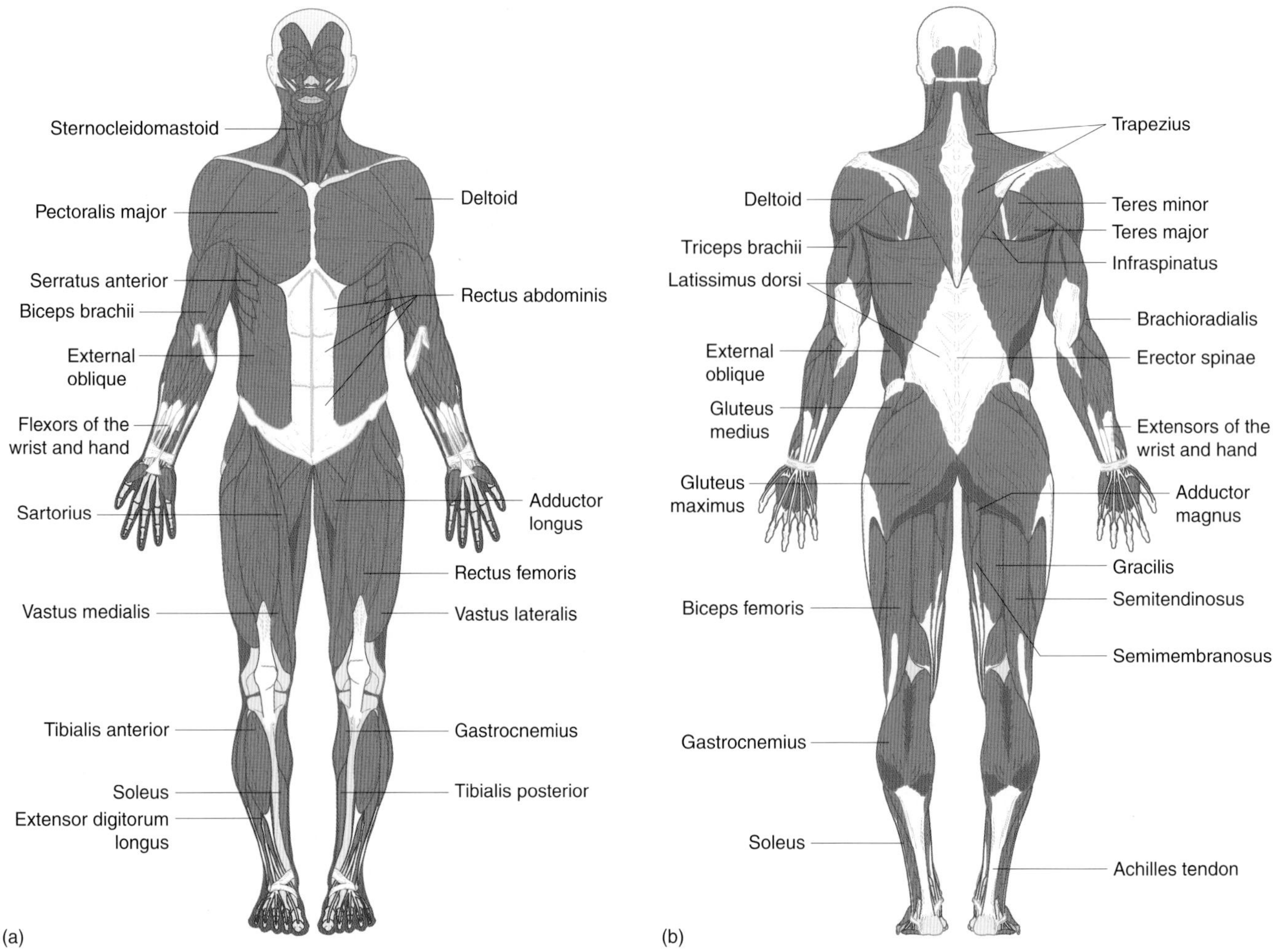


**Figure 5.18** Skeletal muscles of the human body a) Anterior view b) Posterior view

## Activity 10

1. Using sticky labels, label the muscles on a partner's body. Try to label as many as you can without looking at your textbook.
2. Collect as many pictures of bodybuilders as you can and label/identify the defined muscles.

## EXAMINER'S TIP

You must make sure that you know the names of the muscles and the function each muscle performs (i.e. what movement patterns or joint actions they cause).

## EXAMINER'S TIP

Make sure you can name the four muscles of the quadriceps group and the three muscles of the hamstring group.

Table 5.4 Major muscles, their origins and insertions, and actions performed

| Major muscle/group | Origin | Insertion | Actions performed during a weights session |
|---|---|---|---|
| Trapezius<br>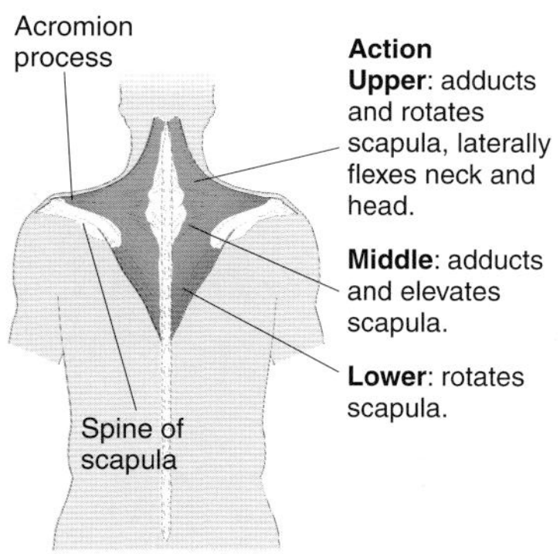<br> | Base of the skull<br>Thoracic vertebrae | Acromion process<br>Clavicle<br>Scapula | Shoulder shrugs<br>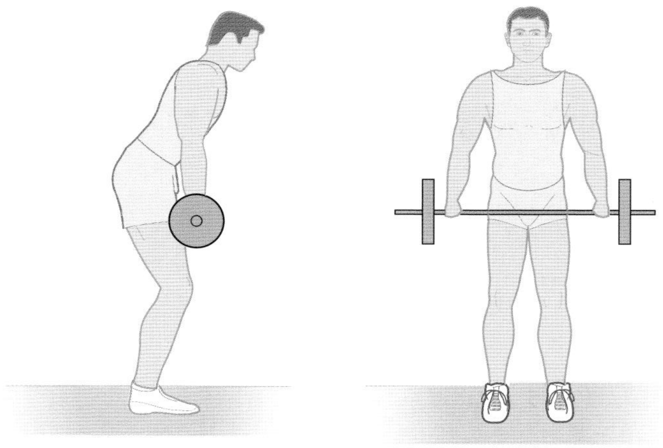 |
| Pectoralis major<br>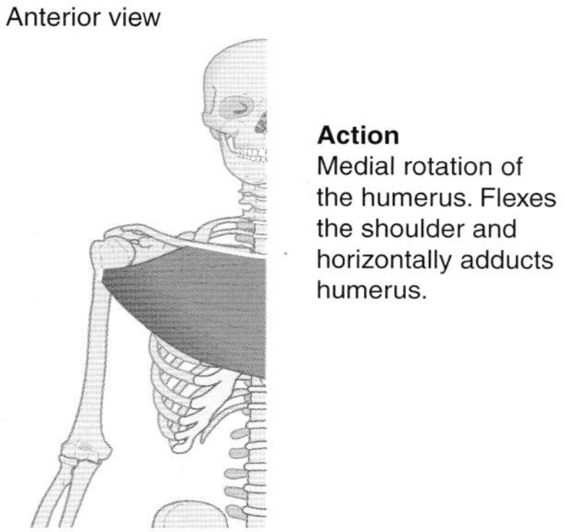<br> | Sternum<br>Clavicle<br>Rib cartilage | Humerus | Barbell chest press<br>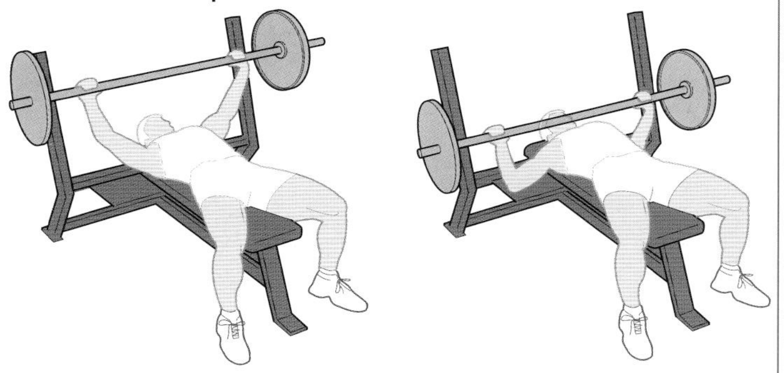 |

Continued

Table 5.4 *Continued*

| Major muscle/group | Origin | Insertion | Actions performed during a weights session |
|---|---|---|---|
| Deltoids 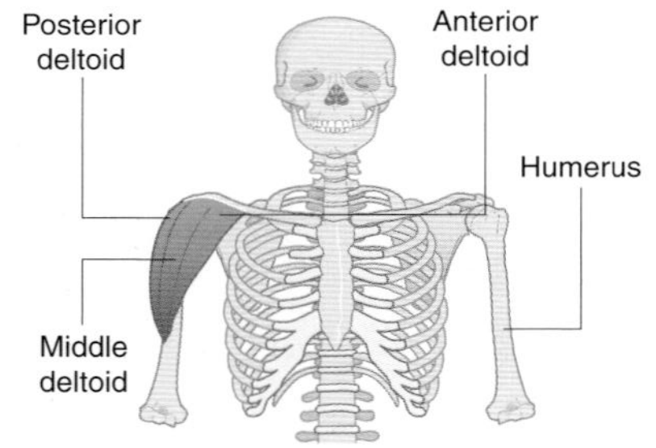  **Action** Anterior deltoids–flexion of shoulder<br>Middle deltoid–abduction of shoulder<br>Posterior deltoid–extension of shoulder | Clavicle<br>Scapula<br>Acromion process | Humerus | Deltoid 'fly' 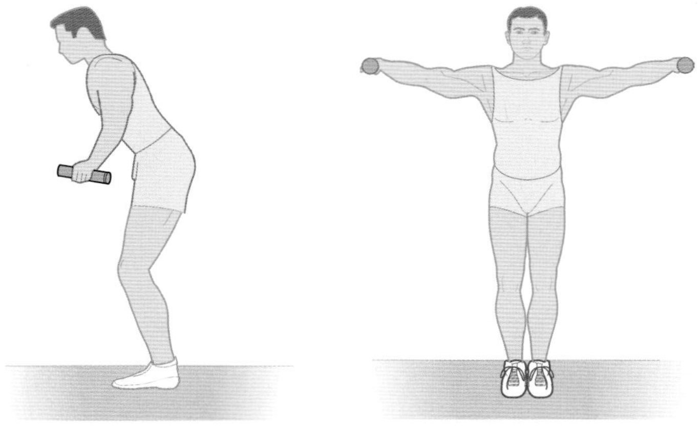 |
| Triceps brachii 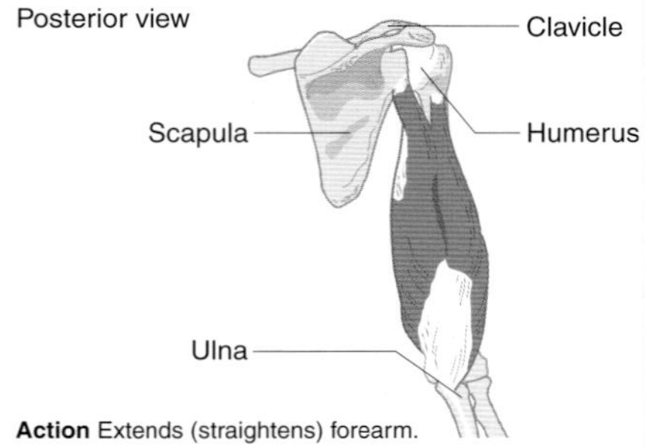  **Action** Extends (straightens) forearm. | Humerus<br>Scapula | Ulna (olecranon process) | Triceps extension 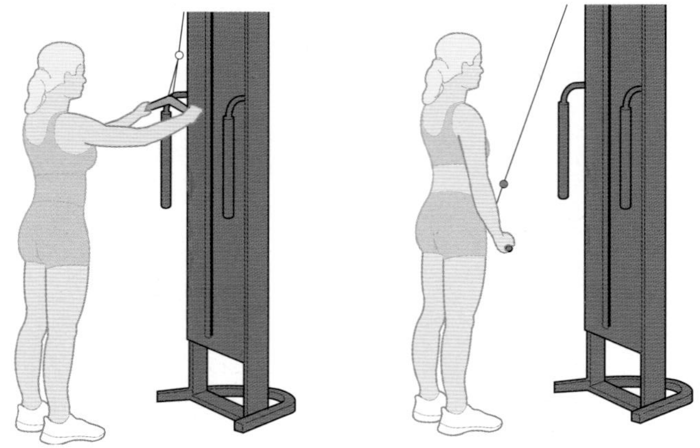 |

| Major muscle/group | Origin | Insertion | Actions performed during a weights session |
|---|---|---|---|
| Latissimus dorsi<br>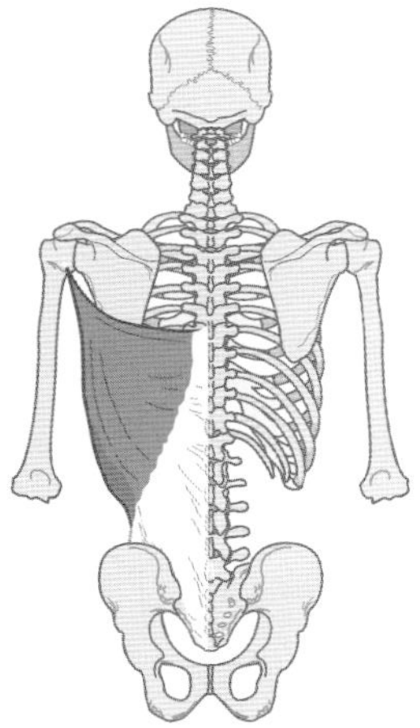<br>**Action** Adduction of humerus. | Thoracic vertebrae<br>Lumbar vertebrae<br>Iliac crest | Humerus | 'Lat' pull-down<br>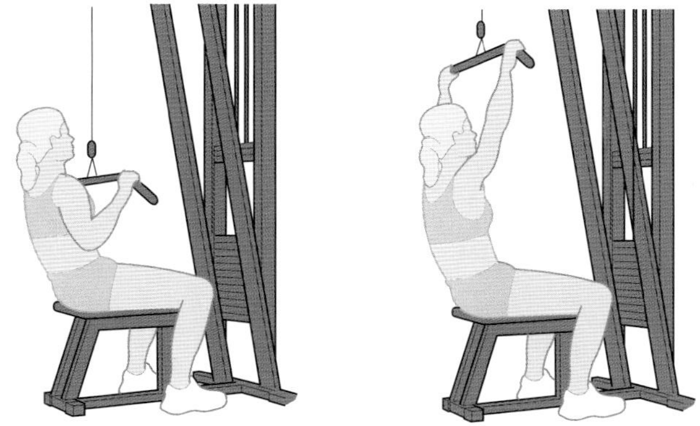 |
| Rectus abdominis/obliques<br>**Action**<br>**Transverse**: constricts abdominal contents, assists in forcing air out of lungs<br>**Rectus**: gives anterior support to lumbar spine, holds rib cage and pubis together.<br>**Internal/external obliques**: flex, rotate and side-bend trunk.<br>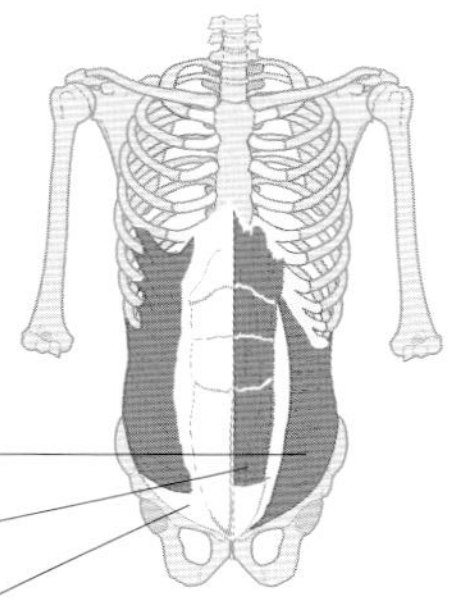<br> | Ribs | Ilium pubis | Swiss ball abdominal crunches<br>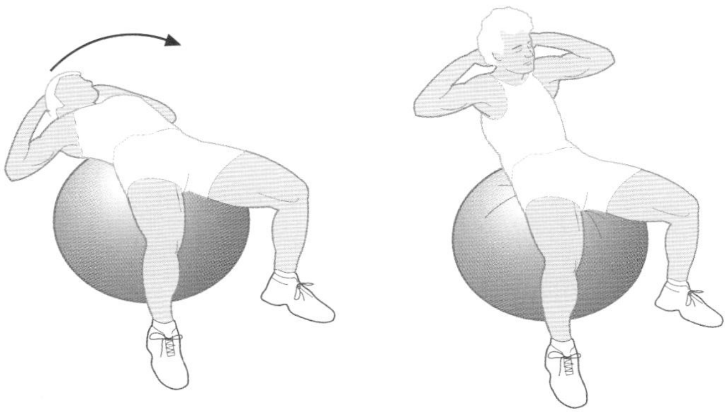 |

*Continued*

Table 5.4 *Continued*

| **Major muscle/group** | **Origin** | **Insertion** | **Actions performed during a weights session** |
|---|---|---|---|
| Gluteus maximus 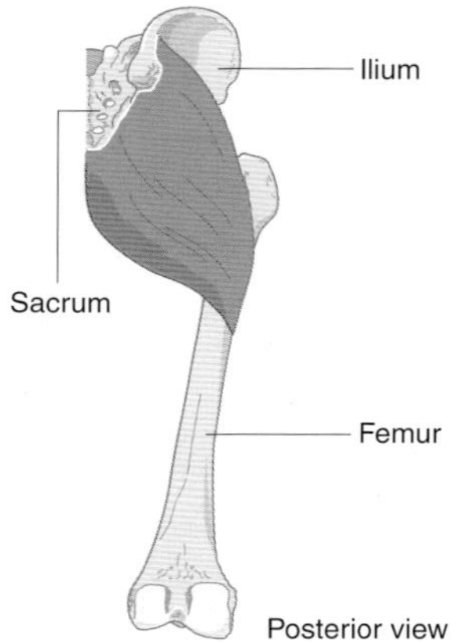  **Action** Extends hip, laterally rotates femur. | Ilium<br>Vertebrae<br>Femur | Femur | Hip extensor 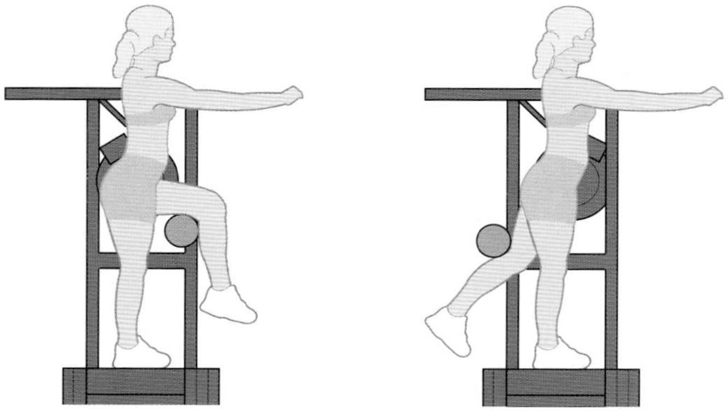 |
| Gluteus medius/minimus 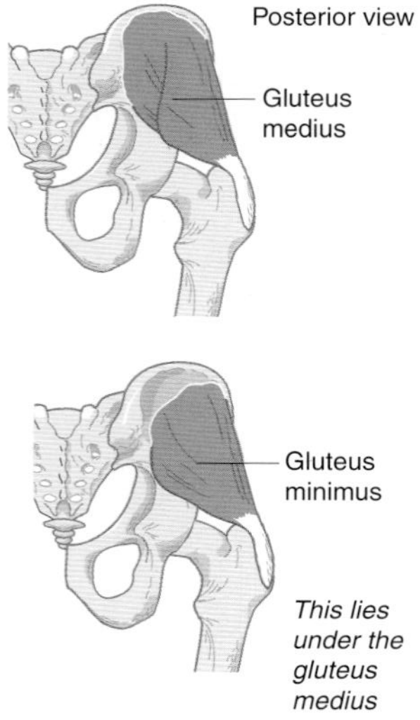  **Action** Abduct femur, medial rotators. | Ilium | Femur | Hip abduction 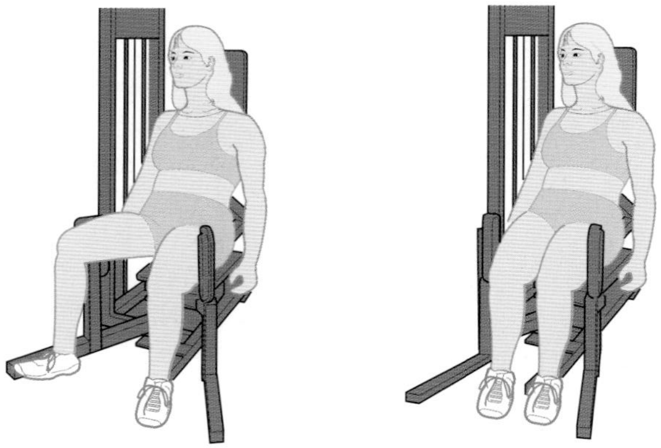 |

| Major muscle/group | Origin | Insertion | Actions performed during a weights session |
| --- | --- | --- | --- |
| Adductors<br>**Action**<br>Adduction of hip flexion and lateral rotation of the femur.<br>**Origin**<br>Front part of pubic bone and lower part of hip bone (ischial tuberosity). | Pubic bone (ischial tuberosity) | Femur | Hip adduction |
| Biceps brachii<br>Anterior view<br>**Action**<br>Flexes and supinates (turns palm upwards) the forearm. | Scapula | Radius | Barbell biceps curl |

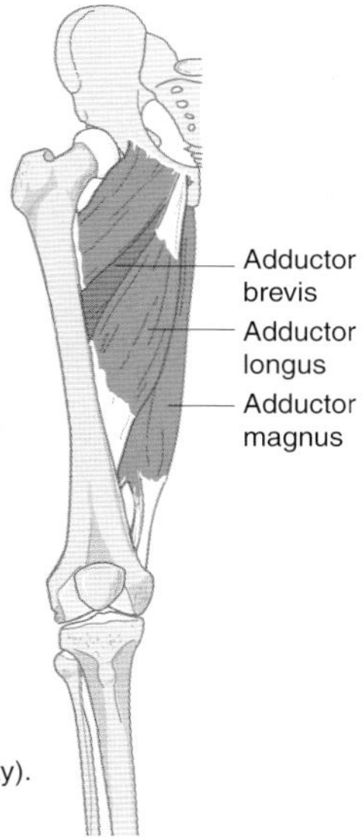


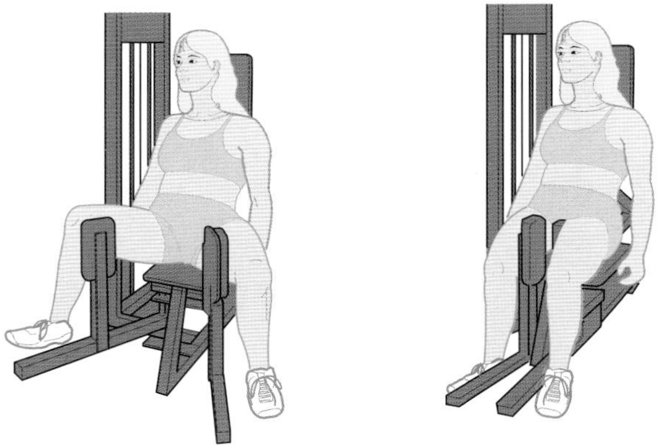

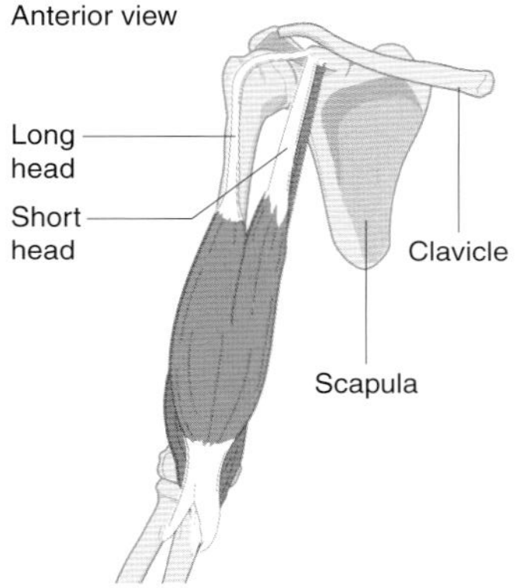


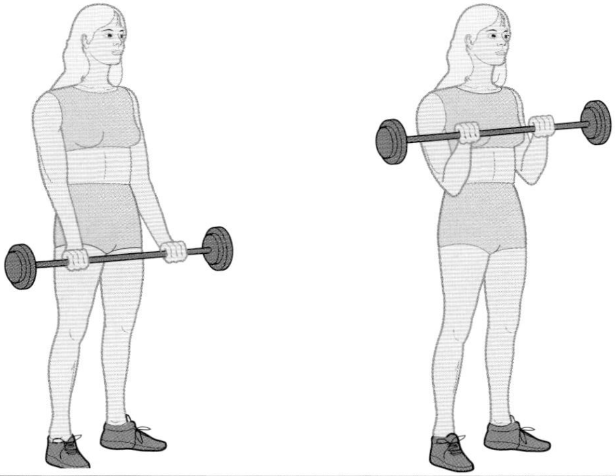

*Continued*

Table 5.4 *Continued*

| Major muscle/group | Origin | Insertion | Actions performed during a weights session |
|---|---|---|---|
| Wrist flexors/extensors<br>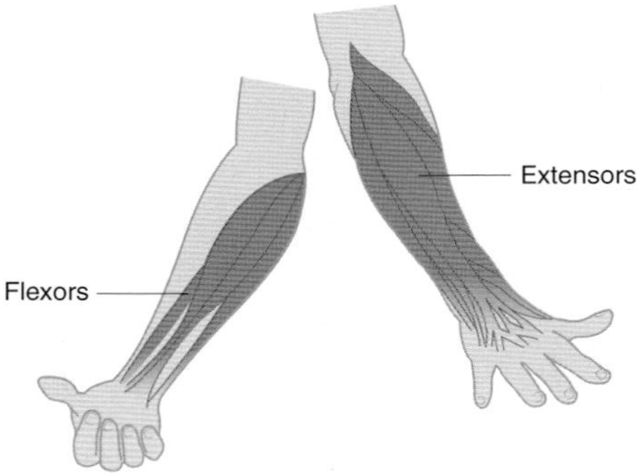<br><br>**Action** **Flexors**: flex the wrist<br>**Extensors**: extend the wrist | Humerus<br>Radius<br>Ulna | Carpals<br>Metacarpals<br>Phalanges | Wrist curls (flexors)<br>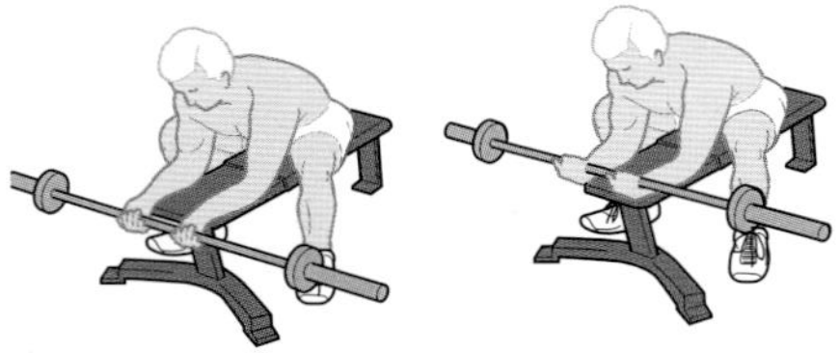<br>Reverse wrist curls (extensors)<br>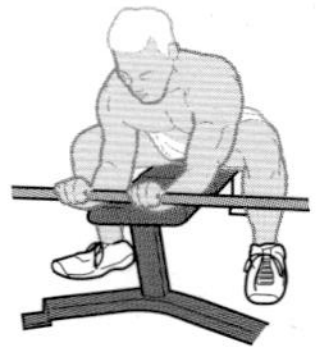 |
| Quadriceps group<br>*The quadriceps are made up of four muscles.*<br>*The rectus femoris acts on* ***both*** *the hip and knee joint.*<br>*The vasti muscles (medialis, intermedialis and lateralis) act on the knee joint only.*<br>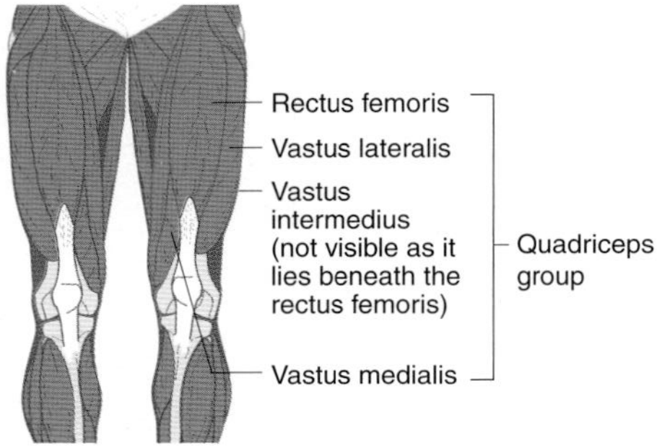<br> | Ilium<br>Femur | Tibia (via patella tendon) | Leg extensions<br>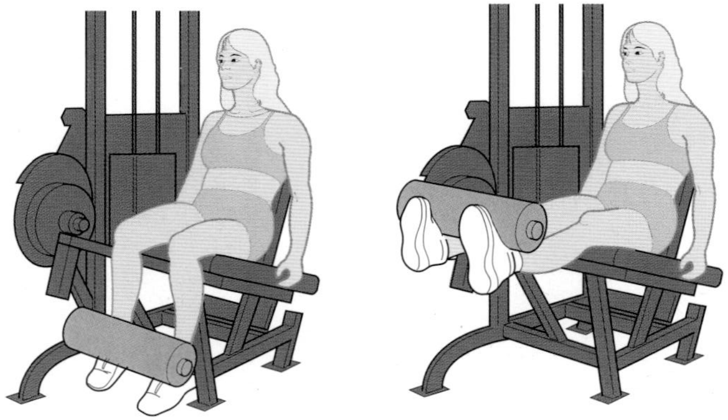 |

| Major muscle/group | Origin | Insertion | Actions performed during a weights session |
|---|---|---|---|
| Hamstring group<br>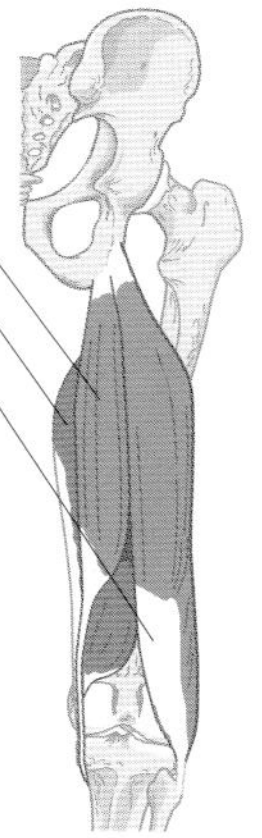<br><br>*The hamstrings consist of three muscles.*<br>**Action**<br>Flexes the knee, extends the femur of the hip. | Pubic bone (ischial tuberosity) | Tibia<br>Fibula | Hamstring curls<br>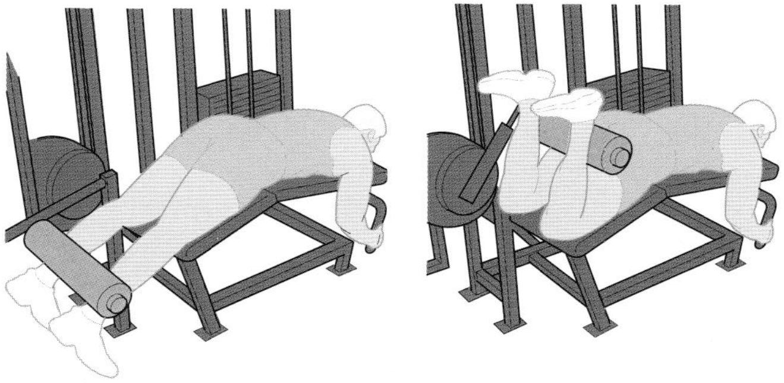 |
| Gastrocnemius/soleus<br>**Action**<br>Plantor flexion of the ankle (pointing the toes at the feet)<br>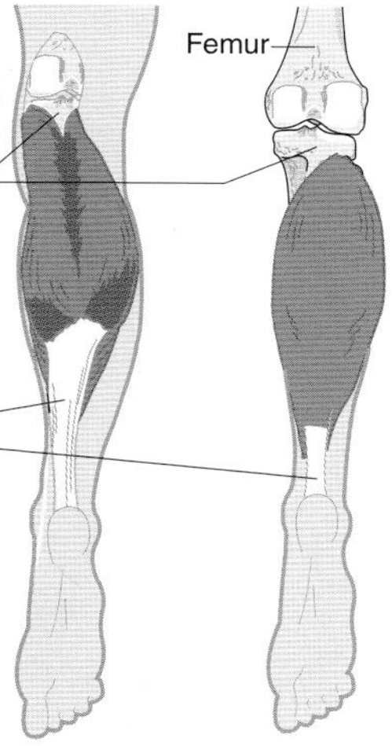<br> | Femur (gastrocnemius)<br>Tibi<br>Fibula (soleus) | Calcaneus | Calf raises<br>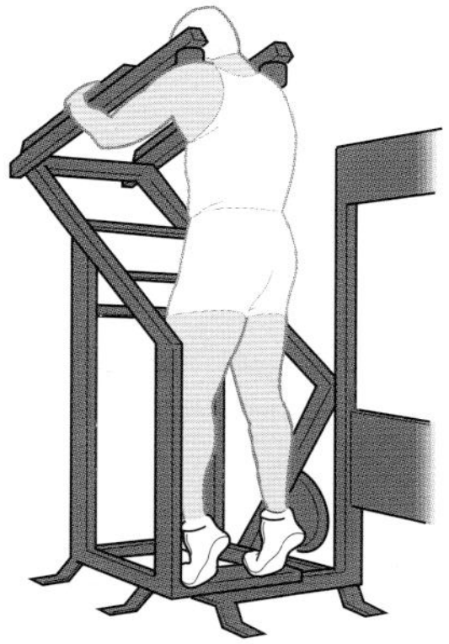 |

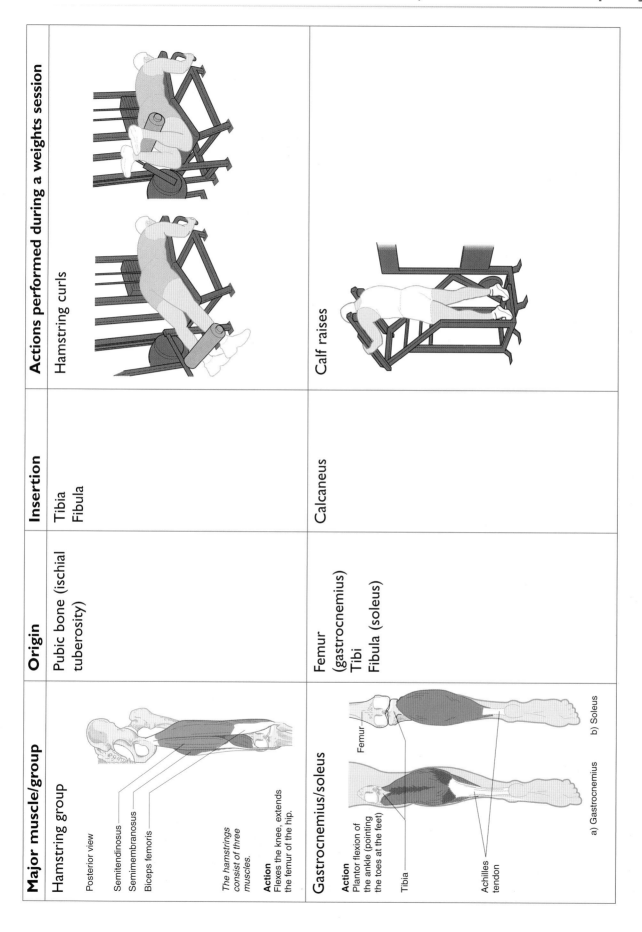

*Continued*

Table 5.4 *Continued*

| Major muscle/group | Origin | Insertion | Actions performed during a weights session |
|---|---|---|---|
| Tibialis anterior<br>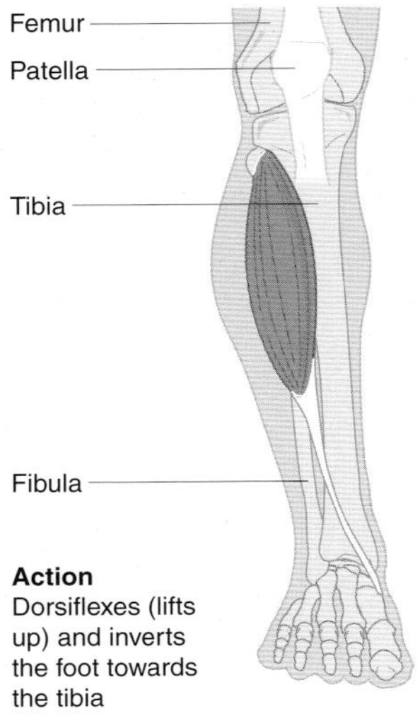 | Tibia | Tarsals/metatarsals | Dorsiflexion<br>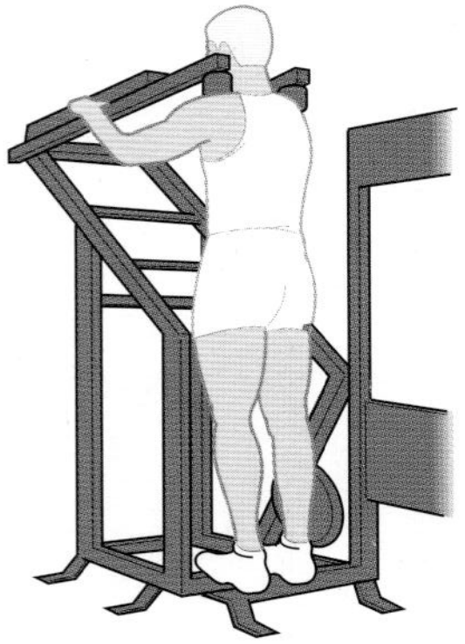 |

# Movement mechanics

## Levers

Efficient and effective movement in the body is made possible by a system of levers. These are mechanical devices used to produce turning motions about a fixed point (called a fulcrum). In the human body, bones act as levers, joints act as the fulcrum and muscle contractions provide the effort to move the lever about the fulcrum.

A basic understanding of lever systems can be used to explain rotational motion, and help athletes develop the most efficient technique for their sport.

There are three types of levers, and each is determined by the relative positions of the fulcrum (F), the point of application of force or effort (E) and the resistance (R) or load (L).

1 First class lever: the fulcrum lies between the effort and the load.
2 Second class lever: the load lies between the fulcrum and the effort.
3 Third class lever: the effort is between the fulcrum and the load.

A simple way of determining the class or order of the lever system operating during a specified movement is to remember the following rhyme,

'For 1, 2, or 3 think F, L, E' to determine the middle component of the lever system, i.e.

- For 1 or first class lever, F is in between L and E
- For 2 or second class lever, L is between F and E
- For 3 or third class lever, E is between F and L.

But beware there may be more than *one* lever system operating at a joint. For example, when flexing the elbow, as in a bicep curl, the effort comes from the point of insertion of the biceps brachii on the radius. This movement involves a 3rd class lever. However, when extending the elbow, as in throwing the javelin, the effort is generated by the triceps brachii via its point of insertion on the ulna. This movement involves a 1st class lever.

The majority of movements in the human body are governed by third class levers.

## Functions of levers

Levers have two main functions:

1 increase the resistance that a given effort can move.
2 increase the speed at which a body moves.

First class levers in the body: can increase both the effects of the effort and the speed of a body; second class levers tend only to increase the effect of the effort force;
third class levers can be used to increase the speed of a body. An example of a third class lever in the body is the action of the hamstrings and quadriceps on the knee joint, which causes flexion and extension of the lower leg. The extent to which this can increase, depends upon the relative lengths of the resistance arm and the effort arm:

1 The resistance arm (RA) is the part of the lever between the fulcrum and the resistance (load). The longer the resistance arm, the quicker the lever system can move. In sport, implements are often used such as rackets or bats to increase the length of the resistance arm which will increase the outgoing velocity of an object such as a ball. However, the optimal length of an implement should be determined by the strength of the person handling it which is why, for example, junior tennis rackets have been designed.
2 The effort arm (EA) is the distance between the fulcrum and the effort; the longer the effort arm, the less effort required to move a given resistance. The effort arm is often increased o overcome a heavy object.

The relative efficiency of the lever system is expressed as the mechanical advantage (MA) which can be determined as follows:

$$MA = \frac{\text{effort arm}}{\text{resistance arm}}$$

Mechanical disadvantage occurs in a lever system where the resistance arm is longer than the effort arm. This means that the lever can be put into action very quickly but is not as effective at moving heavy loads or overcoming resistance.

Mechanical advantage occurs in a lever system where the effort arm is longer than the resistance arm. This means that the lever system is very effective at overcoming and moving heavy loads. The efficiency of levers in the body is illustrated in Figure 5.19.

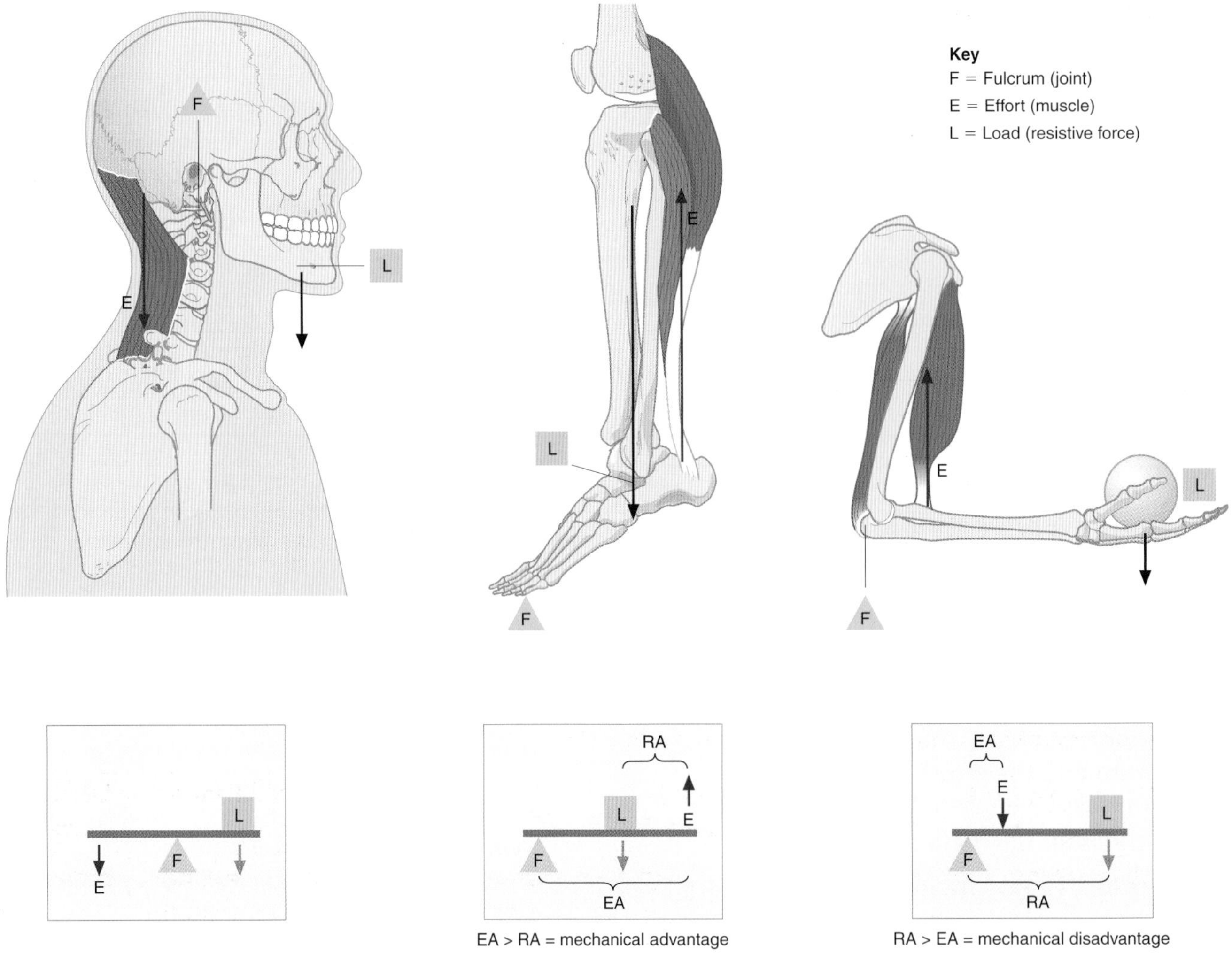


(a)

(b)

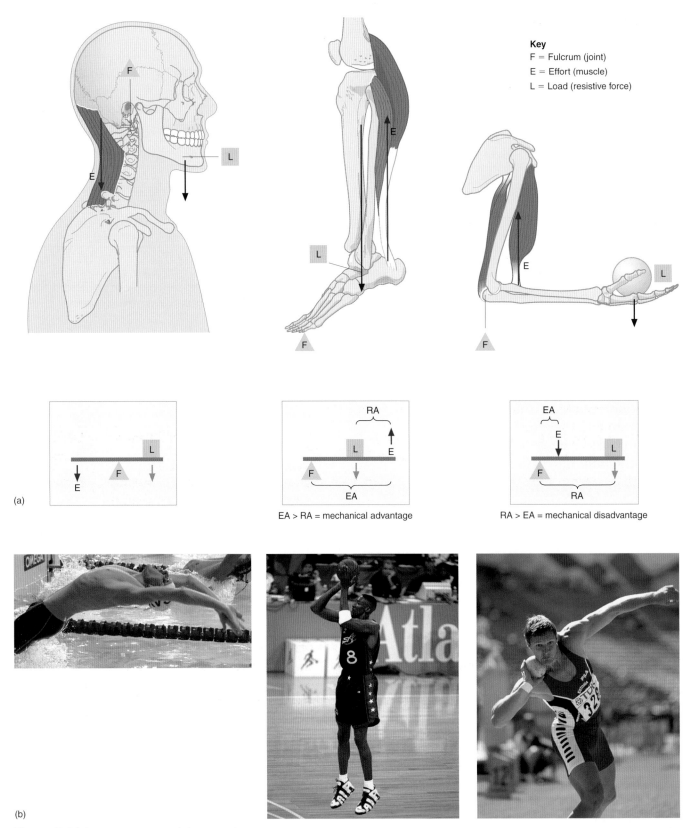

**Figure 5.19** Lever systems and their application

NB: The effort is produced via the muscle insertion.

## Movement analysis of physical activity – putting it all together

Kinesiology is the study of body movement, and thus includes muscle action. When studying this unit it is helpful to consider the following:

- the function of the muscles contracting;
- how the muscle is contracting (e.g. concentric or eccentric);
- the movement patterns occurring at joints as a result of the movement;
- the plane in which the movement occurs;
- the axis about which the movement occurs;
- the lever system in operation.

### Activity 11

Table 5.5 shows one joint movement used in basketball. Think of other 5 sporting situations, then copy and complete the table accordingly. You will find it useful to study the various tables throughout the chapter.

### Activity 12

For each of the following joints, state which muscles are used for the movement patterns shown in brackets:

- knee (flexion and extension);
- hip (flexion, extension, abduction, adduction);
- shoulder (flexion, extension, abduction, adduction);
- ankle (plantar flexion, dorsiflexion, inversion, eversion).

**Table 5.5** A movement analysis of the knee joint when performing a jump shot in basketball

| Sport | Action | Movement pattern | Muscles working | Type of contraction | Plane | Lever system |
|---|---|---|---|---|---|---|
| Basketball | Jump shot | Extension at knee | Quadriceps group: rectus femoris vasti muscles | Concentric | median/ sagittal | 3rd class |

### Activity 13

For your course you need to be able to complete a full movement analysis for a range of skills, including:

1 The shoulder and elbow action during a push up, overarm throwing and forehand racket strokes.

2 The hip, knee and ankle action whilst running, kicking, jumping and performing squats.

On page 121 there are some skills from a variety of activities. In each case, study the movement that has occurred from phase 1 to phase 2 and complete a full movement analysis on the joints specified. Use the format of Table 5.6, and don't forget to cover all aspects of the movement. Table 5.6 show a complete movement analysis of throwing (at the shoulder and elbow). Study this before having a go at the sporting actions pictured on page 121.

Table 5.6 An analysis of the arm action when throwing the javelin

| Joint | Phase of movement | Plane | Axis | Movement pattern | Muscle responsible | Role of muscle | Type of contraction | Lever system |
|---|---|---|---|---|---|---|---|---|
| Elbow | Preparation | Sagittal | Transverse | Flexion | Biceps brachii | Agonist | Isometric | 3rd |
| | Execution | Sagittal | Transverse | Extension | Triceps brachii | Agonist | Concentric | 1st |
| Shoulder | Preparation | Horizontal/ Transverse | Longitudinal | Horizontal extension/ abduction | Trapezius Rhomboids | Agonist | Concentric | 3rd |
| | Execution | Horizontal Transverse | Longitudinal | Horizontal flexion/ adduction | Pectoralis Major | Agonist | Concentric | 3rd |
| Hip | Preparation | Sagittal | Transverse | Flexion | Gluteal Muscles Illiopsoas | Agonist | Eccentric Concentric | 3rd |
| | Execution | Sagittal | Transverse | Extension | Gluteal Muscles | Agonist | Concentric | 3rd |
| Knee | Preparation | Sagittal | Transverse | Flexion | Quadriceps group Hamstring group | Agonist | Eccentric Concentric | 3rd |
| | Execution | Sagittal | Transverse | Extension | Quadriceps group | Agonist | Concentric | 3rd |
| Ankle | Preparation | Sagittal | Transverse | Dorsi flexion | Tibialis anterior Gastrocnemius | Agonist | Concentric Eccentric | 3rd |
| | Execution | Sagittal | Transverse | Plantar flexion | Gastrocnemius Soleus | Agonist | Concentric | 2nd |

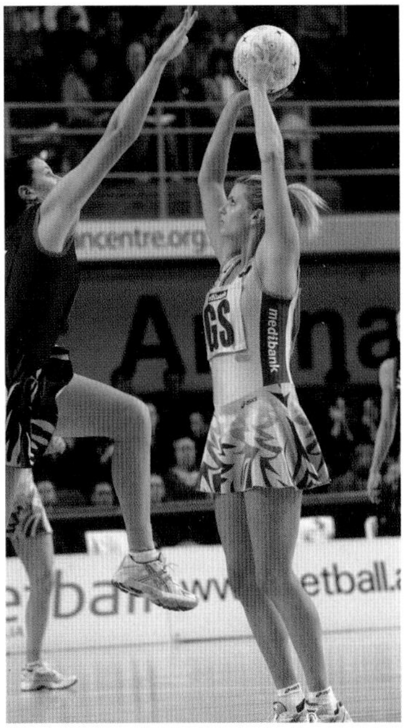


Figure 5.20 Netball shooting – knees, ankles, elbows

(a) (b)

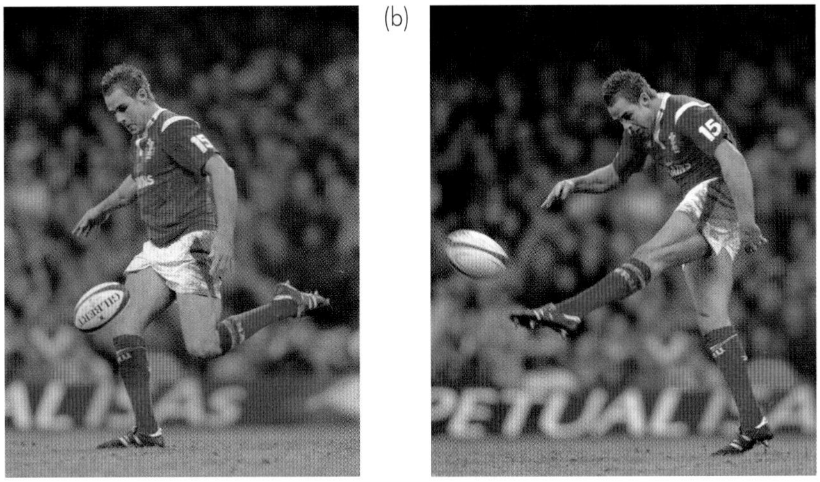

Figure 5.21 Kicking – hip, knee, ankle

(a) (b)

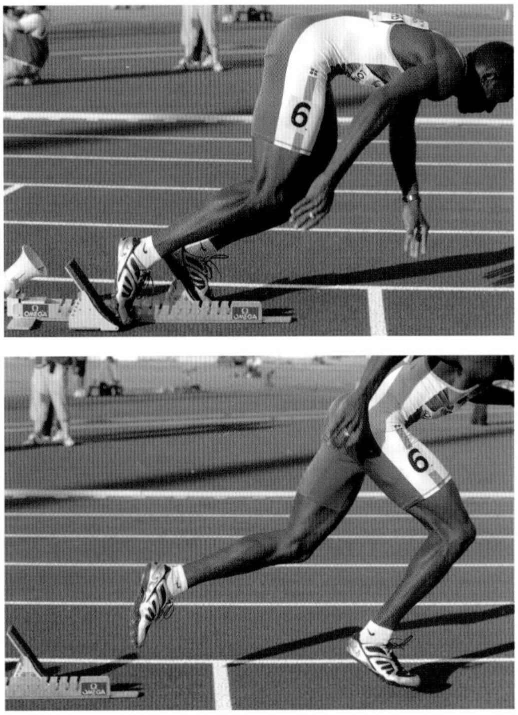


Figure 5.23 The sprint start – hip, knee, ankle

(a) (b)

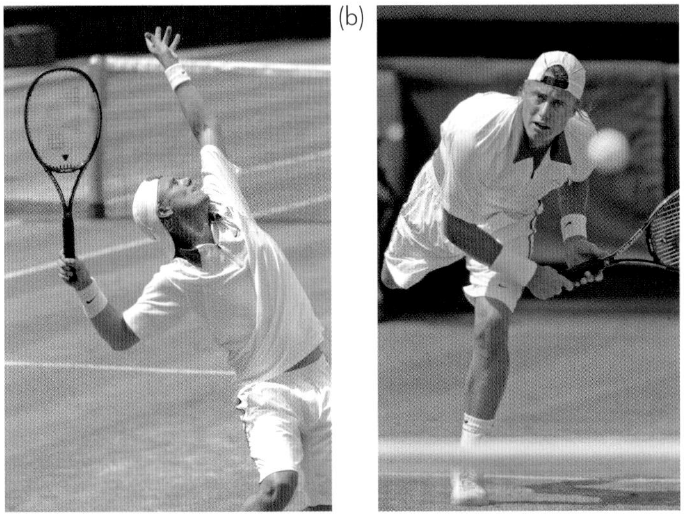

Figure 5.22 The tennis serve – shoulder, elbow, wrist

(a) (b)

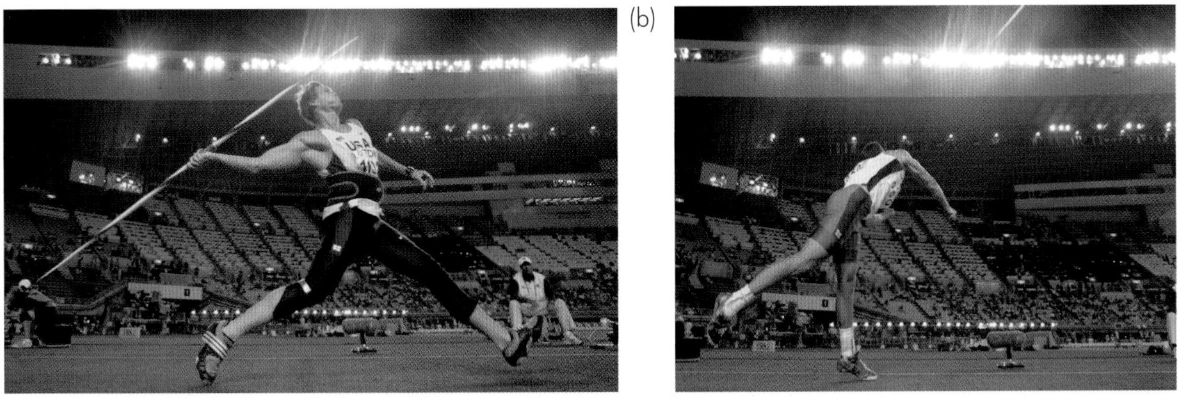

Figure 5.24 Throwing the javelin – shoulder, radio-ulnar, wrist

## Exam-style questions

**1** Identify the joint action, main agonist and type of muscle contraction at the hip and ankle joint in the upward phase of a squat jump.

| | **Hip** | **Ankle** |
|---|---|---|
| Joint action | | |
| Agonist | | |
| Type of muscle contraction | | |

**2** i) Name the agonist and main antagonist acting at the elbow joint when a performer moves from an 'up position' to a 'down position' when performing a press-up.

ii) Name the types of muscle contraction that occur during the press-up:

- At the up position whilst the performer is stationary;
- As the performer moves from the 'up position' to the down position.

iii) Through which plane and about which axis will the elbow action take place?

Table 5.7 summarises the key movement patterns and muscle actions. With this information you should be able to apply your knowledge to a wide range of sporting activities.

**Table 5.7** The musculoskeletal system: movement analysis

| **Joint** | **Action** | **Plane** | **Muscles used** | **Diagram** | **Example** |
|---|---|---|---|---|---|
| Hip | Flexion | Median<br>Horizontal | Psoas<br>Iliacus<br>Rectus femoris | 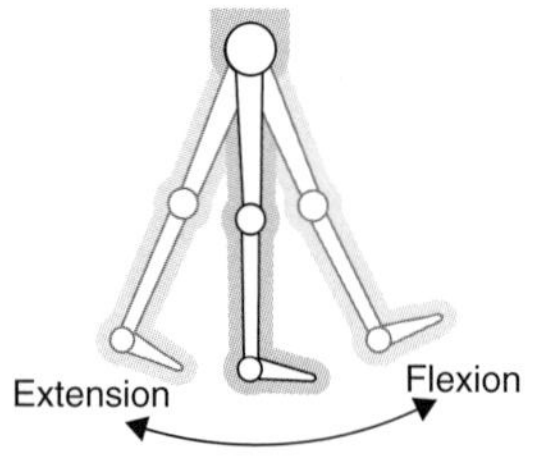 | eg, performing a 'tuck' jump in trampolining |
| | Extension | Median | Gluteus maximus<br>Biceps femoris<br>Semimembranosus<br>Semitendinosus<br>Gluteus medius (posterior) | | eg, preparation to kick a football |
| | Abduction | Frontal | Gluteus medius<br>Gluteus minimus<br>Tensor fasciae latae | 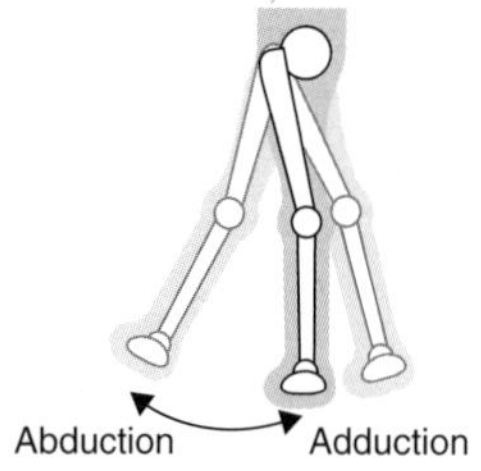 | eg, performing a cartwheel |
| | Adduction | Frontal | Adductor magnus<br>Adductor brevis<br>Adductor longus<br>Pestineus<br>Gracilis | | eg, the kick action in breaststroke |
| | Medial rotation | Horizontal | Gluteus medius<br>Gluteus minimus<br>Tensor fasciae latae | 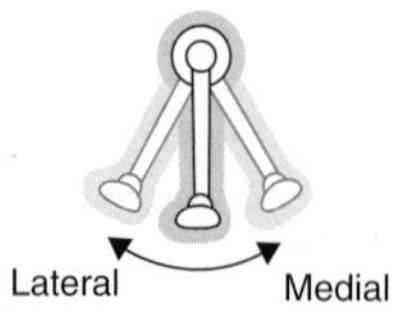 | eg, rotational movement when throwing the discus |
| | Lateral rotation | Horizontal | Gluteus maximus<br>Adductors | | eg, a side foot pass in football |

*Continued*

Table 5.7 *Continued*

| Joint | Action | Plane | Muscles used | Diagram | Example |
|---|---|---|---|---|---|
| Knee | Flexion | Median | Semitendinosus<br>Semimembranosus<br>Biceps femoris<br>Popliteus<br>Gastrocnemius | 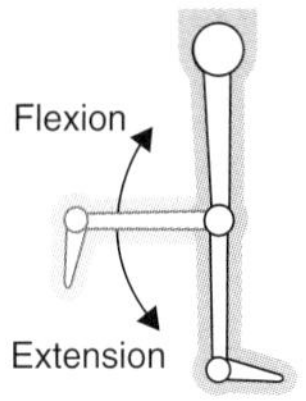  | eg, preparing to kick a conversion in rugby |
| | Extension | Median | Rectus femoris<br>Vastus medialis<br>Vastus lateralis<br>Tensor fasciae latae | | eg, rebounding in basketball |
| | Medial rotation (when flexed) | Horizontal | Sartorius<br>Semitendinosus | 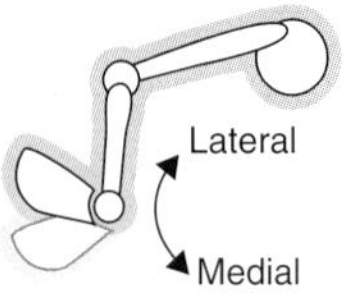  | eg, breastroke 'kick' phase |
| | Lateral rotation (when flexed) | Horizontal | Tensor fasciae latae<br>Biceps femoris | | e.g. breastroke recovery |
| Ankle | Dorsi flexion | Median | Tibialis anterior<br>Extensor digitorum longus<br>Peroneus tertius | 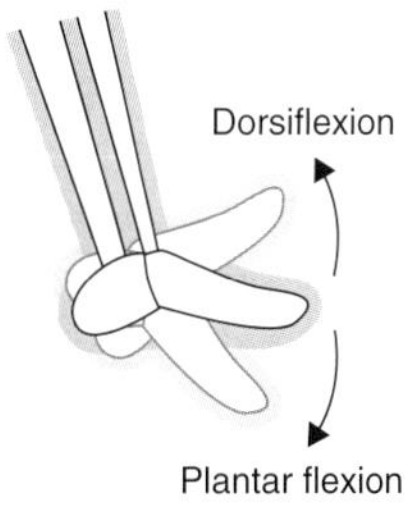  | eg, landing from a lay up in basketball |
| | Plantar flexion | Median | Gastrocnemius<br>Soleus<br>Peroneus longus<br>Peroneus brevis<br>Tibialis posterior<br>Flexor digitorum longus | | eg, pointing toes when performing a handstand |
| | Inversion | Frontal | Tibialis anterior<br>Tibialis posterior<br>Gastrocnemius<br>Soleus | 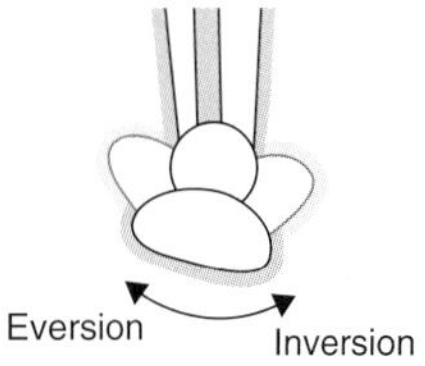  | eg, line kicking in rugby<br>(kicking a ball with outside of the foot) |
| | Eversion | Frontal | Peroneus longus<br>Peroneus brevis | | eg, kick phase in breastroke |
| Shoulder | Flexion | Median | Anterior deltoid<br>Pectoralis major<br>Coracobrachialis | 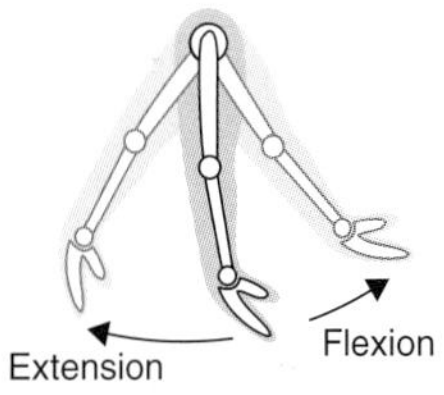  | eg, blocking of the net in volleyball |
| | Extension | Median | Posterior deltoid<br>Latissimus dorsi<br>Teres major | | eg, butterfly arm pull |

*Continued*

Table 5.7 *Continued*

| Joint | Action | Plane | Muscles used | Diagram | Example |
|---|---|---|---|---|---|
| Shoulder | Adduction | Frontal | Latissimus dorsi<br>Pectoralis major<br>Teres major<br>Teres minor | 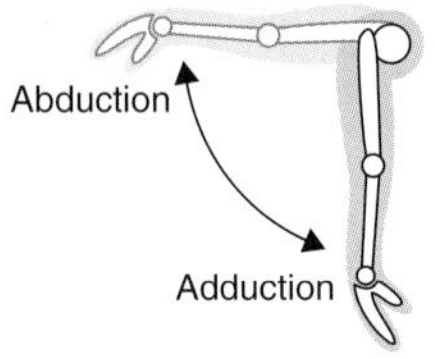 | eg, landing phase of a straddle jump in trampolining |
| | Abduction | Frontal | Medial deltoid<br>Supraspinatus | | eg, straddle jump in trampolining |
| | Horizontal abduction | Horizontal | Posterior deltoid<br>Trapezius<br>Rhomboids<br>Latissimus dorsi | 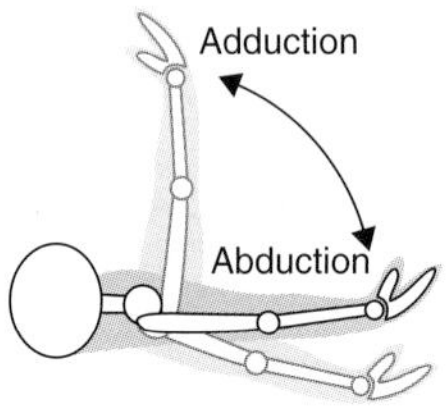 | eg, preparing phase of throwing the discus |
| | Horizontal adduction | Horizontal | Pectoralis<br>Major anterior deltoid | | eg, execution phase of throwing the javelin |
| | Medial rotation | Horizontal | Subscapularis | 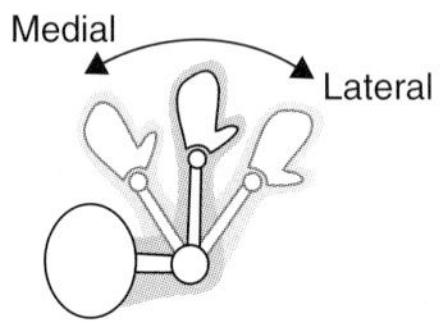 | eg, butterfly armpull |
| | Lateral rotation | Horizontal | Infraspinatus<br>Teres minor | | eg, preparing for a forehand drive in tennis |
| Elbow | Flexion | Median | Biceps brachii<br>Brachialis<br>Brachioradialis | 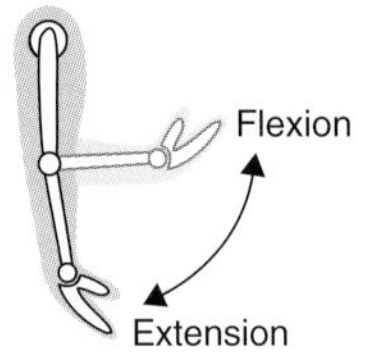 | eg, preparation for a set shot in basketball |
| | Extension | Median | Triceps brachii | | eg, execution of a set shot in basketball |
| Radio-ulnar | Pronation | Horizontal | Pronator teres<br>Pronator quadratus<br>Brachioradialis | 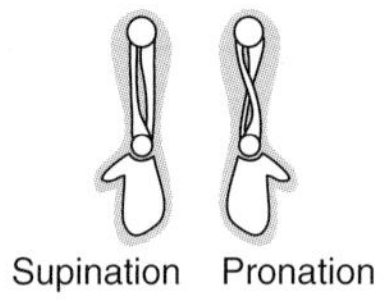 | eg, putting top spin on a tennis ball |
| | Supination | Horizontal | Biceps brachii<br>Supinator | | eg, recovery phase of the arms in breastroke |
| Wrist | Flexion | Median | Wrist flexors | 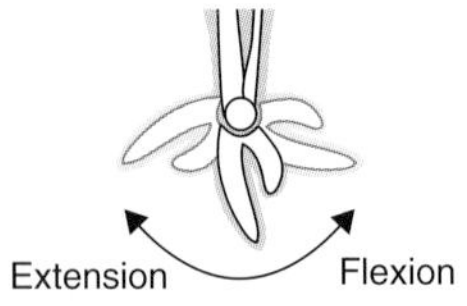 | eg, wrist snap in basketball shot |
| | Extension | Median | Wrist extensors | | eg, initial grip of a shot against neck |

*Continued*

Table 5.7 *Continued*

| **Joint** | **Action** | **Plane** | **Muscles used** | **Diagram** | **Example** |
|---|---|---|---|---|---|
| Movement of the trunk | Flexion | Median | Rectus abdominus<br>Internal obliques<br>External obliques | 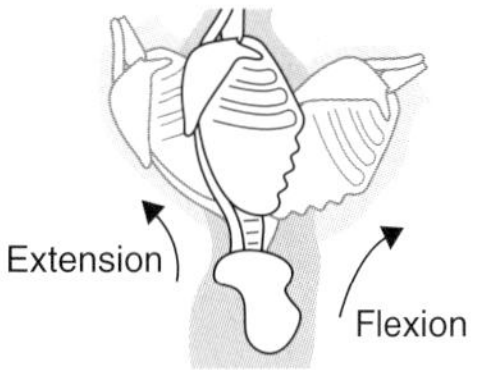 | eg, crouching at start of a swimming dive |
| | Extension | Median | Erector spinae<br>Iliocostalis spinalis | | eg, a backflip in gymnastics |
| | Lateral flexion | Frontal | Internal oblique<br>Rectus abdominis<br>Erector spinae<br>Quadratus laborum | 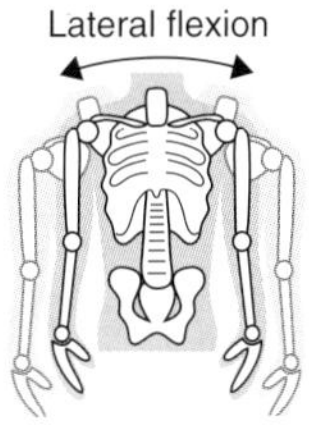 | eg, a cartwheel |
| | Rotation | Horizontal | External oblique<br>Rectus abdominis<br>Erector spinae | 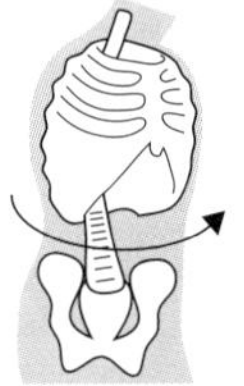 | eg, follow through on a tennis serve |
| Movement of the scapulae | Elevation | Frontal | Levator sapulae<br>Trapezius<br>Rhomboids | 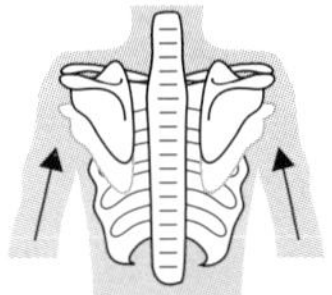 | eg, recovery phase of butterfly armpull |
| | Depression | Frontal | Trapezius (lower)<br>Pectoralis minor<br>Serratus anterior (lower) | 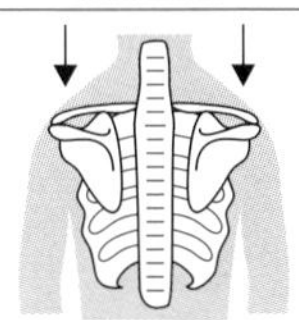 | eg, thrusting off a horse when performing a handspring |
| | Protraction | Frontal | Serratus anterior | 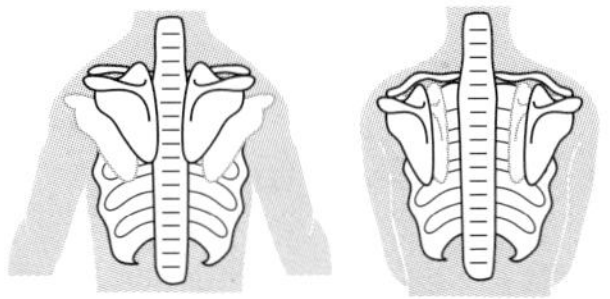 | eg, recovery phase in breastroke |
| | Retraction | Frontal | Rhomboids<br>Trapezius | | eg, pull phase in breastroke |
| | Upward rotation | Frontal | Trapezius (upper)<br>Serratus anterior | 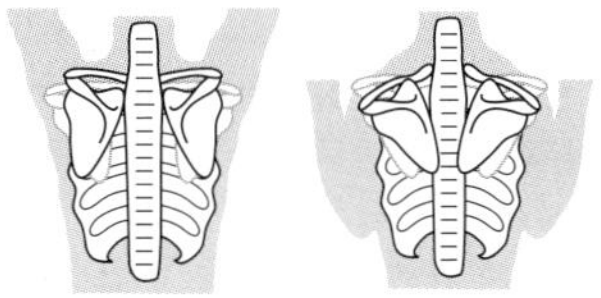 | eg, recovery phase in front-crawl |
| | Downward rotation | Frontal | Rhomboids<br>Levator scapulae | | eg, front-crawl arm pull |

## The impact of different types of physical activity on the skeletal and muscular systems

The benefits of exercise are well documented. Table 5.8 highlights some of the benefits of regular physical activity on the skeletal and muscular systems.

Many studies have shown that children who are active throughout their teenage years have a greater chance of being healthy adults. Exercise has proven beneficial in the avoidance and prevention of certain skeletal disorders, such as osteoporosis and osteoarthritis.

> **EXAMINER'S TIP**
>
> You must be able to critically evaluate the impact of different types of physical activity on the skeletal and muscular systems.

Table 5.8 Benefits of regular physical activity on the skeletal and muscular systems

| Skeletal system | Muscular system |
|---|---|
| • **Increased bone density.** Skeletal tissues become stronger since exercise imposes stress on the bones, which encourages the laying down of bony plates and the deposition of calcium salts along the lines of stress. This reinforces the criss-cross matrix of cancellous bone and improves the tensile stress of the bone. Strength training will be particularly beneficial in developing the strength of skeletal tissues.<br>• **Articular cartilage thickens**, which aids the cushioning of the joint, and therefore protects the bones from wear and tear.<br>• Flexibility and mobility training may enable ligaments to stretch slightly to enable a **greater range of movement at the joint**. | • **Increased muscle mass due to hypertrophy (enlargement) of muscle fibres**. Slow-twitch fibres respond well to activities such as jogging and cycling, while fast-twitch fibres respond well to strength-training activities, such as weight training.<br>• **Tendons thicken** and can withstand greater muscular forces.<br>• **Improved flexibility** due to increased extensibility of muscle fibres.<br>• **Increased force of contraction** due to hyperplasia (splitting) of muscle fibres and increased elasticity. |

### What you need to know

* The skeleton has five basic functions: support, protection, movement, blood production and mineral storage.
* The axial skeleton consists of those bones that provide the greatest support, including the skull, the vertebral column and the ribcage.
* The appendicular skeleton consists of the bones of the limbs and their respective girdles.
* Bones can be categorised as either long, short, flat, irregular or sesamoid.
* Joints are classified according to the degree of movement allowed. There are three basic types of joint: fixed or fibrous joints, cartilaginous joints and synovial joints.
* Movement at synovial joints can be classified as flexion, extension, abduction, adduction, horizontal flexion, horizontal extension, rotation, pronation, supination, circumduction, plantar flexion, dorsiflexion, inversion and eversion.

* The whole of the skeletal system can be strengthened through performing exercise.
* Skeletal muscle properties include extensibility, elasticity and contractility.
* Functions include movement, support and posture, and heat production.
* Muscles are attached to bones via tendons. The origin of a muscle is the attachment to a stable bone, usually the nearest flat bone. The insertion is the muscle attachment to the bone that the muscle puts into action.
* Muscles often work together in order to produce coordinated movements: antagonistic muscle action. A muscle directly responsible for joint movement is the agonist. An antagonist often lengthens in order for the agonist to shorten.
* Muscles can contract in several ways: isotonic (shortening or lengthening), concentric (the muscle shortens), eccentric (the muscle lengthens). A muscle can also contract without any visible movement (isometric).
* There are 3 classes of lever in the body, most of which are 3rd class.
* To determine the class of lever work out the middle component: F = 1st class L = 2nd class E = 3rd class.
* Mechanical advantage in a lever system enables effective movement of heavy loads.
* The analysis of muscle contraction and joint action is called kinesiology.
* Essential information when analysing movement includes
  - name and functions of muscles working
  - bones articulating
  - movement patterns occuring
  - plane and axis of the movement
  - lever system in operation.
* The benefits of exercise to the skeletal system include increased bone density, thickening of articular cartilage and a greater range of movement at joints.
* The benefits of exercise on the muscular system include increased muscle mass and force of contraction, increased strength of tendons and improved flexibility.

## Review Questions

1 Name the bones that articulate at the following joints:
- knee;
- hip;
- shoulder;
- elbow.

2 How is the knee joint structured for stability?

3 Explain how it is possible for us to bend down and touch our toes. What movement patterns are brought about during this action?

4 What is the function of articular cartilage?

5 How is the shoulder structured to enable the different types of movement patterns of which it is capable?

6 State the functions of the following:
- bursae;
- cruciate ligaments;
- patella;
- carpals.

7 Outline the benefits that training has on the skeletal tissues.

8 Analyse the action of a tennis serve. State the movement patterns and joint actions that occur at the shoulder and elbow.

9 Explain how the properties of skeletal muscle enable it to perform its function when sprinting. Use the correct names of muscles, where appropriate.

10 When performing a jump shot in basketball, many different muscles work in the lower body. Identify the muscles working on the hip, knee and ankle joints, and state the specific roles that each of these muscles have (i.e. are they agonists, fixators, etc.?).

11 What are the essential ingredients to successful analysis of movement? Use these to analyse an overhead clear in badminton, with particular reference to the shoulder, elbow and wrist actions.

12 Identify one stroke in swimming. State the muscles that are contracting in each phase of the stroke (e.g. either the kick or recovery phase in the leg action), and state the type of contraction taking place in each muscle.

13 Outline the benefits of exercise on the muscular system.

# Skill Acquisition

SECTION

B

CHAPTER 6

# Skills and ability – characteristics and classifications

## Learning outcomes

**By the end of this chapter you should be able to:**

- understand the term 'skill';
- understand skills and explain how they influence performance;
- explain the different classifications of skills; identify specific sporting examples and justify your decisions for placing them on a specific continuum;
- understand the term 'ability' and explain its characteristics;
- explain the difference between 'gross motor abilities' and 'psychomotor abilities';
- identify sporting examples where specific gross motor abilities and psychomotor abilities are required, and justify your decisions;
- outline the relationship between 'skill' and 'ability'

## CHAPTER INTRODUCTION

Since the second half of the twentieth century the status of sport and physical education within society has increased tremendously. This has been linked, in the main, to developing media, commercial and political interest and has resulted in increased pressure and demands being placed on sports performers. While this in turn has led to major improvements in both technological and physiological preparation it has also meant that more recognition has been given to the need to prepare performers psychologically.

It has long been recognised that even if a performer is physically trained to near perfection and supported by the best equipment and technology available, this does not guarantee an excellent performance or victory. Since the early 1960s research has been carried out by sports psychologists in order to help us to:

- understand – learning/behaviour/performance and situations in sport
- explain – learning/behaviour/performance or factors that influence performance/events in a systematic manner
- predict – potential learning/behaviour/events or outcomes/performance
- influence/control – potential learning/behaviour/performance or events.

When observing sport, commentators and the media often use simplistic terms to explain why certain things happen. Phrases like 'there has been a psychological shift in the game', a performer is 'coping with pressure', a performer has been 'psyched out of the game', a performer has the 'wrong temperament' are all used, along with many others, to explain variations in performance.

Although such phrases are used often without a real understanding of what they mean, they do at least indicate the importance and influence of psychological factors within the context of sport and physical education. During this section of your studies you will begin to gain a clearer understanding of the various strategies that sports psychologists have used to help develop and prepare performers individually or in groups (teams) to cope with the increased pressures of modern sport. It is generally recognised that the traditional approach to sport psychology (the pre-competition 'rousing pep-talk', the 'up and at them' approach) is of very little 'real' long-term value and in some cases could even be considered counterproductive, perhaps leading to poor performance in the short term.

In the same way that an athlete's physical and skills preparation cannot be developed overnight, psychological preparation needs to be developed over a prolonged period of time in order to be effective and retain long-term value. Developing your knowledge of sports psychology should give you a better understanding of the 'causes' and 'effects' of various psychological phenomena which underpin learning and performance in sport.

After reading this section on skill acquisition and sports psychology you will begin to gain a better understanding of:

1 The variety of factors, principles and theories that can affect the learning process during skill development
2 The factors that determine how a performer interprets information and produces skilled movement
3 Strategies that can be employed to develop and refine skill.

## Nature of skilled performance

The terms 'skill' and 'ability' are frequently used to describe sporting performance, but are their full meanings understood and used in the correct context?

As a sporting performer, you will have developed numerous skills and experienced a variety of practice methods to refine those skills in a sporting situation. If skills are to be maximised, both performer and coach must understand the different nature of skills, the abilities required to execute particular skills, and the different methods of manipulating practice sessions to allow for the effective use of time and the refinement of those skills.

We have learned and developed a wide range of skills which we use daily without consciously thinking about it. For example, writing your name, using a mobile phone to send text messages and using money to pay for goods. All these are skills which have developed through practice over time. The aim of every sports performer is to refine their skills, allowing them to execute these with precision and consistency whenever the situation demands it. This can only be achieved through practice. Your aim by the end of this chapter should be to answer the question: What makes one performer more skilled than another, and how can we recognise high quality skills?

### Activity 1

With a partner, make a list of the following:

1 five skills that you use daily;
2 five skills commonly used in many sports (generic skills);
3 five skills required for a specific sport.

Compare lists with another pair. Discuss any similarities and differences.

### What is a skilled performance?

In discussion with your fellow students you will all have been able to suggest various examples of skilled performances, perhaps identifying similar points to the following examples:

- A concert pianist may be said to be performing skilfully.
- A ballet dancer's coordination and timing are skilful.
- A perfect pass by a quarterback in American football is skilful.
- A long-range three-point score in basketball is skilful.
- A well-executed off drive in cricket is skilful.
- A gymnast performing a vault in the Olympic Games is skilful.
- A pole-vaulter completing a vault is skilful.
- A potter using a potter's wheel is skilful.

In other words, we can all recognise the outcome or the end product of a skilful performance. However, as students of physical education and sport you need to know:

- how this end product comes about;
- what process underlies the acquisition of skill and control of movement;
- how skill is acquired;
- what factors influence the attainment of skill and how it is retained.

There are no right or wrong ways to learn skills, as every performer is different and will respond accordingly. The skill of the coach or teacher is to recognise individual characteristics and to structure the learning environment to maximise the chance of learning taking place. Think about your own experiences when attempting to learn a new skill; some methods may have worked while others have failed. Why is this?

## Using the term 'skill'

You may have noticed in the list of examples given above (or in your own discussions) that the word 'skill' can be used in two slightly different ways. We can use the word when referring to skill as an act or task, such as a rugby player converting a penalty or an athlete hurdling. It can also be used as an indicator of quality of performance, such as a gymnast completing a floor routine, or when comparing the performance of one hockey player to another during a game.

### Skill as an act or task

In this context, the word is used to denote an act or a task which has a specific aim or goal; for example, a gymnast performing a vault. Further examples are shown in Figures 6.1, 6.2 and 6.3.

If we were to observe players engaged in any of these examples on a regular basis, and they were achieving a high percentage success rate, we would consider them skilful players. The use of the word in this context refers to a physical movement, action or task that a person is trying to carry out in a technically correct manner, involving some or all of the body. Thus skill can be seen as **goal-directed behaviour**.

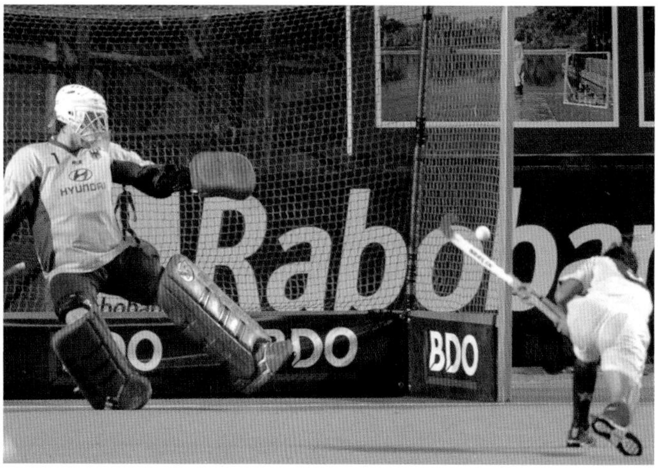


**Figure 6.1** Taking a penalty flick in hockey

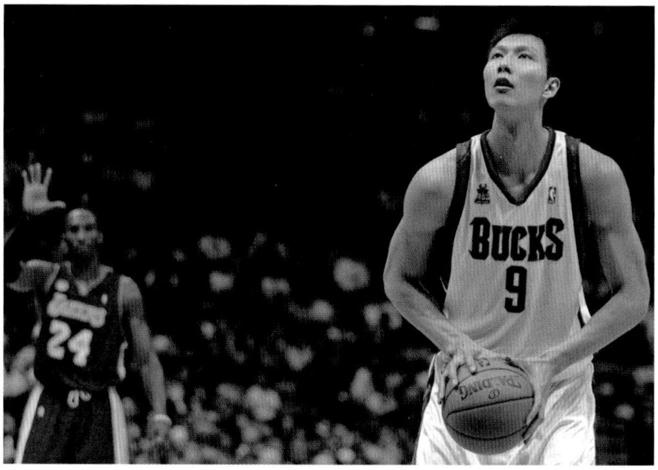


**Figure 6.2** Shooting a free shot after a foul in basketball

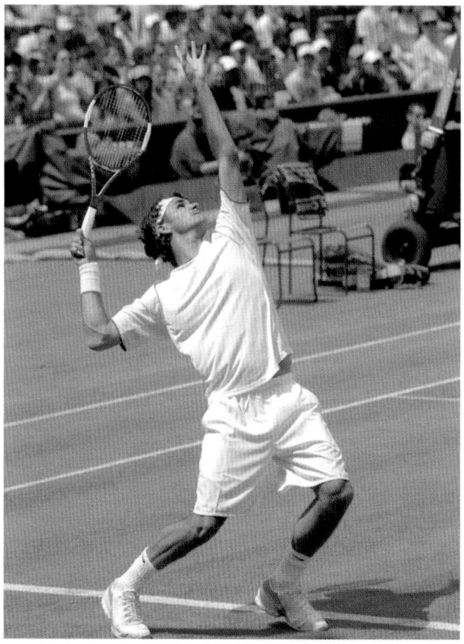

**Figure 6.3** Serving in tennis

## Skill as an indicator of quality of performance

The word in this context is probably a little more ambiguous than skill as an act or task. The word 'well' added to the description of the skill infers a qualitative judgement (by you as the observer) of the skill being made. For example, you might remark on a well-executed off drive during a cricket match. Very often we make judgements by comparing players' performances, looking at players' achievements in the context of the class or school team, or against set criteria. Thus we measure or assess in either relative or absolute terms. However, what we need to understand is what makes it a *well*-performed skill.

**Key term**

**Qualitative:** An opinion or judgement of an individual, which is not supported by facts or data.

## Acquisition of skill

In the phrase 'acquisition of skill', the word 'acquisition' implies that skill is something which you can gain, as opposed to something you already have.

> Skill is said to be gained through learning. Skill is said to be learned behaviour! (B. Knapp)

### Activity 2

1 Select two well-known performers from different sports, or watch a video clip of a sporting event. List five words to describe the athletes' performance. Compare lists with other students.
2 Consider your own performance compared to the performers you have analysed. What are the differences between you? Are they more 'skilled' than you? Justify your answer.

## Definitions and characteristics of skill

You will have a better understanding of the nature of skill if you consider a variety of definitions and see how these have developed. There are numerous definitions of the term 'skill', several of which are outlined below. As you read each one, try to highlight similar characteristics to those you identified in Activity 2 (above).

> Skill is the learned ability to bring about predetermined results with maximum certainty, often with the minimum outlay of time or energy or both. (B. Knapp)

> Skill is an organised, coordinated activity in relation to an object or situation which involves a whole chain of sensory, central and motor mechanisms. (A.T. Welford)

> While the task can be physical or mental, one generally thinks of skill as some type of manipulative efficiency. A skilled movement is one in which a predetermined objective is accomplished with maximum efficiency with a minimum outlay of energy. A skilful movement does not just happen. There must be a conscious effort on the part of the performer in order to execute a skill. (M. Robb)

**EXAMINER'S TIP**

You will not be expected to remember definitions, but you must be able to explain the terms in your own words using relevant examples to support your answer.

Using the definitions set out above, and your own discussions, we can say that the characteristics of skill are:

- *excellent performance* – high quality;
- *goal-directed* – the intention to do it (it is not just luck – there must be a conscious decision and effort);
- *learned* – learning through practice and experience to use the appropriate innate abilities;
- *predetermined* – you have an aim to achieve;
- *consistent* – you are able to execute the action with maximum certainty depending on the environmental conditions;
- *efficient* – there is a minimum outlay of time and energy;
- *aesthetic* – it looks pleasing to the eye, appearing controlled and effective;
- *recognisable* – often the technique can be named and compared either to set criteria or other performers.

The performance of skilled movement involves:

- *sensory mechanisms* – taking in information via the various receptor systems (e.g. senses);

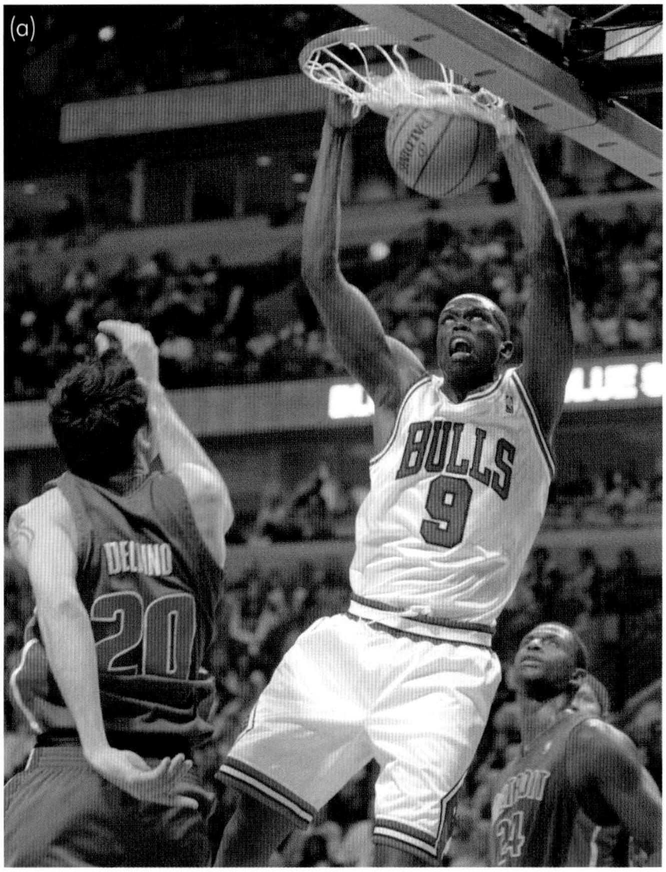


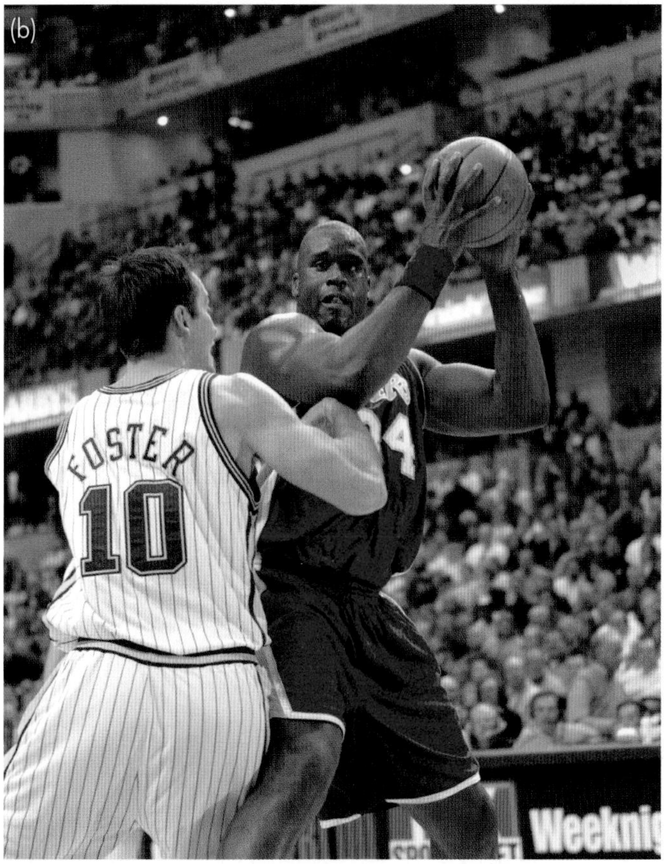


**Figure 6.4** A basketball player has to master numerous skills

- *central mechanisms* – brain (interpretations and decision making);
- *motor mechanisms* – nerves and muscle systems being used to create movement.

Basically, skills involve the use of the senses to detect and take in information; the brain to interpret the information and make decisions according to what you know about the situation; and the nervous system, together with muscles, to work the various parts of the body in order to carry out the action.

## Types of skill

Psychologists have considered different types of skill, trying to differentiate between motor skills and verbal skills, for instance. Examples of three different types of skill are:

1. Intellectual skills or cognitive skills – skills which involve the use of a person's mental powers, for example, problem solving, verbal reasoning (verbal skill). Within a sporting context, this may involve planning strategies and tactics to outwit an opponent, or calculating the split times required to run a race in a certain time.
2. Perceptive skills – interpreting and making sense of information coming in via the senses. For example, during a basketball match a player will have to analyse their own location and that of other players on court, the flight of the ball, the options available and the rules before making a decision on which skill to attempt.
3. Motor skills – smoothly executing physical movements and responses, for example, the completion of a pass, dribble or shot resulting in a successful basket or defensive play.

**Key terms**

**Cognitive skill:** Skill which involves thought process and intellectual ability.
**Perceptual skill:** Skill which involves the detection and interpretation of information from the environment.
**Motor skill:** Skill which involves physical movement and muscular control.

When National League basketball players are performing a 'skilful' dribble and 'driving' to the basket, not only are they showing technically good movements (i.e. showing motor skill), but in carrying out the action the player has also had to make many decisions, including:

- whether to dribble or pass;
- how to dribble;
- position of opposition;
- position of own teammates;
- context of game;
- situation in game (winning or losing);
- time in game (how long to go?);
- whether to score or keep the ball;
- the odds of making the dribble, drive and possible shot.

This obviously involves a whole host of cognitive and perceptual skills. Only after taking into account all the information (cues, signals, stimuli) being received from around them can a basketball player carry out the necessary motor skill successfully. Therefore, from a sporting point of view, when we talk of 'skill', we usually mean a combination of all three areas. Skill is more than just technical excellence. (In your further reading around this topic you will come across the phrase 'perceptual motor skills', or very often just 'motor skills' – the perceptual or cognitive involvement is usually implied.)

## Classification of skills

In order to maximise the opportunity for learning and refining skills, classification systems are often used to group together different types of skills with similar characteristics. This will allow the most appropriate training or practice method to be used. By classifying skills that are involved in sporting activities:

- a teacher or coach is able to generalise across groups of skills and apply major concepts, theories and principles of learning to types of skills;
- a teacher or coach will not necessarily have to consider each specific skill in a unique way;
- a teacher or coach will be able to select the appropriate starting point for a learner;
- the identification of appropriate types of practice conditions (e.g. whole, part, whole, massed or distributed – see Chapter 13, The application of classification to the organisation and determination of practice) will be easier – similar methods can be applied to skills within the same groupings;
- the timing and types of instruction to be given are clarified (e.g. verbal feedback, ongoing or terminal);
- the detection and solving of any problems the learner may be facing is made easier;
- a teacher or coach would probably not use the various classifications in isolation, but would move from one to another, or combine aspects of all of them at the appropriate time.

### Classification systems

Several different ways of classifying or grouping skills have been developed to assist in our understanding of motor skills. In order to solve the problem of listing skills under certain headings, which could lead to confusion over where to list skills made up of several different aspects, the use of a continuum was devised. This allows for skills to be analysed and placed between two given extremities, according to how they match the analysis criteria being applied.

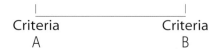

|————————————————|

Criteria A          Criteria B

Many skills have components which may fall into either end of a particular continuum. In such cases, it is advisable to view the skill as a whole movement rather than attempting to identify sub-routines, which can lead to misunderstanding. For example, the entire bowling action of a cricketer should be classified, rather than just the wrist action during the release of the ball.

**Key term**

**Continuum:** A continuum is an imaginary line between two extremes.

**EXAMINER'S TIP**

When classifying a skill, always use a specific example (e.g. do not simply say 'basketball' – name the actual skill, such as the 'lay-up shot').

#### The muscular involvement (gross–fine) classification

This classification is based on the degree of bodily involvement, or the precision of movement needed to execute the skill.

As you can see from Table 6.1 below, some skills do not fall easily into specific categories; nor can they be listed exclusively under exact headings. Darts,

Table 6.1 Gross–fine skill classification

| Gross skills | Fine skills |
|---|---|
| Involve large muscle movements<br>Involve large muscle groups<br>Major bodily movement skills associated with:<br>● strength<br>● endurance<br>● power<br>For example, walking, kicking a football, jumping, running | Involve small muscle movements<br>Involve small muscle groups<br>Small bodily movement skills associated with:<br>● speed<br>● efficiency<br>● accuracy<br>For example, shooting, throwing a dart, a snooker shot, release of the fingers in archery |
| ? ← Darts → ? | |
| ? ← Spin bowling → ? | |
| ? ← Badminton → ? | |

spin bowling and serving in a game of badminton all involve wrist and finger speed and dexterity, along with aiming accuracy, which suggests that they should be taught as a fine skill. In order for these small movements to be made, however, larger movements – particularly in spin bowling – have also had to take place, which suggests that they should be taught as a gross skill.

## Activity 3

Using the gross–fine classification (see Table 6.1), place darts, spin bowling and badminton along a continuum, according to how they match the criteria being applied. Justify your answers.

Gross — Fine

**EXAMINER'S TIP**

When classifying a skill, always justify your answer. Do not simply state where you think the skill should be placed on a continuum.

## The environmental influence (open–closed) classification

This classification is based on the stability of the environment or situation in which the skill is being performed. A performer may only have to focus on their own technique if they are involved in an event in which they are competing individually and the conditions remain virtually the same on each occasion (e.g. a javelin thrower). However, team players may have to take into account the positions of others, the flight path of a ball and the playing surface before adapting and executing an existing skill.

Table 6.2 The open–closed continuum

| Closed skills | Open skills |
|---|---|
| Not affected by the environment | Very much affected by the unstable, changing environment |
| Stable, fixed environment (space/time) predictable | Externally paced environment |
| Internally/self paced predominantly habitual stereotyped movements (e.g. headstand in gymnastics/weightlifting) | Predominantly perceptual movement patterns require adjustment (adaptation) |
| | Very often rapid adjustments, variations of skill needed (e.g. passing/receiving in netball or basketball/tackling in rugby) |

## Activity 4

Draw an open–closed continuum (see Table 6.2) and place the following skills on it:

- free shot in basketball;
- serve in tennis;
- smash in badminton;
- dribbling in a game of football;
- rugby tackle;
- running a 1,500m race;
- sailing;
- backhand defensive shot in table tennis;
- judo.

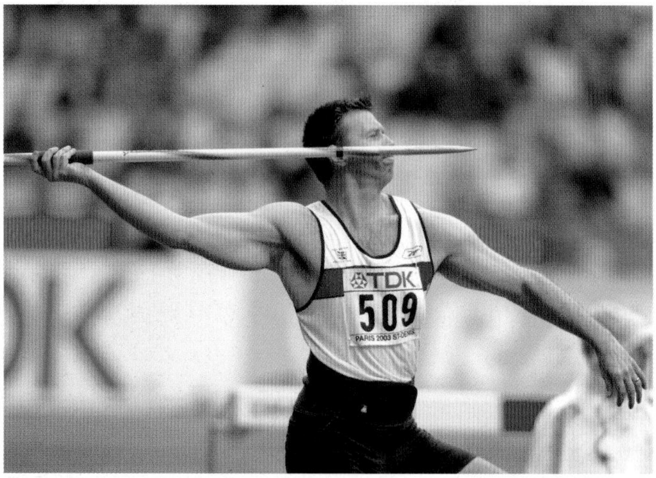


Figure 6.5 The javelin throw is a closed skill

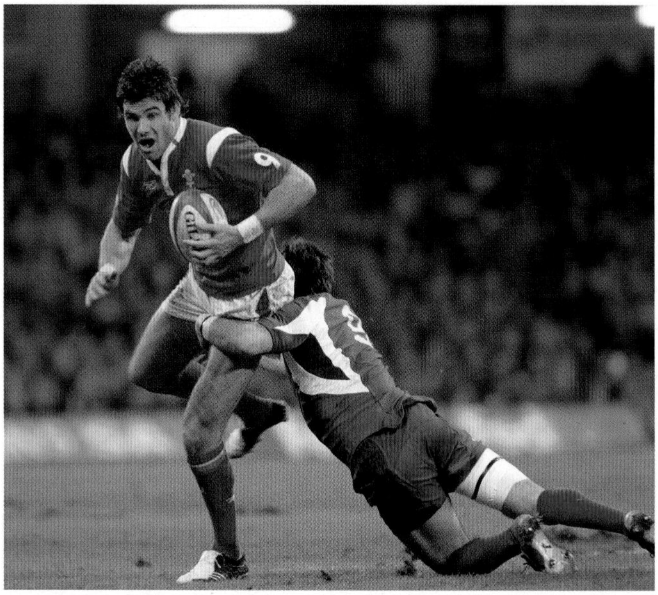

Figure 6.6 The rugby tackle is an open skill

## The continuity (discrete–serial–continuous) classification

**This classification is made on the basis of the relationship between sub-routines, and how clearly defined the beginning and end of the skill are to observers.**

## Activity 5

Using the information in Table 6.3, decide where the following activities fit on the continuum, making sure you can justify your decision in each case:

- hockey pass;
- serve in tennis;
- throw-in in football;
- long jump;
- throwing a javelin;
- penalty flick in hockey;
- dance routine;
- skiing;
- aerobics;
- 1,500m run;
- trampoline routine;
- penalty corner routine in hockey.

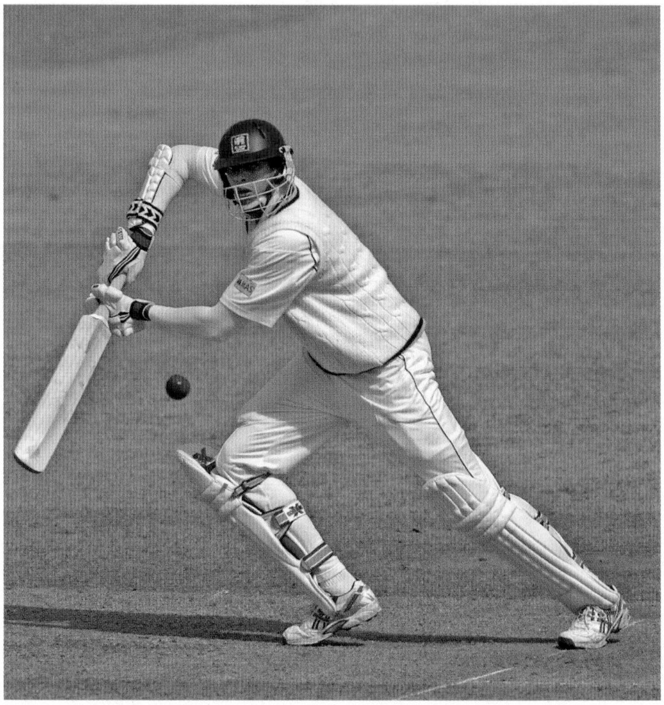

Figure 6.7 A cricket shot is a discrete skill

Table 6.3 The discrete–serial–continuous continuum

| Discrete skills<br>Criteria | Serial skills<br>Criteria | Continuous skills<br>Criteria |
|---|---|---|
| Well-defined beginning and end | A number of discrete skills put together to make a sequence or series | Poorly defined beginning and end |
| Usually brief in nature – a single specific skill | Order in which the distinct elements are put together is very important | Activity continues for an unspecified time (ongoing) |
| If skill is repeated, have to start at beginning (e.g. a basketball free throw/kicking a ball/hitting, catching/diving/vaulting) | Each movement is both stimulus and response (e.g. gymnastic routine/triple jump/high jump) | End of one movement is beginning of next repetition (e.g. swimming/running/cycling) |

## The pacing (self-paced – externally paced) continum classification

This classification is based on the degree of control the performer has over the movement or skill being carried out (i.e. not governed by the actions of others). It refers to the amount of control for both the timing and the speed of the movement. This classification is synonymous with the open and closed classification.

Table 6.4 The pacing continuum

| Self-paced/internally paced skills | Externally paced skills |
|---|---|
| Performer controls the rate at which the activity is carried out | Action is determined by external sources |
| Performer decides when to initiate movement | |
| Involves pro-action | Involves the performer in reaction |
| More closed skill (e.g. shot put/forward roll) | More open skill (e.g. white-water canoeing/receiving a serve in tennis) |

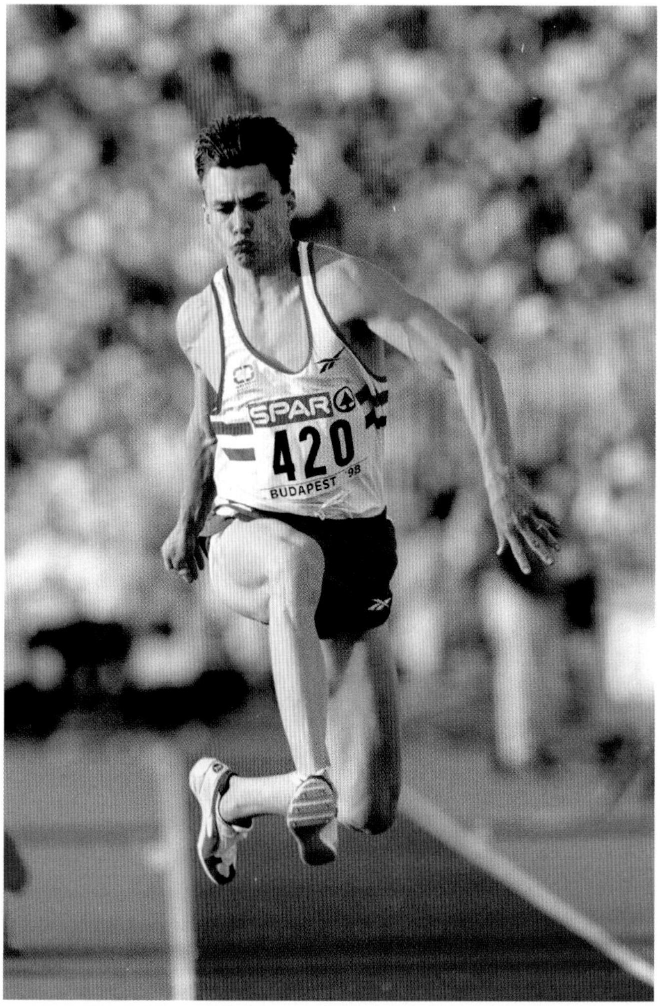

Figure 6.8 A triple jump is a serial skill

### The organisation (low–high) classification

This classification is based on the relationship between the sub-routines of the specific skill.

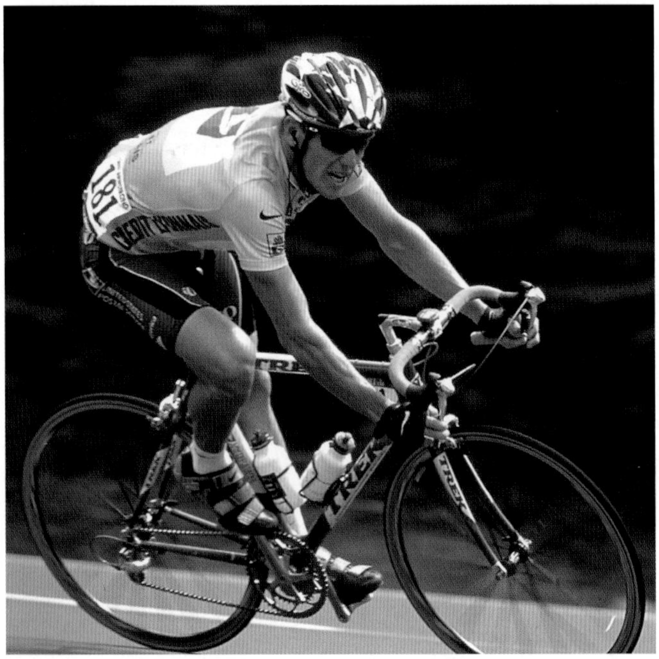

Figure 6.9 Cycling is a continuous skill

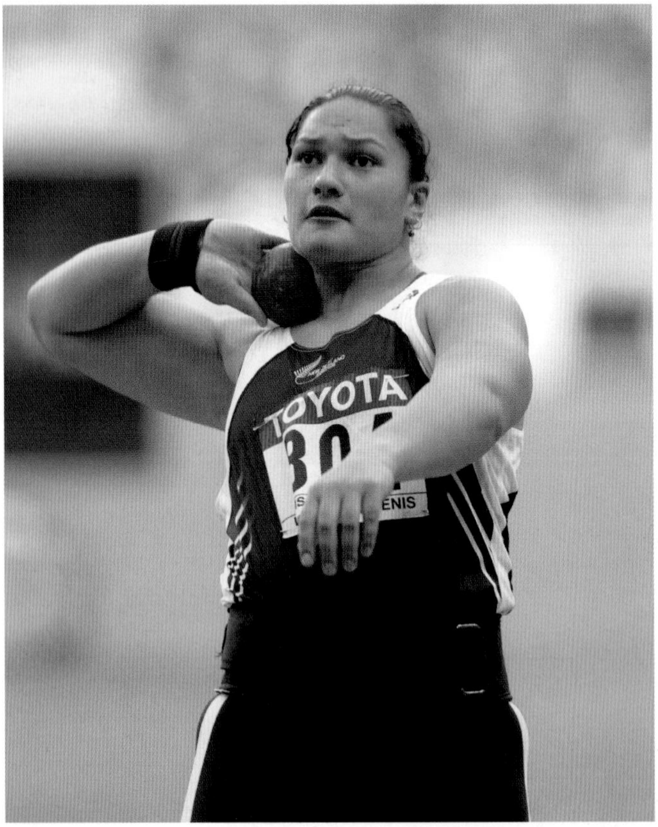


Figure 6.10 Shot put is a self-paced skill

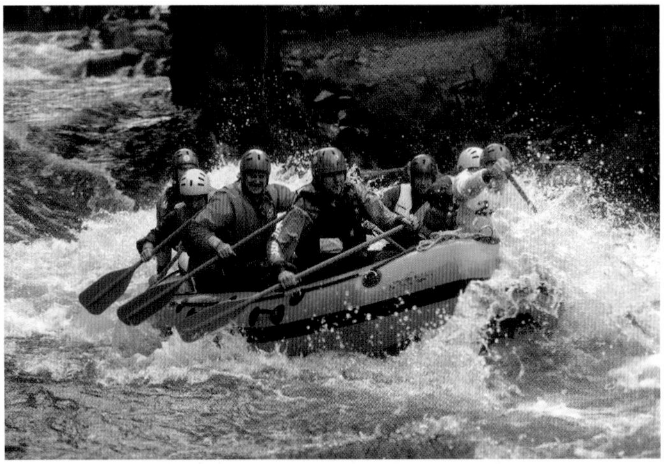

Figure 6.11 White-water rafting is an externally paced skill

## Classification of abilities relating to movement skills

### Using the term 'ability'

It is important at this stage to consider another term which is very often used synonymously with the word 'skill', and is frequently used in definitions of skilled behaviour: *ability*.

In your discussions of what constitutes skill, the term 'ability' may well have been used in the wrong context. In a variety of sports, players from abroad are commonly referred to as having higher levels of ability than our 'home' players, when what we mean is that their skills in terms of technique are of a higher quality. It is the word 'ability' which is being used in the wrong context here. We tend to talk of players having 'lots of ability', when what we mean is that they have developed high levels of skill.

### Definitions and characteristics of ability

It is important to understand the differences between skill and ability. Below are three definitions of ability:

> An inherited, relatively enduring trait that underlies or supports various kinds of motor and cognitive activities or skills. Abilities are thought of as being largely genetically determined. (R. Schmidt)

> Motor abilities are relatively enduring traits which are generally stable qualities or factors that help a person carry out a particular act. (E. Fleishman)

> Motor abilities are innate inherited traits that determine an individual's coordination, balance, agility and speed of reactions. (R. Arnot and C. Gaines)

We can therefore identify particular characteristics of abilities. Abilities are:

- stable and enduring capacities or qualities;
- genetic/innate, inherited traits;
- crucial to underpinning skills – abilities combine to allow specific skills to be performed.

A person trying to perform a sporting activity will learn to use these underlying innate qualities or characteristics in an organised way in order to carry out coordinated movement. It is probably true to say that your innate level of ability will be a major determining factor in your sporting success. For example, if you possess speed and leg power you may be suited to the long jump, but might lack the required slow-twitch fibres and aerobic capacity to excel at endurance-based events.

## Types of abilities

Numerous attempts have been made to classify abilities. One of the most common is that proposed by E. Fleishmann, who subdivided abilities into two categories:

- gross motor abilities (physical proficiency abilities) – which involve movement and are often linked to fitness;
- psychomotor abilities (perceptual motor abilities) – which involve information processing and implementing the selected movement.

### Psychomotor abilities

These include:

1 *limb coordination* – the ability to coordinate the movement of a number of limbs simultaneously;
2 control precision – the ability to make highly controlled and precise muscular adjustments where large muscle groups are involved;
3 *response orientation* – the ability to select rapidly where a response should be made, as in a choice reaction time situation;
4 *reaction time* – the ability to respond rapidly to a stimulus when it appears;
5 *speed of arm movement* – the ability to make a gross, rapid arm movement;
6 *rate control* – the ability to change speed and direction of response with precise timing, as when following a continuously moving target;
7 *manual dexterity* – the ability to make skilful, well-directed arm/hand movements, when manipulating objects under speed conditions;
8 *finger dexterity* – the ability to perform skilful, controlled manipulations of tiny objects, primarily involving the fingers;
9 *arm/hand steadiness* – the ability to make precise arm/hand-positioning movements where strength and speed are minimally involved;
10 *wrist/finger speed* – the ability to move the wrist and fingers rapidly, as in a tapping task;
11 *aiming* – the ability to aim precisely at a small object in space.

**Key term**

**Psychomotor ability:** This usually involves the processing of information and the formation of a decision which is executed as a skill.

### Gross motor abilities

These include:

1 *static strength* – maximum force exerted against an external object;
2 *dynamic strength* – muscular endurance in exerting force repeatedly (e.g. pull-ups);
3 *explosive strength* – the ability to mobilise energy effectively for bursts of muscular effort (e.g. high jump);
4 *trunk strength* – strength of the trunk muscles;
5 *extent flexibility* – the ability to flex or stretch the trunk and back muscles;
6 *dynamic flexibility* – the ability to make repeated, rapid, trunk-flexing movements, as in a series of stand and touch toes, stretch and touch toes;
7 *gross body coordination* – the ability to coordinate the action of several parts of the body while it is in motion;
8 *gross body equilibrium* – the ability to maintain balance without visual cues;
9 *stamina* – the capacity to sustain maximum effort requiring cardiovascular exertion (e.g. a long-distance run).

**Key term**

**Gross motor ability:** This usually involves movement and is related to fitness.

**EXAMINER'S TIP**

When asked to outline the abilities required for a specific skill, always justify why they are needed.

## Ability is task-specific

Certain skills may use different sets of abilities, or they may use the same abilities but have a different priority order. Abilities are not necessarily linked or related; for example, a person having high levels of trunk strength may not have high levels of explosive strength. If a person is good at throwing a cricket ball, there is no guarantee that they will be good at throwing a basketball or a javelin. In other words, the fact that a person does not have the level of abilities necessary to succeed at one activity does not mean that they do not have the potential to succeed in another activity, requiring slightly different abilities or levels. Performers learn to combine and use abilities in specific situations and for carrying out specific skills. For example, high jumpers need high levels of explosive strength.

While there is a certain degree of overlap between the requirements of different activities (e.g. strength, coordination and speed), when you analysed the level and type of abilities required you will have seen that they became much more specific to the sport being considered (e.g. different types of strength). Dynamic strength is used when weight training, but explosive strength is employed in the high jump.

## The implications for teaching and coaching

1 We have to ensure that we do not assume from the above that two people cannot achieve similar standards of performance in a physical activity because of different levels of genetically determined abilities. If one person (possibly with lower levels of specific abilities) is given the opportunity at an early age to use their abilities (e.g. parents take them to the local sports club) and they are prepared to work hard, learning to use their abilities in an appropriate manner, they could achieve a level of proficiency similar to a person who has not had the opportunity or is unwilling to develop innate abilities to higher levels.
2 By analysing the types of abilities needed for specific sports, teachers and coaches could ensure that their students experienced the types of practice necessary for these abilities to be developed more fully. Since balance is an essential ability, required for the

### Activity 6

Using the lists of abilities set out above, make a list of the main abilities required for the following activities:

- badminton;
- hockey;
- gymnastics;
- table tennis;
- weightlifting;
- swimming;
- high jump.

Compare lists with a partner and try to decide on the ability level needed in order to excel in each activity:

- high level;
- reasonable level;
- basic level.

It is important to understand that all individuals possess all the abilities identified above, but we do not possess them at equal, or even similar levels. If a person does not possess the appropriate levels of specific abilities needed for a particular sport, then the odds against them making it to the top in that sport may be high. But this does not mean that such a person has to give up altogether. Practically no one is born with a package of superior abilities large enough to make for an overall athletic ability. Although researchers have tried to identify the possibilities of an 'all-round, general athletic ability', results have tended to support the view that specific skills require specific abilities. However, while we are born with certain levels of abilities, these can be trained and improved in specific situations.

successful completion of a wide variety of complex or difficult skills, it would appear relevant for a PE programme in infant and junior schools to provide the opportunity for children to develop their balance ability in a variety of situations.

3 Teachers and coaches should ensure that children who show a high inherited potential for sports are not disadvantaged from an early age as a possible result of their personality and social environment. Some young children appear to display natural athletic tendencies, often as a result of being bigger and stronger early on. This can result in early success, greater motivation, higher teacher expectations and further development. However, without early success, even children with higher levels of innate ability will avoid continued participation in sport, thus building up what has been termed a skill deficit. This has obvious sociocultural implications for a child's future interest in sport.

4 The role of ability identification as a predictor of potential achievement in learners has to be considered carefully. Think of the implications, both good and bad, if we were able to measure a beginner's abilities and then channel them into the appropriate sport. Prediction studies have shown that abilities which are important at the early stages of learning (cognitive phase) are not necessarily the same as those which are important at more advanced stages of learning (autonomous phase).

5 The ability to take in information and make sense of it, in other words, perceptual ability – involving cue selection, concentration and attention, and vision spatial orientation – is more important at the early stages of learning than later, when learning is replaced more by kinaesthesia.

## What you need to know

* Skills are learned behaviour and are refined through practice.
* Skills are consistent, appear effortless, involve decision making and have a predetermined objective.
* Skills can be cognitive (thinking), perceptual (interpreting and analysing) and motor (movement). Sports skills are often referred to as psychomotor skills.
* Classification systems consider the common characteristics of skills.
* A continuum is a more effective tool in classifying skills.
* Abilities are innate, enduring qualities or capacities.
* Abilities are task-specific. Specific skills need different abilities.
* Abilities underpin skill development.
* Gross motor abilities involve movement and are linked to fitness.
* Psychomotor abilities involve processing information and executing the movement.

## Review questions

1 What are motor skills and perceptual skills?

2 What are cognitive skills?

3 What are complex skills and simple skills?

4 What is an ability?

a) What is a psychomotor ability?

b) What is a gross motor ability?

5 Explain the relationship between skill and ability.

6 Identify three gross motor abilities required for badminton. Justify your answers.

7 Identify three perceptual abilities required for volleyball. Justify your answers.

8 What is meant by classification of skills?

9 Why do we classify skills?

10 What is a continuum and why is it used?

11 Differentiate between gross and fine skills. Give examples.

12 What are discrete, continuous and serial skills? Give examples.

13 What are self-paced and externally paced skills? Give examples.

14 What are high and low cognitive skills? Give examples.

15 What are open and closed skills? Give examples.

# CHAPTER 7

# Information processing

## Learning outcomes

**By the end of this chapter you should be able to:**

- explain the stages of Whiting's model of information processing;
- identify the stages of information processing with reference to practical examples;
- outline the stages of the multi-store memory model;
- explain the characteristics and functions of the short-term sensory store, short-term memory and long-term memory;
- suggest strategies to improve all stages of the memory process;
- define the terms 'reaction time', 'response time' and 'movement time';
- discuss the impact of reaction time on performance and outline the factors which contribute to a performer's reaction time;
- explain the terms 'psychological refractory period', 'single-channel hypothesis', 'choice reaction time', 'Hick's law' and 'anticipation'.
- explain the term 'motor programme';
- outline the relationship between motor programmes and the long-term memory;
- discuss the different forms of motor control, including open-loop control and closed-loop control;
- explain how motor control varies, depending on the skill and ability of the performer;
- evaluate the different types of feedback used to detect and correct errors.

## CHAPTER INTRODUCTION

Information processing is a key topic and is central to your understanding of many other areas of your course. A sports performer uses information from the current situation, previous experience and their memory systems in order to reduce uncertainty and help them to decide how to act. Information processing is an approach which sees the development of human motor behaviour (motor learning) as a process rather than a specific stimulus-and-response relationship. It has developed under the umbrella of cognitive psychology.

Much of the terminology used in the various models is reflective of the post-war computer age in which it developed. The models appear to make comparisons between the ways in which computers function and process information, and the ways in which humans 'achieve, retain and transform knowledge' (Bruner 1972).

Although research and the many models produced tend to suggest that the process learners go through is basically the same, the information-processing approach recognises the individuality of the learner.

Traditionally, the information-processing approach has been based on two assumptions:

1. That the processing of information can be broken down into various sub-processes or components/stages.
2. That each of these components has limitations in terms of capacity or duration which affect the amount of information that can be processed.

Information processing emphasises that the following all play an important part in the overall learning process:

- perception;
- attention;
- memory;
- decision making;
- feedback.

# Information-processing models

Various psychologists have put forward graphical representations (models) of how they see the various parts of the cognitive process relating to each other. These models are intended to aid understanding by helping teachers/coaches in their task analysis. The learning process, however, is a changing, complex and multidimensional one, and such models must be seen as hypothetical and flexible. Two of the better-known models which are generally referred to are Whiting's and Welford's, and can be seen in Figure 7.2 and 7.3.

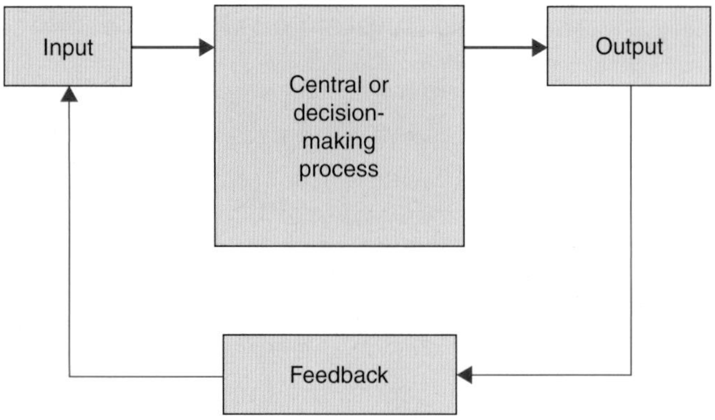


**Figure 7.1** Simplistic information-processing model

The basic process includes:

- Stimulus identification stage/input stage.
- Response identification/selection stage/ central stage.
- Response programming stage/output stage.

## Stimulus identification stage (input)

This stage is mainly a sensory stage where the stimulus (e.g. a ball) is detected, along with speed, size, colour, direction of movement, and so on, from the display.

### The display

This is the physical environment in which the learner is performing. The display for the player shown in Figure 7.4 would be her own teammates, the opposition, the pitch, the ball, the goal posts, the crowd and whatever else is going on in the vicinity of the game, whether important or not.

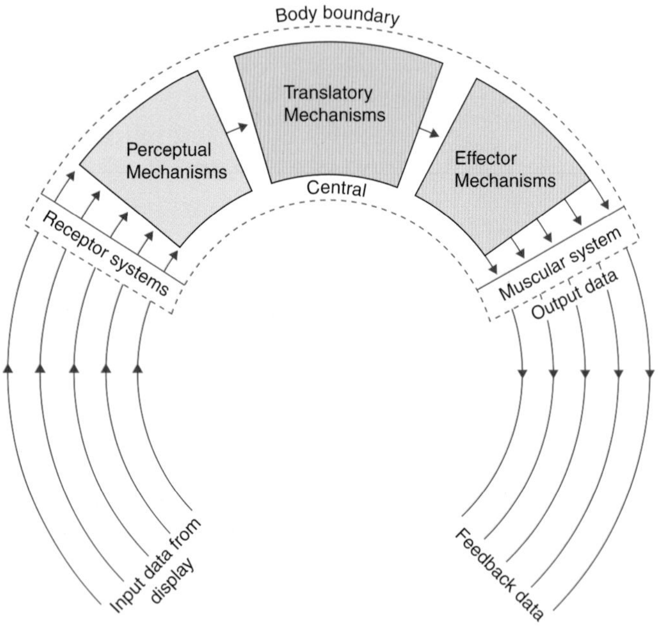


**Figure 7.2** Whiting's model is a well-known illustration of the information-processing theory
*Source*: Adapted from H.T.A. Whiting (1969) *Acquiring Ball Skill*, Bell & Son

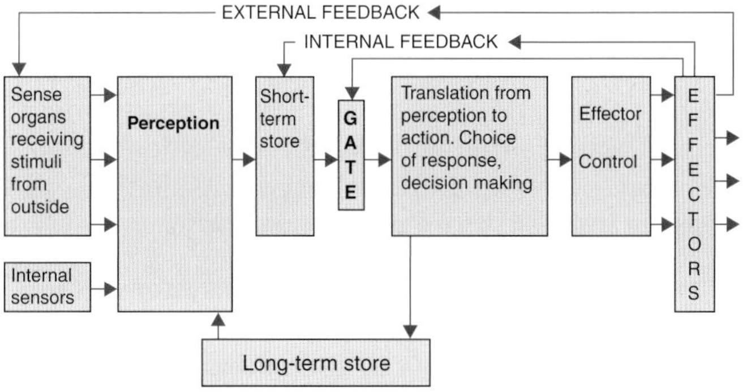


**Figure 7.3** Welford's information-processing model
*Source*: Adapted from A.T. Welford (1968) *Fundamentals of Skill*, Methuen

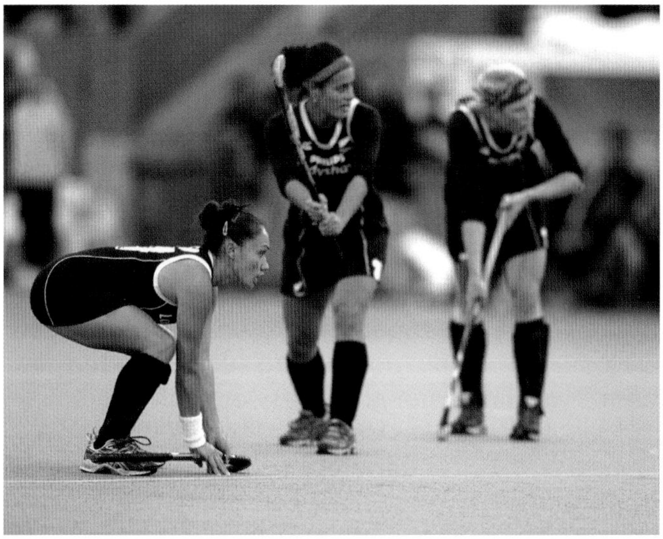

**Figure 7.4** The stimulus identification stage: a player hears her teammates call, sees the ball, feels her grip on the stick and braces her legs in ready position to receive the ball

## Stimuli and cues

These are specific aspects of the display that are being registered by the learner's sense organs (e.g. a ball being passed to them, or players calling for the ball).

## Sense organs, sensory systems and receptors

These are the receptors which take in the sensory information. There are three types or categories of receptors:

1 Exteroceptors – receive extrinsic information from outside the body (from the display):
- visual;
- auditory;
- touch;
- smell;
- taste.

2 Proprioceptors – nerve receptors within the body in muscles, joints, and so on, providing intrinsic information regarding what class of movement is occurring. Kinaesthetic information is also provided about the feel or sense of movement. The inner ear also provides proprioceptive information (e.g. are you balanced?).

3 Interoceptors – information from the internal organs of the body (heart, lungs, digestive system, etc.). This information (e.g. how fast the heart is beating, register fatigue) is passed to the central mechanism of the brain via the body's sensory nervous system.

### Activity 1

1 Play an invasion game of your choice, but alter the amount and type of information entering the sensory system to limit the amount of information received. For example, wear earplugs, an eye-patch, blinkers, thick gloves, and so on. Do not restrict all your senses at once!

2 Change the type of sensory inhibition after several minutes. Discuss the effects and implications on performance with a partner.

### Activity 2

For each of the major sensory exteroceptors (vision, auditory and touch), suggest ways in which the intensity of the stimulus may be altered to aid the detection of the stimulus and processing of information.

## Perception

This process involves the interpretation of the sensory input, along with discrimination, selection and coding of important information that may be relevant to the decision-making process. The process of selective attention and use of memory are important at this stage.

**Key term**

**Perception:** 'the process of assembling sensations into usable representations of the world.' (D. Coon 1983)

## Response selection stage (central stage)

Having identified information from the display, this stage involves deciding on the necessary movement in the context of the present situation (e.g. does the hockey player receive the ball and pass, change direction and dribble, or hold the ball?).

### Translatory/decision-making mechanism

This involves an individual having to use the coded information received to recognise what is happening around them in order to decide on and select the appropriate motor programme to deal with the situation. Perception, selective attention short-term memory and long-term memory are all involved.

**Key term**

**Selective attention:** A process that filters irrelevant information which has been gathered by the sensory system. Information is prioritised, which can help speed up the decision-making process.

## Response programming stage (output)

In this final stage the motor systems are organised in order to deliver the chosen plan of action.

### Effector mechanisms/effector control

Motor programmes or schemas (plans of action; see pages 157 and 185) are selected and developed, involving short-term and long-term memory. These plans, in the form of coded impulses, are sent via the body's effector or motor nerves to the appropriate muscles, telling them what action to perform.

**Key term**

**Motor programme:** An organised series of sub-routines which have to be performed in the correct order to execute the skill effectively.

### Muscular system/effectors

The muscles receive the relevant 'motor programme' or plan of action in the form of coded impulses; they initiate the movement and the action is performed.

### Feedback

As a result of whatever action has been carried out, the receptor systems receive information in various forms. There are many different types of feedback, but it can be either extrinsic (from outside the body) or intrinsic (from within the body).

It can be seen that the body's control system (brain), through a series of receptors and effectors, controls our physical movements by evaluating the need for action and then executing it when and where it deems necessary. How effective this processing of information is depends on many variable factors, which will be dicsussed in detail in Chapter 13.

# Memory

The memory is seen as a critical part of the overall learning and performance process. It is central to our ability to receive the relevant information, interpret it, use it to make decisions and then pass out the appropriate information via the body's effector systems.

There has been much debate about the structure, organisation and capacity of the memory process, with many modifications being suggested to the basic 'two-dimensional process' or 'multi-store' model of memory as described by Atkinson and Shiffrin (1968). It is generally suggested, however, that there are two main aspects of memory: short-term memory (STM) and long-term memory (LTM). These two parts of memory are in some way preceded by a third area, known as the sensory system or short-term sensory store (STSS), which involves a selection and attention process.

The STSS receives all sensory information provided by sensory receptors. It can hold large amounts of information (it is virtually limitless). Information usually lasts in the STSS for a fraction of a second (maximum 1 second). Unless it is reinforced it will be lost – scanning is a way of reinforcing information.

## Selective attention

Owing to the apparent limited neurological capacity of the short-term memory suggested by many single-channel models (e.g. Broadbent 1958; Norman 1969, 1976), it is acknowledged that there is some form of selection system in order to prioritise information, although there are

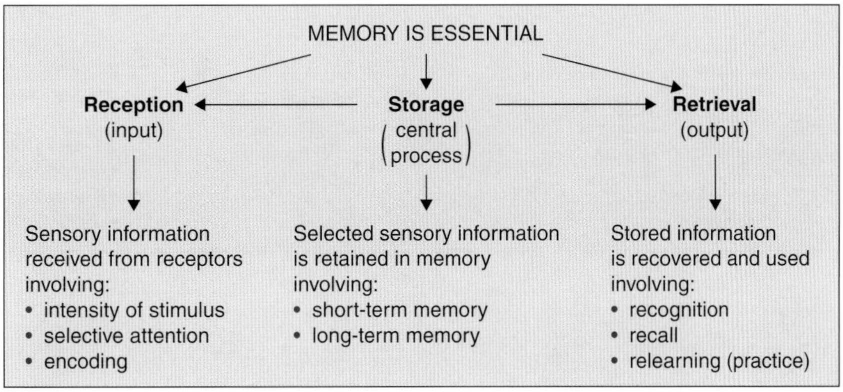


Figure 7.5 Memory is essential

disagreements about the positioning of this filtering system.

The process of selective attention is responsible for selecting relevant from irrelevant information from the display. This allows a tennis player, for example, to focus on the specific cues being presented by their opponent when receiving serve (the grip, throw-up of the ball, angle of racket, position in relation to service court, etc.) and to ignore other aspects of the environment (display) which may distract them (e.g. crowd, noise from the next court, ball boys), thus helping to prevent potential information overload. As well as increasing the time that a stimulus can remain in the STM, effective selective attention can help to reduce reaction time.

The efficiency of the short-term sensory store and the selective attention process is influenced by several factors:

- experience – an experienced tennis player will know what to look for when facing an opponent;
- arousal – the more alert you are, the more likely you are to choose the appropriate cues; in cricket, a batsman who is alert is able to pick up on the spin, speed and direction of the ball;
- quality of instruction – as a beginner, you do not always know what to respond to; the coach or teacher can direct your attention verbally, visually and mechanically;
- intensity of stimulus – the effectiveness of the senses (e.g. short-sighted, poor hearing) when detecting speed, noise, size/shape, colour, and so on.

Selective attention can be improved by:

- lots of relevant practice;
- increasing the intensity of the stimulus;
- use of language associated with or appropriate to the performer in order to motivate and arouse;
- use of past experience/transfer to help explanations;
- direct attention.

## Short-term memory

Because the short-term memory appears to function between the STSS and the LTM, receiving and integrating relevant coded information from both areas and passing on decisions via the body's effector systems (processing and storing information), it is often referred to as the 'working memory' or 'workspace' (Atkinson and Shiffrin 1971). The information in our STM at any one time is said to be our 'consciousnesses'.

### Capacity of STM

Compared with the other two aspects of memory, the STM has very limited capacity, hence the need for the process of selective attention (when only relevant information is encoded and passed to STM). Seven plus or minus two items (7 +/– 2) appears to be the maximum amount of information 'chunks' that any one person can hold. It has been suggested, however (Miller 1956), that by practising a process called 'chunking', or grouping together many items of information, a person can remember seven chunks of information rather than just seven individual items. Thus a games player, with practice, may be able to remember seven different tactical moves or options happening around them, rather than the seven aspects of a specific skill or strategy. In

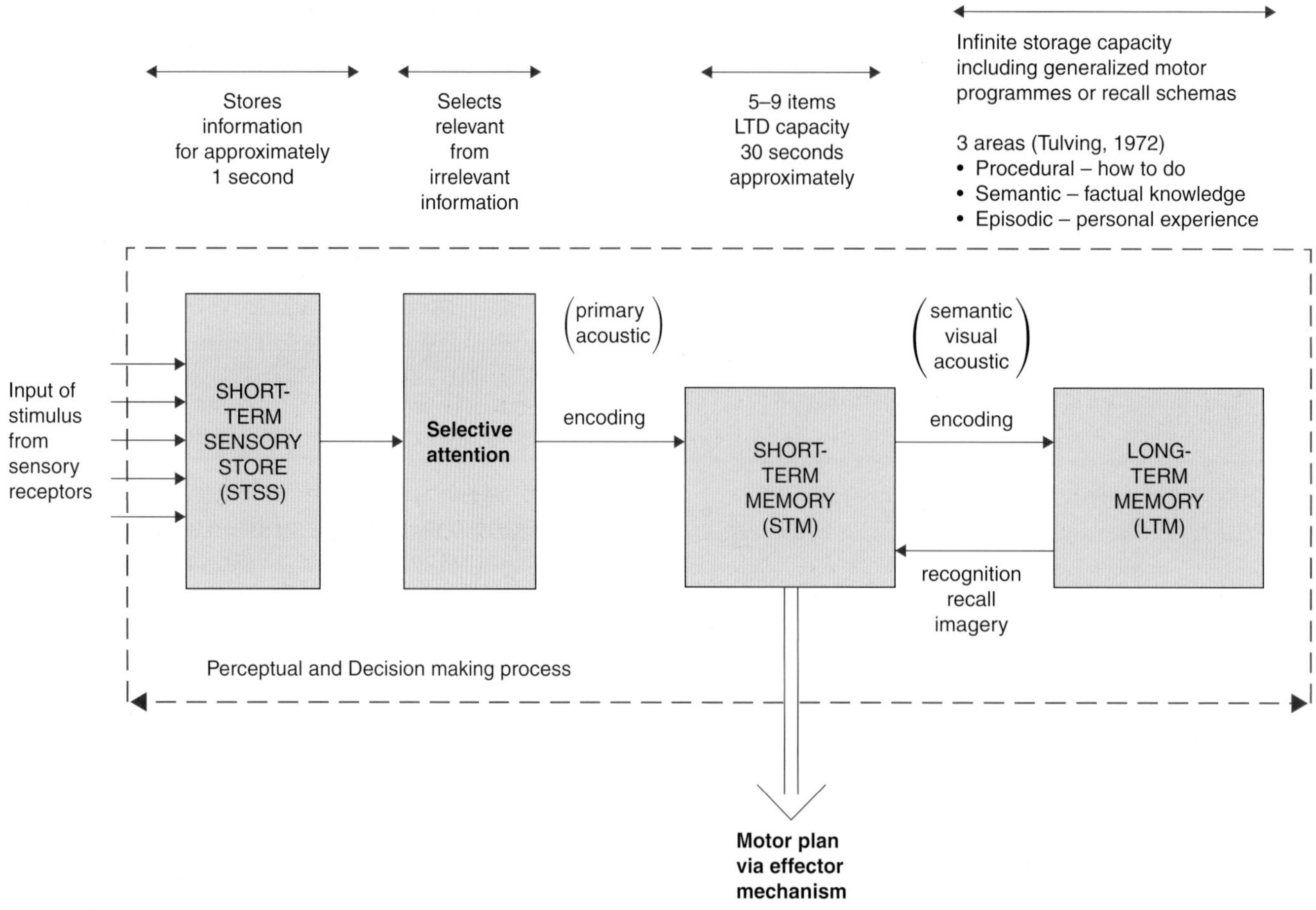


**Figure 7.6** Memory stores and the memory process

addition, a performer, by linking together various aspects of a particular skill, such as a tennis serve, will see it as a whole, once learned, rather than as the various sub-routines of the service, grip, stance, throw-up, preparation of racket, point of contact, follow-through and recovery.

## Duration of STM

It is generally accepted that unless the 7 +/– 2 items of information within the STM are reinforced in some way by practice, repetition or rehearsal, they will only remain in the STM for a relatively short period of time: approximately 30 seconds. If 'attention' is directed away from the information being held in the STM, it tends to be forgotten. In order to keep information 'circulating' within the STM, research has suggested that it is more effective for a person to repeat it verbally. Visual imagery, although slower, can also be used. Important areas of information are passed on to the long-term memory for retrieval and use at a later date.

### Activity 3

1. Compile a list of random numbers, the first comprising 4 digits, the next 5 digits, and so on, until there are 12 digits in the sequence.
2. Read each number in turn to your partner, who must recall and record the sequence immediately. Check the answers and then change roles, using a new set of numbers.
3. Compare your results – who has the best short-term memory?

## Long-term memory

The long-term memory is what is generally thought of as someone's 'memory'. Information about past experiences is stored, including learned knowledge, perceptual skills, motor skills, and so on. In short, all classes of information associated with learning and experience are retained in the LTM.

### Capacity of LTM

The long-term memory is thought to have unlimited capacity. It enables a performer to deal with present situations or tasks by using information (either behavioural or factual) that has been specifically learned, or information gained from general past experiences.

### Duration of LTM

Information, once learned and stored in the long-term memory, is thought to be there indefinitely, perhaps permanently. The main problem with information stored in the long-term memory is one of retrieval. Once information has been rehearsed, reinforced and linked together in the appropriate manner within the STM (coding), it is passed to the LTM for storage. It is generally thought that once learned and stored in the LTM, motor skills in particular are protected from loss. There is evidence to suggest that retrieval is more effective with skills that have been 'over-learned' (practised continually) and have become autonomous. Skills that are linked or associated in a more continuous way (cycling, swimming), rather than individual skills (handstand, headstand), can also be retrieved more effectively.

### Retrieval of information

Retrieval of information that has been stored in the LTM for future use can take several different forms. The more common forms are recognition, recall and relearning.

- Recognition: when a tennis player sees something familiar with regard to a style of serve by their opponent and has to adapt their own movement to it, or a defender in soccer sees several things happening in front of them and has to make up their mind which is the most dangerous, having 'recognised' certain cues or signals (retrieval cues).
- Recall: when a performer has to actively search their memory stores for certain previously learned skills or information that may help to solve a problem in the present.
- Relearning: if something has previously been learned and then forgotten, it may be easier to learn a second time round.
- Imagery: when a performer is able to 'hook' their present cognitive or motor situation onto some form of visual image of a previously well-performed situation, skill or strategy (mental rehearsal); movement memory is aided by verbal labels which can produce a mental image of the correct movement.

To ensure that important information stays in the LTM, a teacher/coach/performer will need to:

- rehearse/reinforce/repeat;
- link or associate information with familiar information;
- make information meaningful/relevant;
- make stimuli more recognisable/intense;
- group or 'chunk' information together;
- use imagery.

### Activity 4

1 Draw a blank model of the memory process.
2 Select a skill you perform during a game situation.
3 Complete each stage of the model, using practical examples to explain how the final decision is made before it is passed to the effector mechanism.

## Decision making, reaction time and response time

In adopting an information-processing approach to analysing how a performer uses present

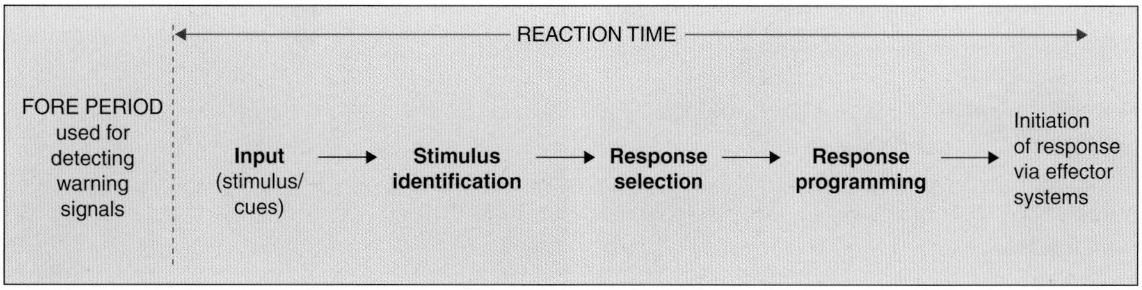


Figure 7.7 Reaction time

information in the form of cues and signals from the environment (display), in conjunction with previously learned or experienced information or movement skills in order to carry out some form of response (decision making), you will have realised by now that this process takes time. Being able to select the correct plan of action (make a decision) quickly, is obviously critical in many sports, particularly those classified as using open skills, where adapting to continually changing situations is important (e.g. tennis, basketball, hockey). It therefore follows that the quicker a performer can go through the whole process, the greater advantage this should have for the motor action being carried out: anticipation becomes possible.

Reaction time is seen as an important performance measure, helping researchers to find out exactly what happens prior to a response being made (response preparation time) and what factors can affect the speed and effectiveness of the response.

- Reaction time is defined as 'the time between the onset of a signal to respond (stimulus) and the initiation of that response' (R.A. Magill).

This is different to another time zone very often associated and sometimes confused with response time, namely 'movement time' response.

- Movement time is 'the time from the initiation of the first movement to the completion of that movement'.
- Response time is the time from the onset of a signal to respond (stimulus) to the final completion of the response or action (reaction time plus movement time).

Individuals differ considerably in their speed of reactions (reaction time – RT), or what has been termed 'response preparation time'. There are many important factors that can affect a performer's reaction time, usually associated with one of the following:

- stimulus (type or amount);
- individual performer;
- requirements of the task.

Response preparation time (decision making) can be affected by various factors associated with the amount of information and the number of decisions that have to be made.

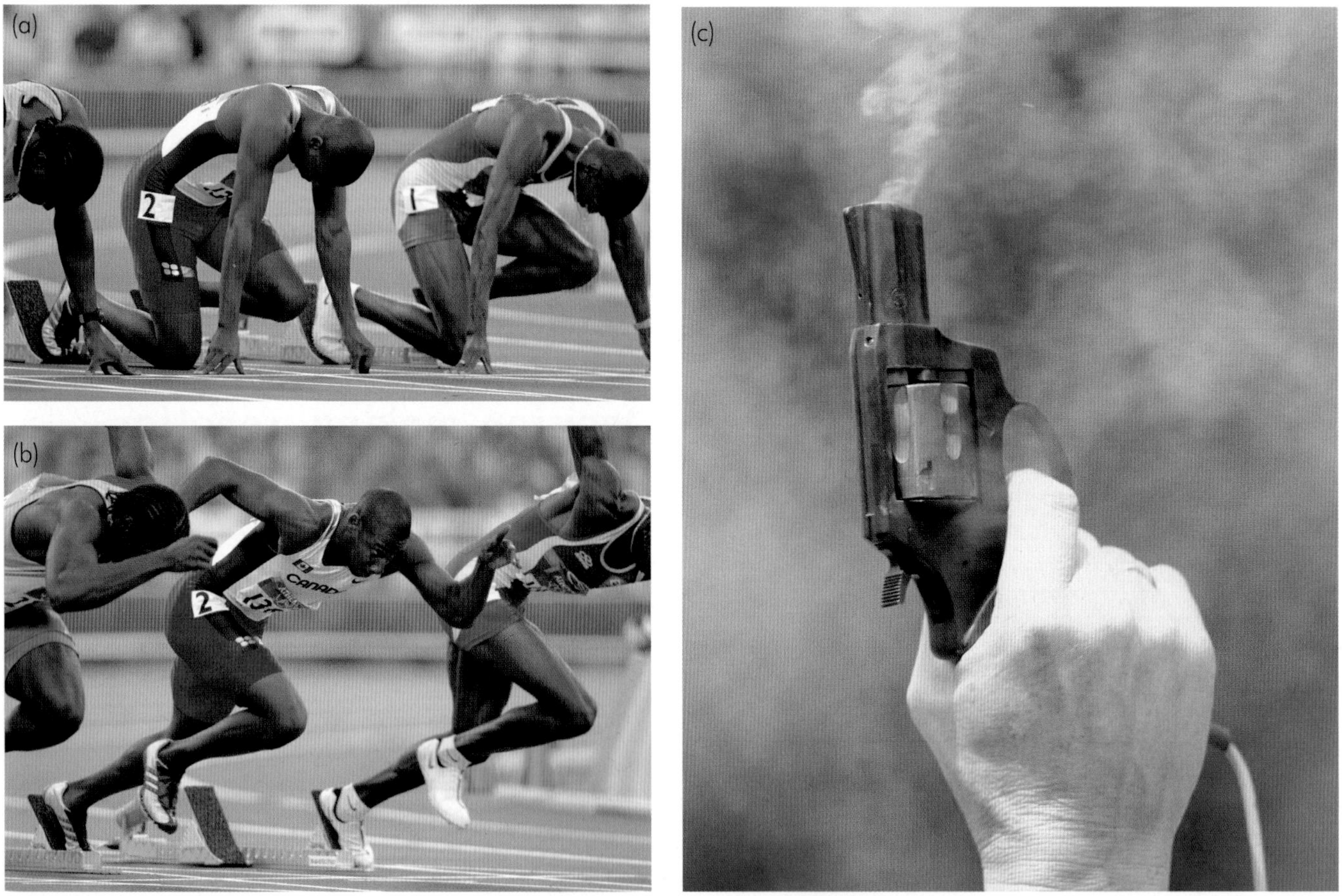


**Figure 7.8** A sprinter in the blocks, and leaving the blocks after the gun has fired

## Activity 5

Complete the missing labels in the diagram below.

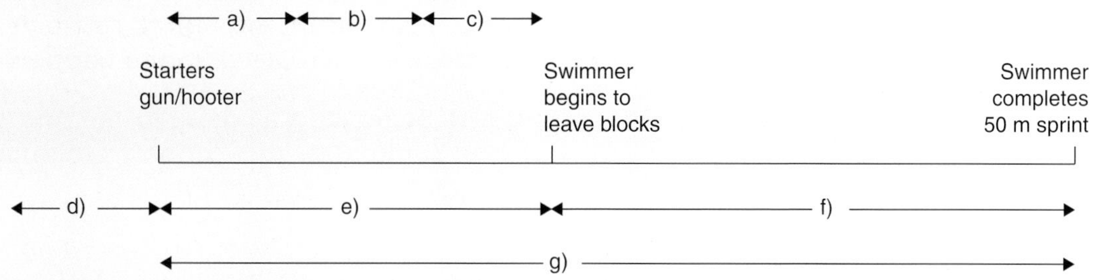

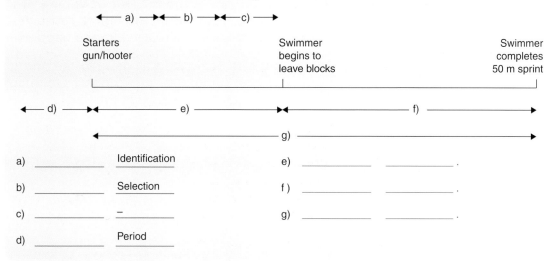

a) ____________ Identification

b) ____________ Selection

c) ____________ – ____________

d) ____________ Period

e) ____________ ____________ .

f) ____________ ____________ .

g) ____________ ____________ .

## Simple response time

This is a specific reaction to a specific stimulus (one stimulus – one response), such as reacting to a starter at the beginning of a race.

## Choice response time

This is when there are a number of alternatives: either a performer has to respond correctly when faced with several stimuli all requiring a different response, or they have to respond correctly to a specific stimulus from a choice of several stimuli. Generally, the more choices a performer has to face with regard to either the number of stimuli there are to deal with, or, more importantly, the number of optional responses, the more information they have to process and the longer or slower the reaction time. This general rule of thumb is based on Hick's Law (1952), which states that: 'Reaction time will increase logarithmically as the number of stimulus response choices increases.'

The linear relationship implies that response time increases at a constant rate every time the number of response choices is doubled. This has obvious implications for a performer when trying to outwit an opponent. A bowler in cricket is better placed to dismiss a batsman if they have more types of delivery at their disposal and can use them at various times to create a feeling of uncertainty in the batsman's mind – RT can be increased by over 50 per cent.

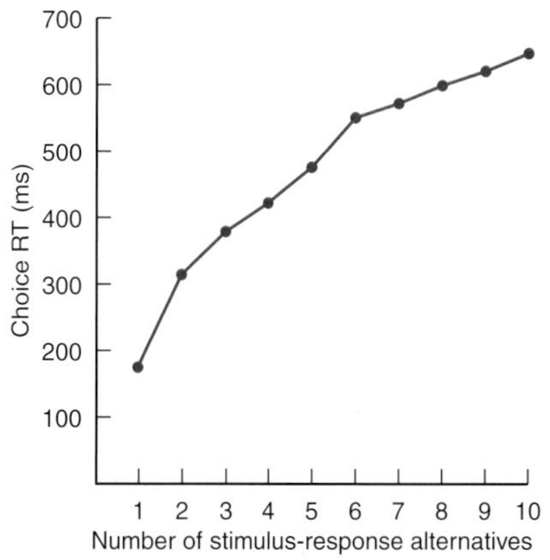


**Figure 7.9** Response time curve illustrating Hick's Law

## Activity 6

For this activity you will need a pack of playing cards and a stopwatch. In pairs, one person records the time and the other completes the tasks below; then swap roles.

1 Divide the cards into two piles of red and black.
2 Divide the cards into four piles, one of each suit.
3 Divide the cards into eight piles, with picture cards and numbers of each suit.
4 Plot a graph and discuss the results. Compare your graph to that in Figure 7.9 showing Hick's law.

## Psychological refractory period (PRP)

A performer using previous experience in order to help them anticipate certain moves or actions depends heavily on making the correct predictions in order to reduce the time needed to prepare a response. One way a performer can try to increase the RT of their opponent is by presenting false information – a certain stance or movement of the racket in tennis or stick in hockey which implies to the opponent that a certain shot or movement will occur (predicting). The opponent then processes this information in order to prepare and initiate a response. As the opponent's response to the first dummy or fake action is initiated, the player changes the move or shot, causing the opponent to re-evaluate the situation and react to the second set of stimuli. The processing of the new information (e.g. a drop shot in badminton rather than the anticipated overhead clear) takes time, creating a slight time delay. This delay in being able to respond to the second of two closely spaced stimuli is termed the psychological refractory period (PRP) as shown in Fig 7.10. In practice, if timed correctly, the opponent in tennis or badminton, or defenders in hockey or basketball, are made to look foolish as, by the time they have reorganised their movement to deal with the second stimulus, the point has been won or they have been beaten by the attack.

### Single-channel hypothesis

Theoretically, the delay is created by the increased processing time caused by a hold-up or 'bottleneck effect' (Fig 7.11) within the response programming stage. Within this stage, it is suggested that the brain can only deal with the initiation of one action or response when presented with two closely following stimuli. This is known as the single-channel hypothesis. A PRP will only occur, however, if the fake or dummy move or action is significant enough to cause the opponent to think it is actually going to happen.

There must also be no lengthy delay in carrying out the second stimulus or 'real' action, as this may negate the whole significance of the PRP.

### How to make use of 'deception' in sport

- Deception makes use of the psychological refractory period.
- The response to one stimulus must be completed before the response to a second stimulus can begin.
- Therefore, by introducing a second stimulus before the response to the first stimulus is completed, the performer playing the dummy gains time.
- For example, when setting a dummy in team ball games, the ball player pretends to pass/run one way/direction; when the opponent responds to that movement, the ball player changes direction/passes the other way.
- More time is gained because the opponent must finish the first movement before reacting and readjusting to the second stimulus.
- Deception creates uncertainty/insecurity.

#### Activity 7

Copy and complete the diagram of the psychological refractory period (Figure 7.10) with a practical example you have experienced yourself.

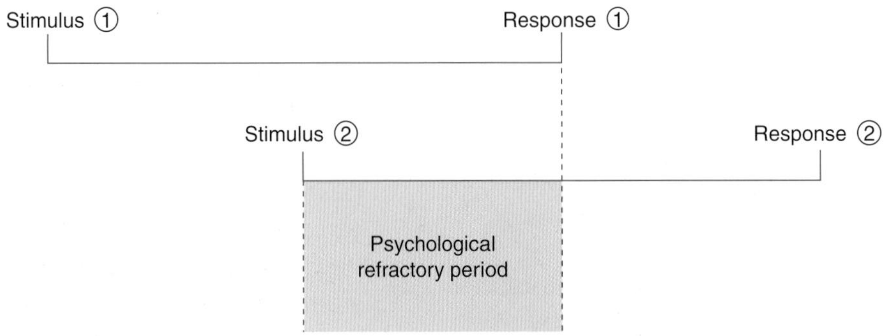


**Figure 7.10** Psychological refractory period

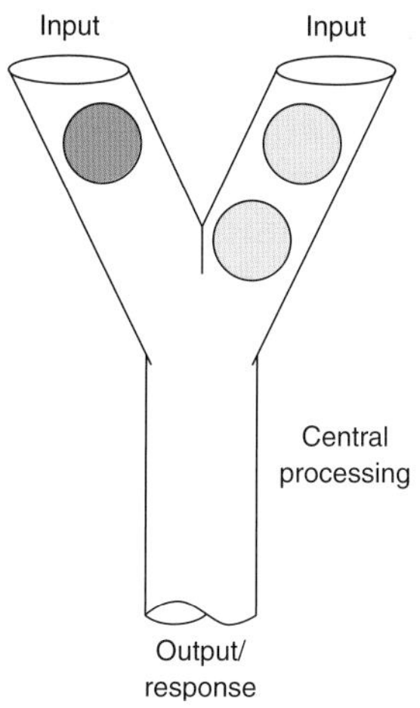


Figure 7.11 The single-channel hypothesis

### Strategies to deceive opponents

- Delay movements as long as possible.
- Disguise relevant cues.
- Emphasise non-important cues.
- Present false information (e.g. fast early action, then soft contact – 'selling a dummy'):
  - This will create uncertainty.
  - The opponent will slow down if alternatives are presented (should s/he tackle/try to intercept a pass, etc.?).
  - Attention of opponent will be distracted by the uncertainty.
  - Reactions of opponent will be delayed by the second movement.

## Anticipation

Anticipation is linked very closely to experience. Anticipation, where a performer is able to initiate movement programmes or actions with 'perfect timing', relies very much on them using signals and cues, and recognising certain stimuli early, thus predicting what is going to happen. The defender in hockey or football who always appears in the right place at the right time to make the tackle or intercept the attacking pass is using their previous experience.

An experienced tennis player receiving a second serve would have picked up on their opponent's angle of racket and subtle positioning of feet, and so on, to recognise that a top-spin serve, causing the ball to kick up high and wide to the forehand, was probably coming over the net. He or she then prepares accordingly; thus processing has begun earlier. An inexperienced beginner, on the other hand, would not understand what a top-spin serve can do to the ball or be able to recognise the warning signals/cues (selective attention). Thus they would be totally unprepared for the high bouncing ball when it arrived. Beginners need more processing time in order to organise, prepare and initiate a response.

### Types of anticipation

Two types of anticipation have been recognised:

- Spatial or event anticipation is when a performer can judge or predict what is actually going to happen and therefore prepares appropriate actions accordingly, enabling the response to be initiated almost immediately the actual shot occurs (e.g. blocking in volleyball).
- Temporal anticipation is when a performer knows what is going to happen but is unsure of when it will happen, and attempt to predict the timing of action.

While temporal anticipation is useful, having *both* temporal and spatial anticipation is much more effective. The fact that many sports performers, particularly in 'open' activities involving rapid changes in actions, rely heavily on anticipation means that as well as using anticipation to their own advantage, they can use the principles behind it to disadvantage their opponents (see PRP above).

Factors affecting anticipation are:

- predictability of stimulus;
- speed of stimulus;
- time stimulus is in view;
- complexity of response;
- practice;
- age.

## Factors affecting response time

There are numerous factors that may influence the reaction time of a performer, some of which are discussed below.

### Stimulus–response compatibility

The compatibility of a stimulus and response (S–R) is related to how naturally connected the two are. If a certain stimulus occurs, what response does it usually cause? The more natural, or usual, the response, the quicker the reaction time.

The converse obviously applies. For example, in hockey, a player's natural response to a ball played down their left-hand side is to reach over with the stick in the left hand and lay the stick down, taking the ball on the reverse (stimulus–response compatibility). However, if the coach wants a player to move across and take the ball on the open stick in order to be 'strong on the ball' after receiving, this, for most beginners, is S–R incompatibility (unnatural), therefore RT would be increased considerably.

Experienced sailors can reduce their reaction time to almost zero as they move the tiller of the boat in relation to wind changes (S–R compatibility). It appears almost natural.

## Predictability of stimulus occurring

The more predictable a stimulus is, the more effective the response can be in terms of time and accuracy. If a performer can predict in advance what is going to happen by being able to pick up on various cues and signals or advance information, then RT can be reduced dramatically. This pre-cueing technique, as it is sometimes called, has the reverse relationship caused by Hick's Law regarding choice reactions.

A player's RT can only be reduced, however, if they pick up on the correct cues and predict the correct stimulus.

### Activity 8

In discussion with a partner, consider a badminton or tennis situation. What pre-cueing information might you be looking for when facing a serve? What might this enable you to do?

## Previous experience/practice

The more experienced a performer is and the more practice they have had of making choices, and relating the compatibility and probability of certain responses to certain stimuli, the more likely it is that their RT will be faster. The effect is obviously greater where choice RT rather than simple RT is involved. Hence the experienced badminton player, when placing the shuttle in various parts of the court, knows, through a good deal of appropriate practice, that only certain types of shot can be played by their opponent from this position. This will allow them almost to pre-select plans of action (see Motor programmes and control of movement, page 159), that is, to anticipate, thus reducing their reaction times and response times to what appears to be almost instant processing.

## Intensity of stimulus

There is evidence to support the view that as intensity of stimulus increases (e.g. larger, brighter rackets or balls), RT decreases, for beginners in particular.

## Age

It is generally accepted that while being relatively limited in early childhood, RT improves rapidly through the developing years up to the optimum level, which is thought to be the late teens/early twenties. After this, it levels off, slowing down considerably as old age approaches. Lack of experience on which to base quick and effective decisions has been suggested to explain children's limited RT. Practice and experience will delay the effect of age.

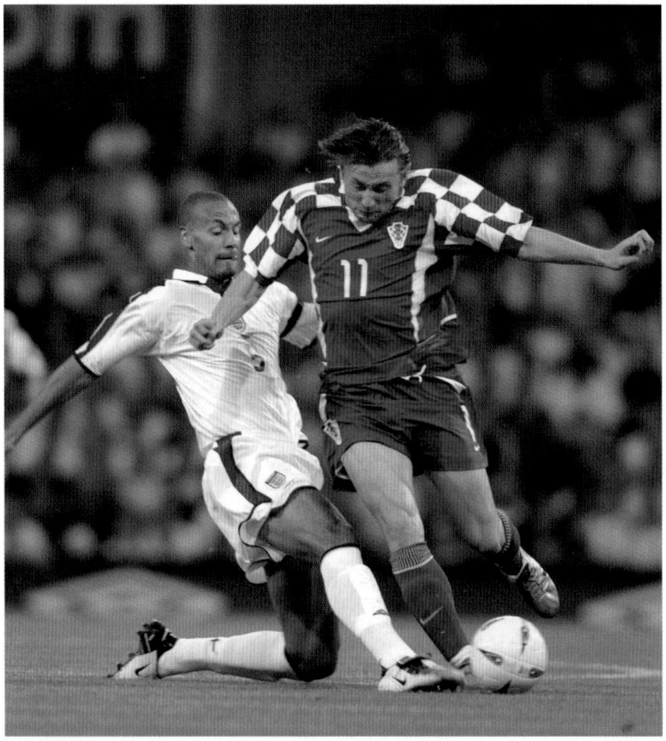

**Figure 7.12** Experienced defenders can pick up on the appropriate cues/signals and anticipate attackers' movements/actions

### Gender

Research has tended to support the view that males have shorter reaction times, although female reaction times deteriorate less with age. The factors already discussed, however, have much more of an influence than gender.

### Arousal

The level of arousal of a performer is seen as a significant influencing factor on their ability to make decisions quickly (response preparation time). As an introduction to the concept, arousal can be viewed as the energy or excitement levels of the individual, generated at the time the performance is taking place. These levels can vary from extremely high, almost agitated behaviour, to the lowest level, sleep. Clearly neither of these extreme states is recommended for the performer in sport, as they do not create the optimum state of mental readiness for effective decisions to be made.

### Fatigue

As the performer becomes tired, their levels of concentration often decline. As a result, they may not detect relevant cues and their RT will slow.

### Presence of a warning signal

If the performer has the opportunity to be prepared for the expected stimulus, their RT can improve. For example, a sprinter will receive the instructions, 'take your marks' and 'set' before the starting pistol is fired. During a game situation, teammates will often call or make a gesture to indicate where the ball may be placed or be expected to arrive from. Similarly, the use of calls for set moves prepares the player for what may happen in the immediate future.

## Strategies to improve response/ reaction time

- Mental rehearsal – going over responses in your mind.
- Concentration/ignoring irrelevant signals.
- Practise reacting to specific stimuli/signals/cues (groove the response).
- Improve physical fitness.
- Anticipate.
- Concentrate on warning signals and early movements.

# Motor programmes and control of movement

The traditional view of a motor programme was that it was a centrally organised, pre-planned set of very specific muscle commands which, when initiated, allowed the entire sequence of movement to be carried out, without reference to additional feedback. The term 'executive motor programme' refers to a sequence of linked movements which are stored in the long-term memory and retrieved when required. This view helped to explain how performers sometimes appear able to carry out very fast actions that have been well learned (particularly closed skills), without really thinking about the action, almost like a computer. In other words, they use very little conscious control. This has obvious links to Fitts and Posner's autonomous stages of learning, see Chapter 8.

**Key term**

**Executive motor programme:** A series of sub-routines organised into the correct sequence to perform a movement.

Each executive motor programme has a series of sub-routines which have to be performed in the correct order if the skill is to be completed effectively. Figures 7.13 and 7.14 illustrate two skills and their respective sub-routines.

In relating this notion of automatic movement to information processing, you can appreciate that the limited capacities of the memory process would easily be overloaded, and would take considerable time if every part of every action had to pass via the short-term memory. The notion of a motor programme being decided on and initiated from the short-term memory appears to solve the overload problem, where, in relatively stable situations, movement can be carried out without the need for modification. This type of control of movement is called open-loop control, without feedback.

**EXAMINER'S TIP**

Ensure you are able to evaluate the motor programme theory and its limitations.

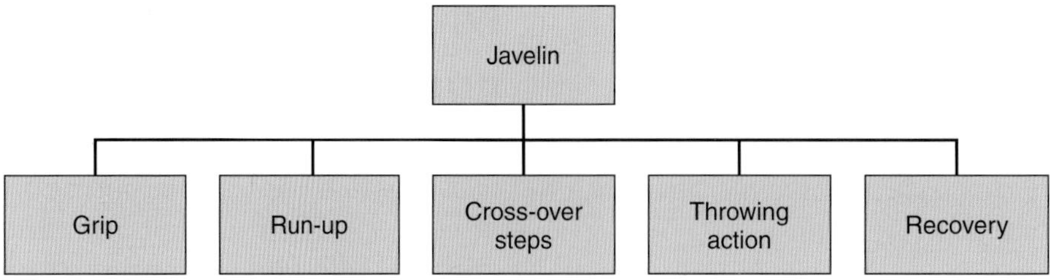


**Figure 7.13** Possible sub-routines for a javelin throw

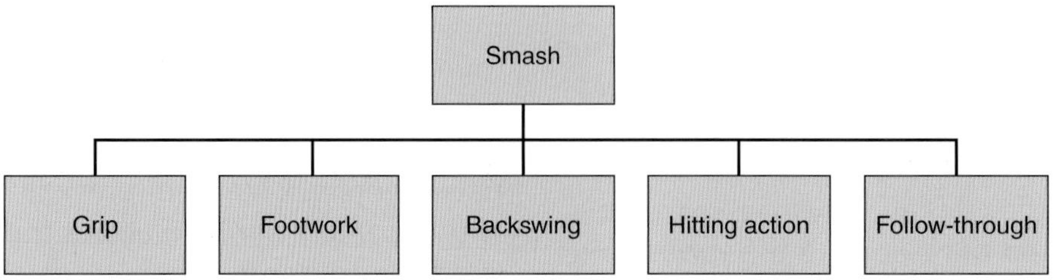


**Figure 7.14** Possible sub-routines for a badminton smash shot

## Activity 9

1 Identify the core skills required in your chosen practical activity (refer to the syllabus).
2 For each core skill, identify the sub-routines and highlight two key points of technique for each one.

## Open-loop control

Motor programmes, or pre-learned mastered movements initiated on command, are thought to be developed through practice. A series of movements is built up, starting with very simple ones, until certain actions are stored as complete movements. These complete movements or motor programmes can be stored in the long-term memory and retrieved at will; the whole movement to be carried out can then be initiated by one complete command. It is suggested that such skills are built up in a hierarchical or schematic way are then recalled and executed without the need of feedback as illustrated in Figures 7.15 and 7.16.

## Closed-loop control

Within the closed-loop model, the loop is completed by information from the various sensory receptors feeding back information to the central mechanism, as illustrated in Figures 7.17 and 7.18.

While it is accepted that there are many types of feedback, in this view of feedback control, the feedback is internal (kinaesthetic), allowing the performer to compare what is actually happening during the movement with the point of reference, namely the correct or currently learned and stored motor performance. This evaluation of the movement currently being undertaken means that any errors can be detected and acted on. All feedback goes back through the processing system, which means that the process of detecting and correcting errors is relatively slow.

Research has shown that the closed-loop system of movement control generally works more effectively with movements taking place over longer periods of time (continuous skills such as running) or with skills requiring slower limb movements (e.g. headstand or handstand). Closed-loop models are not thought to be effective for controlling quick, discrete movements; in such cases, open-loop control of movement appears to be a better explanation for what happens.

In practice, while in certain actions one specific mode of control may dominate, the fact is that most sporting activities involve fast, slow, simple and complex movements in a whole variety of coordinated ways. This suggests that performers are continually moving between open-loop and closed-loop control, with all systems of control being involved in controlling the performer's actions.

J.A. Adams suggested that the motor programme was made up of two areas of stored information:

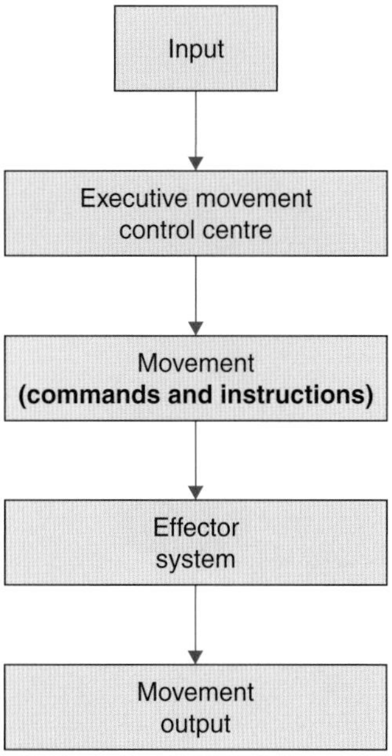


Figure 7.15 Simplified model of open-loop control

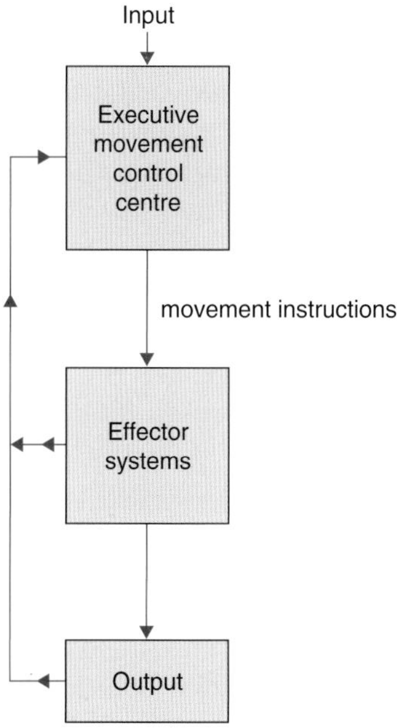


Figure 7.17 Simplified model of closed-loop control

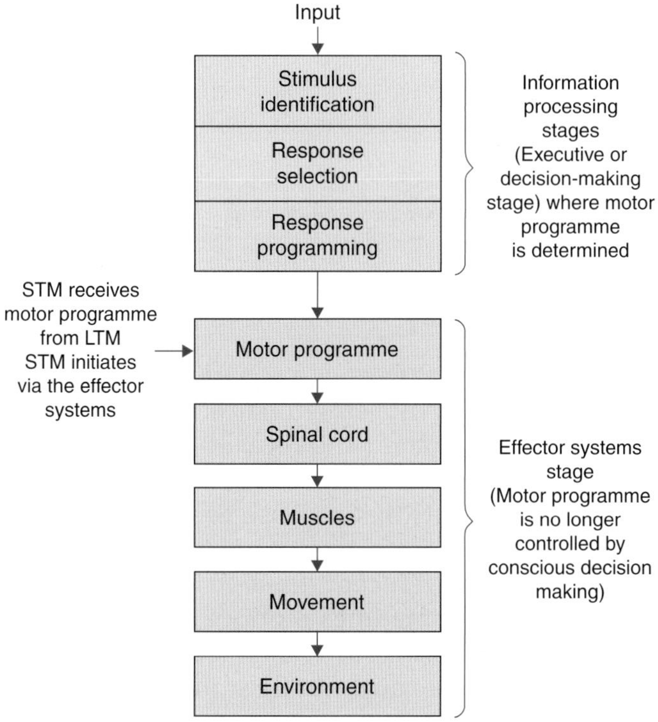


Figure 7.16 Expanded model of open-loop control

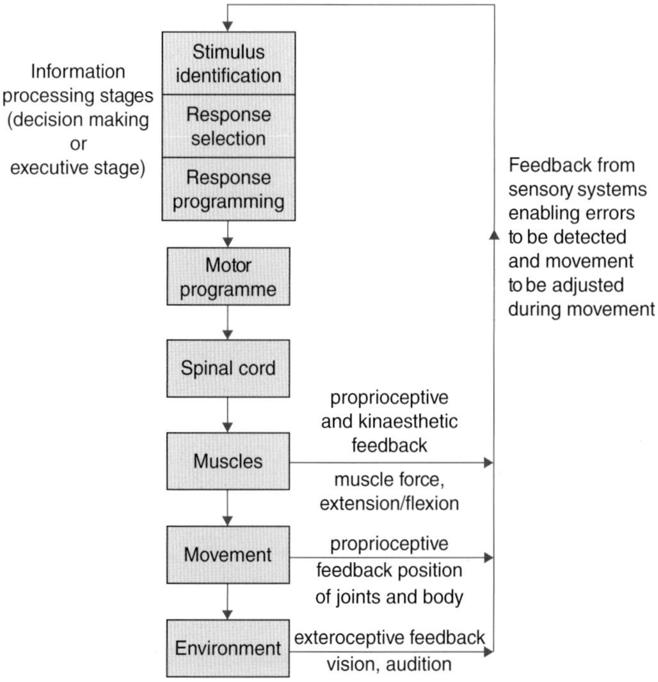


Figure 7.18 Expanded model of closed-loop control

1. Memory trace – used for selecting and initiating movement, operating as an open-loop system of control prior to the perceptual trace. It does not control movement.
2. Perceptual trace – used as the point of reference (memory of past movements) and to determine the extent of movement in progress. Thus the perceptual trace is operating as a closed-loop system of control, making the ongoing adjustment where/when needed.

For example, a trampolinist during a routine will initiate a series of movements using the memory trace. During the sequence, the feedback gained via their kinaesthetic awareness will allow them to adjust their movements (perceptual trace) based on their previous experience. If they are moving away from the centre of the trampoline, they can make the relevant changes. Similarly, if they are losing height during the routine, they can attempt to gain additional height on the next bounce.

### EXAMINER'S TIP

Make sure you can explain the difference between open and closed-loop theory, as well as outline the role of the memory trace and the perceptual trace.

The quality or strength of all these traces is built up and developed through practice, with the performer using both intrinsic and extrinsic feedback, particularly knowledge of results (KR), which in the early cognitive stages is very often provided by the teacher or coach. Once the perceptual trace, in particular, is strong and well developed, the performer is able to carry out his/her own error detection and correction. (Performer moves from associative phase to autonomous phase and learning.)

### Activity 10

For each of the skills listed below, decide if the movements involved are under open-loop or closed-loop control:

- continuous netball chest pass;
- forward roll to balance;
- hockey penalty flick;
- walking along an upturned bench;
- running 200m in 40 seconds, with the aid of a stopwatch to monitor your time;
- side-stepping between a series of cones;
- badminton rally;
- five basketball free throws.

Discuss the results with a partner.

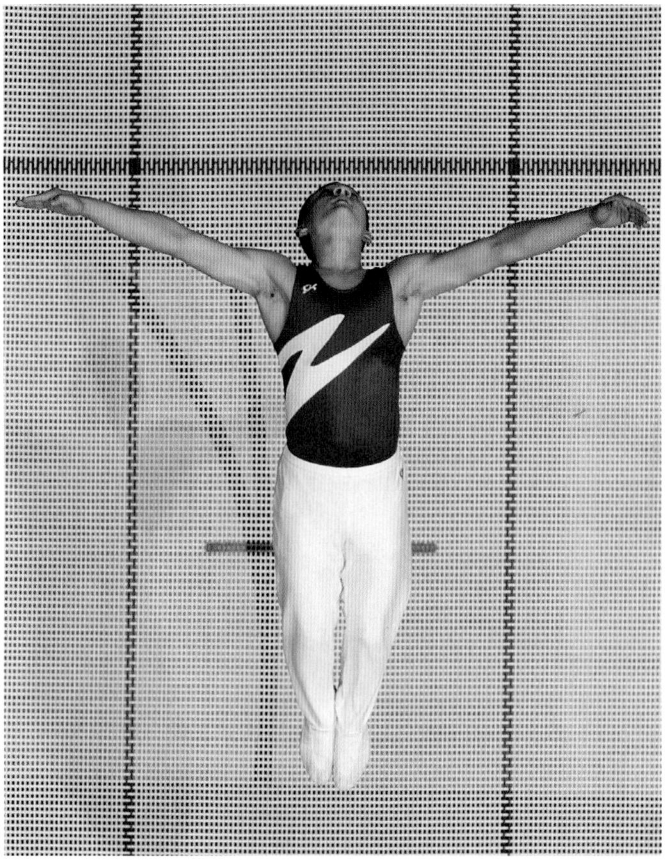

**Figure 7.19** A trampolinist will adjust their position based on feedback from their perceptual trace

However, there are several criticisms of the motor programme theory:

- It assumes that there is a separate memory trace for each movement pattern, which has to be accommodated and recalled from the long-term memory.
- It also suggests that practice should be accurate and that variance would hinder learning, which recent research has refuted.
- Performers sometimes produce movements that are spontaneous and unusual, for which a memory trace could not be stored.

## What you need to know

* The human motor system can be viewed as a processor of information, with sensory information passing through various stages.
* The performer is involved in gathering data, processing the relevant stimuli to form a decision, which is then executed by the muscular system.
* The process consists of three basic stages:
  - stimulus identification (input);
  - response selection (decision making);
  - response programming (output).
* The effectiveness with which a performer processes various forms of sensory information often affects overall performance.
* The memory process involves the short term sensory store, short term or working memory and the long term memory.
* The faster the memory process the faster the reaction time.
* The memory process can be improves by 'chunking', chaining and practice.
* Reaction time is an important measure of information-processing speed, and is affected by many factors.
* Response Time is Reaction Time plus Movement Time.
* In order to assess the effectiveness of the decision and completed actions, feedback is obtained from a variety of sources, either internally or externally.
* Feedback provides information about errors to help make corrections and improve performance. It can act as reinforcement for correct actions and help to develop motivation.
* The quality of feedback information is important to ensure that learning is effective.
* Performers at different stages of learning will use various forms of feedback in different ways.
* Motor programmes are pre-planned sets of muscular movements, stored in the memory, which can be used without feedback.
* Motor programmes are organised in a hierarchical structure, with sub-routines making up executive programmes.
* Sub-routines, for example:

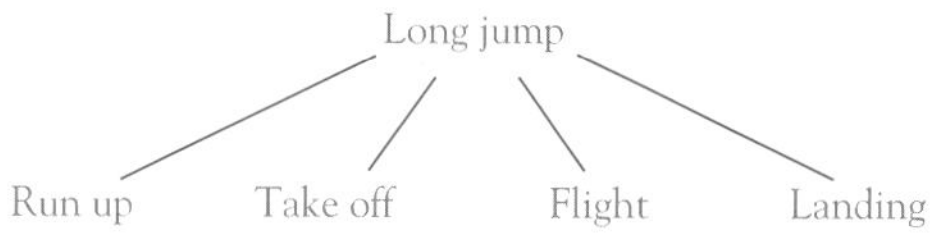


* Sub-routines are short, fixed sequences which, when fully learned, can be run off automatically without conscious control.
* Open-loop explains how we perform fast movements without having to think about them (subconsciously).
* Pre-learned mastery of motor programmes is essential for open-loop control; feedback is not integral in motor control.
* Feedback and kinaesthesis are imperative in closed-loop control.

## Review questions

1 What is meant by information processing?

2 Draw a simple model of information processing and give practical examples from tennis or badminton for each of the parts.

3 What are receptors? Explain the different types.

4 What happens within the three stages of stimulus identification, response selection and response programming?

5 Draw and label Whiting's model of information processing and explain the terms.

6 What are the various parts of the memory process?

7 Draw a simple model to show your understanding of how the different parts of memory link together.

8 What is the process of selective attention?

9 What is response preparation time better known as?

10 Explain the difference between simple reaction time and choice reaction time.

11 How does Hick's law relate to response preparation time?

12 What other factors affect a performer's speed of reactions?

13 What is anticipation?

14 What are the possible postive and negative effects of anticipation?

15 Explain the difference between spatial and temporal anticipation.

16 What does PRP stand for? Explain a situation in a game where it could be used to benefit performance.

17 What is the single-channel hypothesis?

18 What are motor programmes?

19 What are the sub-routines of a tennis serve?

20 Explain open-loop and closed-loop control of movement.

21 Outline the function of the memory trace and the perceptual trace.

22 Suggest two criticisms of the motor programme theory.

# CHAPTER 8 Learning and performance

## Learning outcomes

**By the end of this chapter you should be able to:**

- explain the terms 'learning' and 'performance';
- outline the stages and characteristics of the cognitive, associative and autonomous stages of learning;
- understand the concept of a plateau and outline strategies to minimise the length of a plateau;
- explain the importance of motivation with reference to learning;
- suggest different motivational strategies to ensure active participation in physical activity;
- outline the drive reduction theory;
- outline the various theories of learning, including operant conditioning, cognitive/insight learning and social/observational learning;
- explain how reinforcement and punishment can influence learning;
- explain the sources of information used according to the Schema Theory required to produce motor programmes;
- discuss and evaluate the concept of transfer of learning and its impact on learning skills;
- outline the principles of goal setting; and explain different types of goals that can be used to direct behaviour.

## CHAPTER INTRODUCTION

All human beings have tremendous capabilities for learning. As a student of physical education and sport, it is not enough simply to recognise that learning has or has not taken place (the end result or outcome); you should have a more in-depth understanding of the theories and principles associated with the underlying learning process and be able to apply this understanding to the practical learning situation.

It would be very convenient to have a list of absolute truths about the learning and teaching of specific motor skills related to every possible sports performance. However, your own experiences should help you realise that there are no conclusive statements and guarantees that learning will take place.

# Learning and performance

## Definitions of learning

As we discussed in Chapter 6, implicit in the understanding of the term 'skill' is the notion that learning has taken place, that skill is learned behaviour. Becoming skilful involves a person's performance changing in line with certain criteria and characteristics associated with skill.

It is generally accepted that for learning to have taken place there has to be a recognisable change in behaviour, and that this change must be permanent. Thus, the performance improves over time as a result of practice and/or experience becoming more consistent in terms of its:

- accuracy;
- efficiency;
- adaptability.

Learning has been defined as:

> the more or less permanent change in behaviour that is reflected in a change in performance. (B. Knapp)

> a change in the capability of the individual to perform a skill that must be inferred from a relatively permanent improvement in performance as a result of practice or experience. (R. Magill)

> a relatively permanent change in behaviour due to past experience. (D. Coon)

> a set of processes associated with practice or experience leading to relatively permanent changes in the capability of skilled performance. (R. Schmidt)

### Activity 1

In discussion with other students in your group, consider the four definitions provided here and select the main characteristics of learning.

In your discussion of the four definitions you should have concluded, and psychologists generally agree, that:

- learning is *not* a 'one-off' lucky effort/performance;
- learning is *relatively* permanent (this does not mean, however, that the skill is performed 100 per cent correctly each time; it does mean that a learner's capability of performing a particular skill consistently has increased);
- learning is due to past experience and/or practice.

## How do we judge if a skill has been learned?

There are various methods of assessing a performance in order that more accurate inferences can be made about learning. The general methodology would be to:

- observe – behaviour/performance;
- measure/test – behaviour/performance;
- evaluate – behaviour/performance;
- translate – the information gained into meaningful conclusions;
- infer – that learning has or has not taken place.

### Reasons for evaluating if learning has occurred

These include the following:

- To give the learner/performer accurate/meaningful feedback.
- To assess whether goals/targets have been achieved.
- To assess the effectiveness of teaching/coaching strategies.
- To record progress/achievement over time.
- To assess performance potential.
- To carry out match/performance statistical analysis (e.g. accuracy, technique, timing, errors, amount, frequency).

Evaluations can be:

- formative (ongoing – helps to provide feedback);
- summative (provides a summary over time).

## IN DEPTH: Types of learning

As you will have realised in your earlier discussions about types of skill, in order to carry out motor skills at the highest levels, more than just pure physical movement is involved. There is usually some degree of cognitive and perceptual involvement, depending on the skill being carried out. In the same way that motor skills involve more than purely the physical movement of muscles, limbs, and so on, learning can occur in more than just a physical way. There have been many different approaches to the analysis of what form learning can take in relation to the types of skills or situations being experienced.

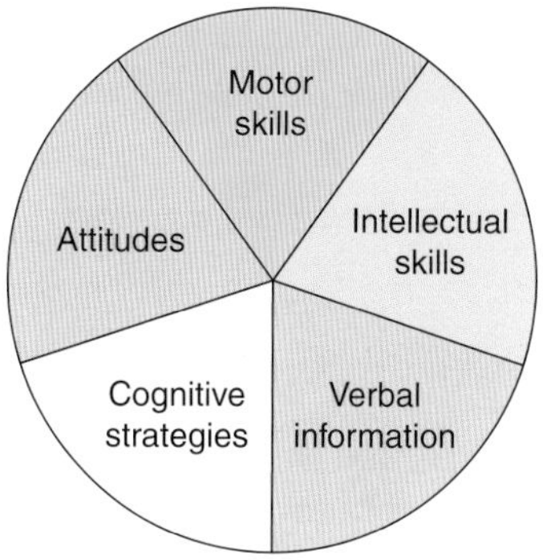


Figure 8.1 The categories of learning

Robert Gagné (1977) suggested that there are five main categories of human performance which may be developed by learning, and that any learned capability, whatever it is called (history, geography, physics, football, swimming, etc.), has characteristics from one or more of these categories:

1. Intellectual skills – Dealing with the environment in a symbolic way (e.g. reading, writing mathematical symbols).
2. Verbal information – Learning to state or tell ideas or information by using oral, written or body language (i.e. communication).
3. Cognitive strategies – Learning to manage one's own learning (i.e. use of memory, thinking, problem solving and analysis).
4. Attitudes – Acquiring mental states which influence choices of personal actions (e.g. choosing badminton rather than hockey as a preferred recreation).
5. Motor skills – Learning to execute movement in a number of organised ways, either as single skills or actions (e.g. catching a ball) or as more comprehensive activities (e.g. playing netball or basketball).

A more simplistic view of learning experienced within physical education and sport can be seen in Table 8.1. When asked to comment on the types of learning experienced within sport and PE, you would need to refer to cognitive, affective and effective.

In dealing with motor learning, it is often difficult to separate the various aspects, as all these will contribute in some way, at some time, to the level of skill. It is therefore necessary to develop all areas in order to make the learning process more meaningful. For example, a sensitive teacher or coach might find that in order to develop a student's high-jumping technique (effective learning), they might have to help the student understand the basic biomechanics of the movement and link this to their ability to analyse their own movement (cognitive learning). In addition, positive attitudes may be needed with regard to specific physical training and psychological aspects, such as confidence and focusing, and holding the moral belief that the use of drugs is cheating (affective learning).

## The nature of performance

While 'learning' is said to be a permanent change in behaviour, as a sports performer it is not always possible to execute each skill correctly every time. This may be due to any number of factors, including over-arousal, interference from opponents, injury and distractions from the crowd, to name just a few. The aim will be to complete the movement as skilfully as possible, but as you will no doubt have

Table 8.1 The three types of learning

| **Cognitive** | **Affective** | **Effective** |
|---|---|---|
| To know | To feel | To do |
| Mental processes, such as:<br>• tactical awareness;<br>• strategies;<br>• problem solving. | Attitudes and values, such as:<br>• ethics;<br>• sportsmanship. | Motor learning, such as:<br>• physical;<br>• catching;<br>• passing. |
| (inclusive of Gagné's categories 1, 2, 3) | (Gagné's category 4) | (Gagné's category 5) |

experienced yourself, this is not always possible. The term associated with the execution of a skill at any given time is 'performance'.

**IN CONTEXT**

**At the 2007 World Athletics Championships, the men's 100m final was won by the American Tyson Gay in a time of 9.85 seconds, while the world record holder (9.77 seconds), Asafa Powell from Jamaica, was third, in a time of 9.96 seconds. However, the following week, Powell's performance improved and he broke the world record again at a Grand Prix meeting, clocking 9.74 seconds.**

# Stages of motor skill learning

Just as there are different types of learning associated with the learning of motor skills, so there are different stages or phases of the learning process. In order to gain a clearer understanding of the learning process, there have been many attempts to identify the various phases, or stages, that students go through when learning motor skills. It has been agreed that whatever the number and names of the phases identified, these are not separate or distinct, but they gradually merge into each other as a person moves from being a novice to becoming proficient.

Having a better understanding of what is happening and what the learner is experiencing during each phase should help you in developing appropriate teaching and coaching strategies to ensure that the learning process is efficient and successful.

**EXAMINER'S TIP**

Be careful not to confuse the three *types* of learning with the three *stages* of learning.

## Three-stage model

Paul Fitts and Michael Posner (1967) identified one of the better-known models, which in its turn has been expanded by others. The three phases identified are:

1. Cognitive;
2. Associative;
3. Autonomous.

While each of these phases has certain characteristics associated with it, movement from one phase to the other is seen as developmental and gradual, along a continuum. The rate at which a performer progresses through the phases is different for each individual.

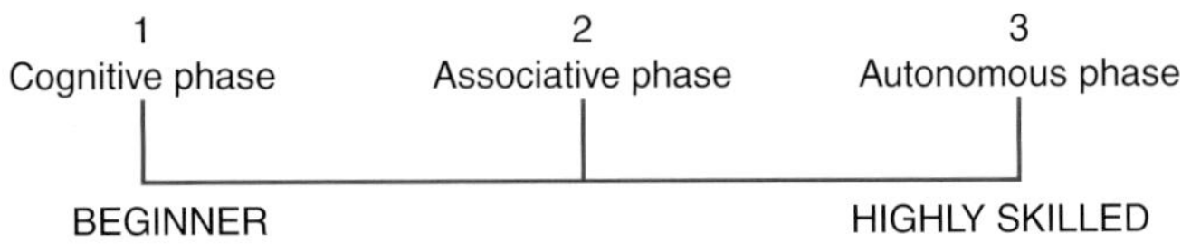


## Cognitive phase

This is the initial phase in the learning process when, as a beginner faced with a new skill or set of skills to learn, you want to be told what you need to know. For example:

- What is required of you?
- What task is to be performed?
- What are the basic rules?

The beginner is trying to get to grips with the basics while dealing with lots of visual, verbal and kinaesthetic information in the form of:

- demonstrations from the teacher or fellow students (visual guidance/mental picture);
- instructions and explanations (verbal guidance to help sequencing);
- initial trials/practice in the form of basic trial/error (kinaesthetic picture).

The emphasis in this phase is very much on early understanding or cognitive involvement (internalising information), allowing a mental picture to be created so that initial plans of action can be formulated. Beginners are directed towards important aspects of the new skill by paying attention to verbal cues. These cues may be highlighted or intensified in order to help concentration (e.g. bigger or brighter bats and balls are often used), and any initial success is reinforced enthusiastically. The length of this phase varies according to the beginner and the strategies being used, but it is generally a relatively short phase.

**Key term**

**Kinaesthetic:** The feeling created during a movement. Proprioceptors located in the muscles detect force and speed of movement, which is transferred to the brain, allowing adjustments to be made.

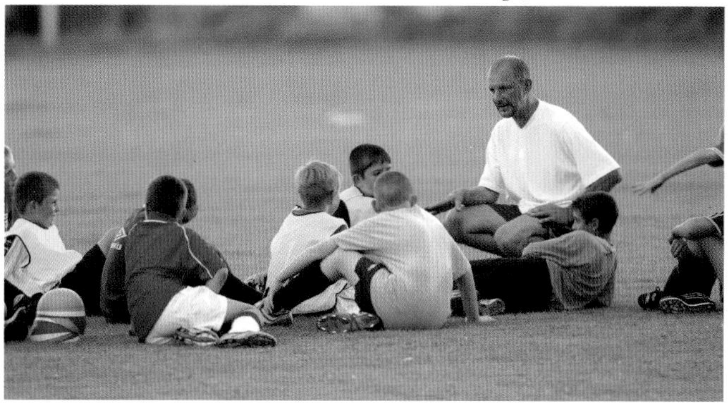

Figure 8.2 In the cognitive phase it is important to keep information clear and simple

## Problems linked to the cognitive phase

- Beginner has difficulty deciding what to pay attention to (selective attention).
- Beginner has difficulty processing information (potential overload).
- Gross errors made (often uncoordinated movements).

Children do not always understand adult words and descriptions. Explanations are too complex for the learner. Therefore teaching/guidance needs to be simple, clear and concise. Demonstrations (visual guidance) are generally seen as being more effective than lots of verbal input at this stage.

As the learner has little idea of what constitutes correct performance, the teacher may have to use manual guidance and physically manipulate the learner's limbs into the correct position. The majority of feedback is extrinsic in nature as the performer does not have the aquired knowledge to correct their mistakes.

## Associative phase

This intermediate or practice phase in the learning process is generally significantly longer than the cognitive phase, with the learner taking part in many hours of practice. The characteristics of this phase are:

- The fundamental basics of the skill required have generally been mastered and are becoming more consistent.
- The mental or early cognitive images of the skill have been associated with the relevant movements, enabling the coordination of the various parts of the skill (sub-routine) to become smoother and more in line with expectations.
- Motor programmes are being developed.
- Gross error detection and correction is practised.
- The skills are practised and refined under a wide variety of conditions.
- There is a gradual change to more subtle and detailed cue utilisation.
- More detailed feedback is given and used.
- There is greater use of internal/kinaesthetic feedback (comparison to ideal by performer).

While the skills are not yet automatic or consistently correct, there is an obvious change in the performance characteristics.

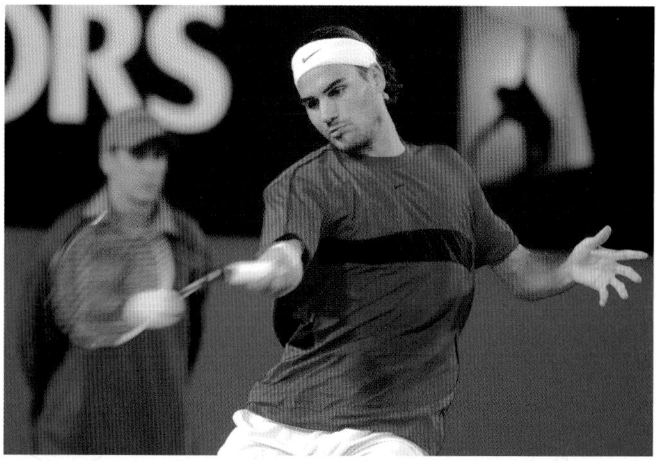


Figure 8.3 To remain in the autonomous phase, regular reference back to the associative phase is essential, even for highly skilled professionals, in order to reinforce motor programmes

## Autonomous phase

After much practice and variety of experience, the learner moves into what is considered the final phase in the learning process, the autonomous phase. The characteristics of this phase are as follows:

- The performance of the skill has become almost automatic.
- The skill is performed relatively easily and without stress.
- The skill is performed effectively, with little if any conscious control – it is habitual.
- The performance is consistent with highly skilled movement characteristics.
- Skills can be adapted to meet a variety of situations.

The performer is able to:

- process information easily, helping decision making;
- concentrate on the relevant cues and signals from the environment;
- concentrate on additional higher-level strategies, tactics and options available;
- detect and correct errors without help.

Once a player has reached this phase of learning, it does not mean that learning is over. Although the performer is very capable, small improvements can still be made in terms of style and form, and the many other factors associated with psychological aspects of performance, which can help develop learning even further; for example:

- self-evaluation of performance;
- mental practice;
- stress management;
- personal motivation.

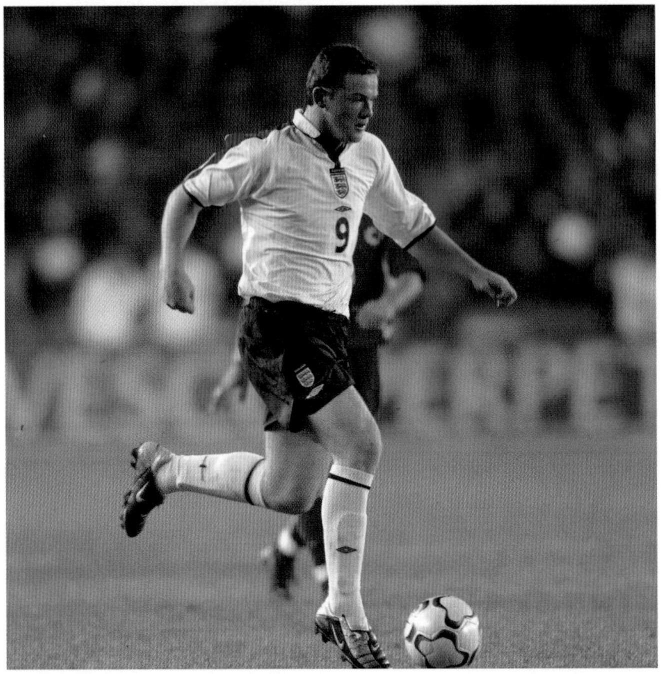

**Figure 8.4** In the autonomous phase, skilled soccer players can dribble the ball habitually, enabling their attentional capacities to consider other aspects of the game at the same time, such as the movements of other players and the options available

## Activity 2

Use the criteria for each phase given above to judge your own level of learning. Place on the continuum where you would classify yourself in relation to your performance of the following skills:

- headstand;
- throwing a cricket/rounders ball;
- kicking a ball;
- shooting a netball;
- jogging;
- backward roll in gymnastics;
- dribbling in hockey.

Cognitive —— Associative —— Autonomous

Make sure you can justify your placements.

## The relationship between learning and performance

As we have already stated, occasional good or 'one-off' performances are not a true indication of learning having taken place. There has to be a relatively permanent change in performance over time, as a result of practice and/or experience. One of the more traditional ways of gathering evidence in order to discover if learning has taken place or not is by comparing practice/performance observations. Performance levels over a certain length of time are recorded and the results are plotted on a graph, producing performance curves. Very often, these curves of performance are referred to inaccurately as learning curves. This is based on the assumption that changing levels of skill closely parallel performance scores. However, it is performance, not learning, that is being measured. By keeping records of skill performance over a period of time (e.g. a lesson, one hour, a term, a season), an individual's, but more often a group's, progress can be plotted. This will provide a graphical representation of the specific aspect of performance being tested. Thus a picture of the relationship between practice and performance is presented, from which inferences can be drawn.

It has been suggested that the validity of performance curves as true representations of learning is problematical, due to the many variables which may have an effect. However, as long as they are not used in total isolation, such curves do act as useful indicators of general trends in learning. Although they may be employed to show changes in an individual's performance of a particular motor skill or skills, performance curves tend to be more widely used to represent composite or group performance.

A performance curve consists of three areas:

- The vertical y-axis of the graph, showing the level of performance being measured.
- The horizontal x-axis of the graph, indicating the amount of time over which the performance has been measured.
- The shape of the curve, from which inferences can be made about the amount of learning taking place.

## IN DEPTH: Types of performance curves

When analysing performance curves, it has been found that graphs are made up of several different shapes within the overall context of the general performance curve. The curves shown in Figures 8.5–8.9 are termed 'smooth curves'. However, as you will have noticed from your own graphs and further reading, curves found in research studies are usually erratic in nature.

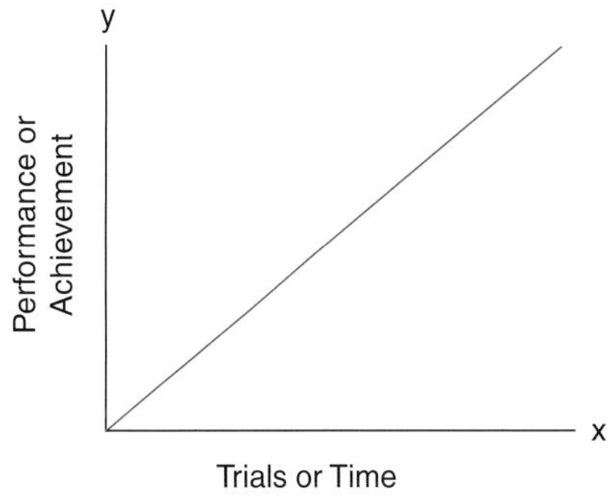


**Figure 8.5** Linear curve of performance

## Activity 3

You are going to undertake a learning experiment in a new skill. It could be a badminton serve with your non-dominant hand, or one-handed ball juggling. You decide on a suitable task. No practice is allowed beforehand or in between attempts.

1 Divide yourselves into pairs.
2 Have ten consecutive attempts at each skill.
3 Count the number of successful attempts each person can manage each time.
4 Log the results on a table, as shown below:

| Attempts | 1 | 2 | 3 | 4 | 5 | 6 | 7 | 8 | 9 | 10 |
|---|---|---|---|---|---|---|---|---|---|---|
| Success | | | | | | | | | | |

5 Plot your own performance and that of a partner on two graphs and compare these.
6 Average out your two scores and draw another graph.
7 Average out all the scores of the members of your group and draw a composite graph for the whole group.
8 What inferences can be drawn from this final graph?
9 What variables may have affected the individual and group performances? How could you make this experiment scientifically more valid?
10 What did you notice with regard to the shape of the curves as you averaged out more by adding more results?
11 A further way to develop your performance curves would be to treat the ten attempts as a block of trials and average this out. Then, over a period of time, repeat the block of ten attempts on a regular basis. This could be done with various skills (e.g. basketball free throws, serving in tennis, target shooting in hockey or football, shooting in netball).

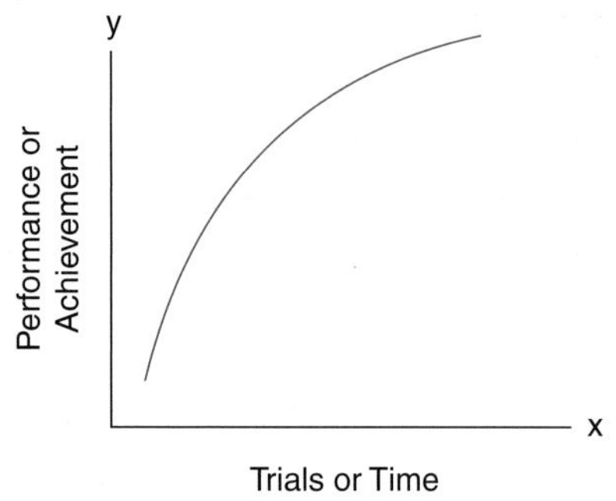


Figure 8.6 Negatively accelerated curve of performance

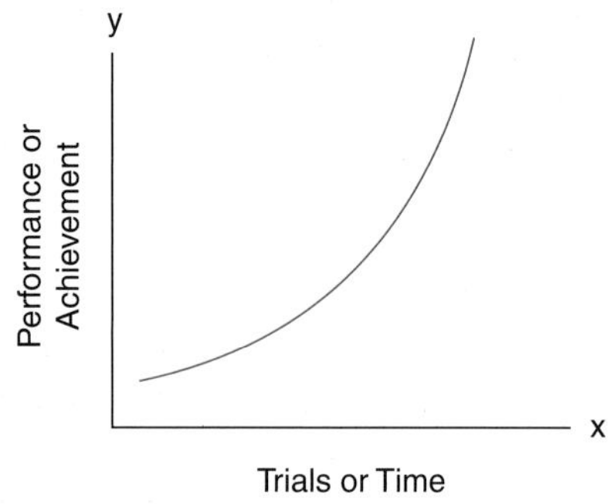


Figure 8.7 Positively accelerated curve of performance

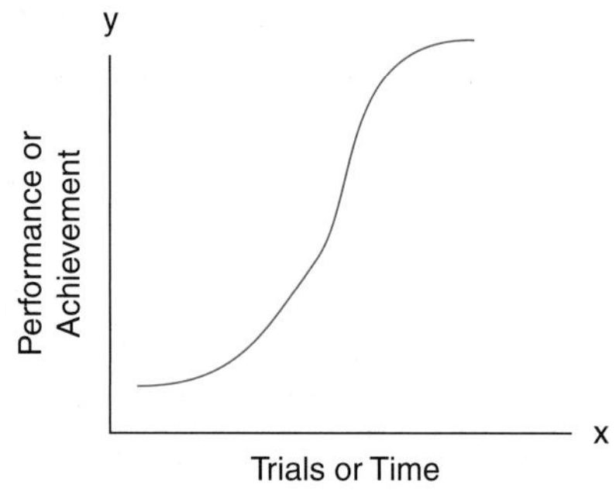


Figure 8.8 Ogive or S-shaped curve of performance

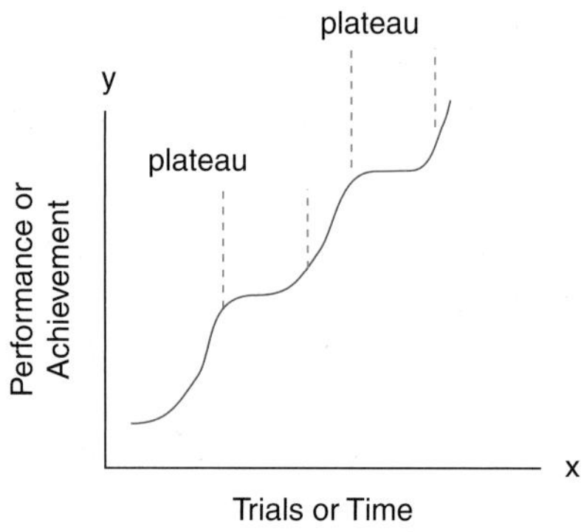


Figure 8.9 Plateau in performance

Figure 8.5 indicates that performance improves directly in proportion to the amount of time or number of trials. In Figure 8.6, the curve of decreasing gain indicates that a large amount of improvement occurred early on in practice; then, although improvement usually continues, it is very slight in relation to the continued amount of time or trials. The inverse curve of increasing gain in Figure 8.7 indicates small performance gains early on in practice, followed by a substantial increase later in practice. Figure 8.8 is a combination of the previous types of curve. The plateaus in Figure 8.9 indicate that during certain periods of practice, or from one particular trial to another, there was no significant improvement in performance.

Plateaus The levelling off in performance preceded and followed by performance gains has been called a plateau. Think of experiences you have had when trying to learn particular skills. There must have been times when initial success was followed by a period when, however hard you tried, no apparent improvement was achieved. Then, all of a sudden, everything 'clicked' and now you cannot even remember what the problem was.

While we may experience plateaus in practice and performance, it has been argued (F.S. Keller 1958) that learning continues, or at the very least that plateaus do not necessarily mean that learning has also plateaued. In terms of learning development, it is generally agreed that if plateaus do exist, they are something that should be avoided, as they can lead to stagnation in performance and a possible loss of overall interest.

Possible causes of plateaus It has been suggested that the following factors have to be considered as possible causes of plateaus:

1 Movement from learning lower-order or simple skills to higher-order or more complex skills may create a situation in which the learner needs to take time to assimilate more involved information and attend to correct cues and signals (transitional period).
2 Goals or targets are set too high or too low.
3 Fatigue/lack of physical preparation.
4 Lack of variety in practice.
5 Lack of motivation/interest due to problems associated with the above.
6 Lack of understanding of plateaus.

7 Physical unreadiness for new skill or next stage.
8 Low level of aspiration.
9 Lack of ability to adapt skills.
10 Bad technique.

**Combating the performance plateau effect** A coach/teacher may have to consider the following strategies to reduce the effect of plateaus:

- ensure that the performer/learner is capable of performing the skill;
- break the practice into shorter/distributed periods;
- re-set goals with agreement of performer;
- offer extrinsic rewards/encouragement;
- use mental rehearsal in practice;
- use appropriate feedback;
- arrange relevant competition against realistic opposition;
- ensure performer pays attention to appropriate cues (selective attention);
- emphasise role in team – enjoyment;
- change role/position/responsibility.

### Activity 4

1. Select a skill which you have mastered, but with which you have experienced a plateau during its development.
2. Consider the possible causes of the plateau and list the practical suggestions made by your teacher or coach to help you progress.
3. Outline what you could have done differently to improve your performance.
4. Present your suggestions to the class and compile a full list of suggestions and strategies.

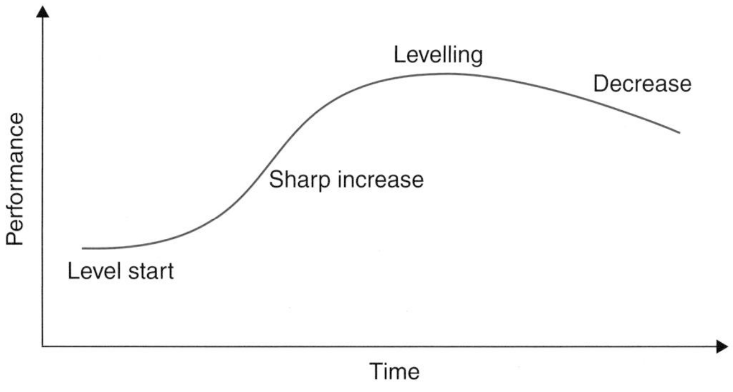


**Figure 8.10** Example of a beginner completing a massed practice of given simple, closed sports skill

Figure 8.10 demonstrates a possible performance curve of a beginner:

- The graph starts at a low level because the beginner has a low skill level.
- At first, progress is slow (shallow slope). The learner is still working out the requirements of the task.
- Early practice produces a sharp increase in performance level.
- The upper level is achieved due to either optimum performance or decreased motivation.
- Levelling out can also be caused by poor coaching/lack of information on how to improve skill level, or fatigue.
- The fall in performance is due to lack of motivation/boredom/fatigue/distraction/faulty technique.

As you can see from your earlier experiment, discussions and reading, there is no one curve of performance. The appearance of these curves is the function of a combination of variable factors. It is important when you interpret the curves and make certain inferences that you are aware of the many factors which can influence learning. If any of these is seen to be a problem in the learning process, the reasons or causes can be recognised, isolated and dealt with in the appropriate manner.

## Motivation

Motivation is a key area of sport psychology. It is recognised as an essential feature in both the learning of skills and the development of performance. In addition, it plays an important role in a learner's preference for and selection of activities. Psychologists all accept that motivation is necessary for the effective learning and performance of skills; however, the enormous amount of motivation-related research has been very diverse, with psychologists posing many questions, including:

- What motivates a learner/performer?
- What motivational factors can influence learning achievement and overall quality of performance?
- Is motivation the same for all people in all activities?
- How can we maintain motivation?
- Why do people take part in certain activities and not others?
- Why do people stop participating in sport?

In evaluating the research we find that there are, once again, no simple answers. What becomes obvious is that in order to gain an understanding of this complex and multifunctional concept, we need to consider a wide variety of research. By taking an integrated approach to analysing motivation we will try to bring together the main aspects of various psychological perspectives. 'Motivation' is the global term for a very complex process.

## Defining motivation

Answering the question 'What do we mean by motivation?' has been one of the fundamental difficulties faced by psychologists, and explanations differ according to the psychological perspective adopted. The term 'motivate' comes from the Latin for 'move', and motives are seen as a special kind of cause of behaviour which energise, direct and sustain a person's behaviour (Ruben and McNeil 1983).

It has been suggested that human beings have both primary motives (e.g. survival and function) and secondary motives, which are acquired or learned, such as the need for achievement and self-actualisation, which are complex, higher-order cognitive behaviours.

Motivation was historically linked with the concept of homeostasis, that is, maintaining the body's physiological balance. In order for a person's body to function correctly, it requires certain essential elements: food, water, heat and rest (primary needs). If these basic elements are not available or are lacking in any way, the body needs to obtain them. Maslow highlighted the basic needs of a person as being a mixture of the physiological and psychological. If the body has developed a need, it will eventually strive to meet that need – it will be driven psychologically to meet its needs. As well as being psychological, the desire to overcome physiological deprivation implies a motivational state.

- Physiological needs result in psychological drives.
- Drives are described as a tendency to fulfil a need.
- Drives result in behaviour.

Maslow (1954) produced a psychosocial model referring to a human being's hierarchy of needs (see Figure 8.11).

- This is a humanistic viewpoint.
- The primary or basic needs at the bottom of the triangle's hierarchy must be satisfied first. The needs at the top of the hierarchical structure are more difficult to achieve. Food and drink (basic) → acceptance → understanding → self-actualisation.
- Each person will achieve self-actualisation in ways individual to themselves.
- The strength of various drives varies occasionally, according to the person and the situation. Personal and social needs have been shown to take over from physiological and safety needs.
- The pursuit of needs/goals that are in the future is one of the unique features of human behaviour. Individuals differ in their ability to set and realise such goals.

Motivation has been defined as:

> the internal mechanisms and external stimuli which arouse and direct our behaviour. (G.H. Sage 1974)

> The direction and intensity of one's effort. (Sage 1977)

> A drive to fulfil a need. (D. Gill 1986)

Defining motivation in this generalised way can have certain disadvantages. Learners and performers may misunderstand the term when advised to 'be more motivated', inferring certain character problems associated with themselves. It can also cause potential problems when motivational strategies are employed.

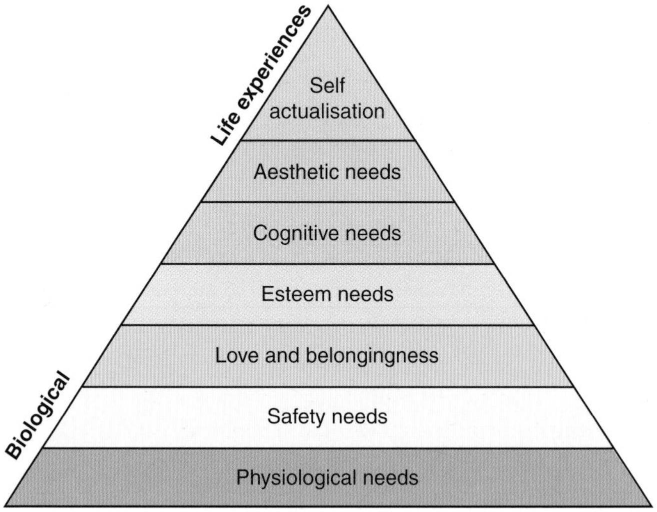


**Figure 8.11** Maslow's hierarchy of needs

In analysing the definition we can see that it involves four main aspects:

1 Internal mechanisms – motivation is linked to and affected by a person's inner drives.
2 External mechanisms – motivation is linked to and affected by external factors that we can experience within our learning/performing situations.
3 Arouse behaviour – motivation is linked to a person's state of arousal that energises and drives our behaviour. The strength of the energised state will determine the degree of intensity of effort used to achieve the goal-related behaviour.
4 Direct behaviour – motivation in its various forms can affect our goals or selection of activities, as well as our maintenance of behaviour in activities (Richard Gross sees motivation as 'goal-directed purposeful behaviour').

Motivation therefore refers to a general energised state which prepares a person to act or behave in some way. Motives relate to the direction that the behaviour will take or the goal which is set.

### Why do performers take part in physical activities?

- The wish/desire/drive to participate in/perform well at a sport.
- Goal-directed behaviour.
- Desire is associated with the expectation that the outcomes will be positive.
- The drive to achieve/will to win.

## Types of motivation

A person's behaviour is affected by many different kinds of motives, derived from both internal and external mechanisms.

### Intrinsic motivation

The study of intrinsic motivation has been linked to cognitive theories. Intrinsic motivation is used to explain how learners/performers strive inwardly, being self-determined in trying to develop competence or excellence of performance. A person who is intrinsically motivated will want to take part in the activity for *its own sake*, for pure love of the sport. They will focus on the enjoyment and fun of competition, try to develop their skills to the highest possible level (pursuit of excellence), and enjoy the action and excitement of seeking out new challenges and affiliations in doing so. A performer pushing themselves hard in difficult circumstances, and feeling a sense of control and pride at achieving a high level of personal skill, is said to be intrinsically motivated. Intrinsic motivation is greatest when learners/performers feel competent and self-determining in dealing with their environment.

**The flow experience** Sports performers sometimes experience a situation when the timing of movements and actions appears perfect. They seem unable to do wrong. Everything they try works! It is one of those perfect days. They are said to be experiencing the ultimate intrinsic experience. Csikszentmihalyi (1975) describes this as the 'flow experience'. In his research he identified the common characteristics of the flow experience as:

- a feeling that the performer has the necessary skills to meet the challenge;
- complete absorption in the activity;
- clear goals;
- the merging of action and awareness;
- total concentration on task;
- apparent loss of consciousness;
- an almost subconscious feeling of self-control;
- no extrinsic motivation (goals, rewards, etc.);
- time transformation (appears to speed up);
- effortless movement.

Many researchers in this area have tended to concentrate on analysing the factors which have a negative impact on intrinsic motivation, whereas Csikszentmihalyi (1990, 1999) has focused on what makes a task intrinsically motivating. Such a peak experience, during which performers are able to lose themselves in the highly skilled performance of their sport, has been likened to Maslow's self-actualisation, explored above. Although it cannot be consciously planned for, the development of flow has been linked to the following factors:

- positive mental attitude (confidence, positive thinking);
- being relaxed, controlling anxiety and enjoying optimum arousal;
- focusing on appropriate specific aspects of the current performance;
- physical readiness (training and preparation at the highest level);

- optimum environment and situational conditions (good atmosphere);
- a shared sense of purpose (team games), good interaction;
- balanced emotional state, feeling good and in control of one's body.

By focusing on aspects of their preparation which can help the development of the above factors, elite performers can increase the probability that the flow experience can occur. Psychological preparation is just as important as physiological performance (Jackson et al. 2001).

Obviously, limitations in any of the above factors can result in disrupted flow. For example:

- injury;
- fatigue;
- crowd hostility;
- uncontrollable events;
- worry;
- distractions;
- lack of challenge;
- non-optimal arousal;
- limited cohesion;
- negative self-talk;
- poor officials;
- poor preparation;
- poor performance.

## Extrinsic motivation

Extrinsic motivation is related to Sage's external mechanisms. If used appropriately, extrinsic types of motivation (contingencies) can serve a very useful purpose in effectively developing certain required behaviours (learning) or levels of sporting performance. Rewards can expedite learning and achievement, serve to ensure that a good performance is repeated, or form an attraction to persuade a person to take part in certain activities (incentive).

While extrinsic motivation is most obviously seen in terms of tangible or materialistic rewards, it can also be intangible.

When using extrinsic rewards and reinforcements to enhance motivation, a teacher or coach needs to be aware of how often they are used (frequency). Should reward or reinforcement be used at every good or successful attempt or every so many times (ratio)? How quickly after the event should reinforcement be used (interval)? What is the most effective type of reinforcement to use? (See Table 8.2.) The value or quantity of the reward is also important (magnitude). In being aware of the above factors, a teacher or coach clearly needs in-depth knowledge of the likes and dislikes of the people being taught. The use of rewards is therefore closely linked to our earlier discussion on reinforcement of learning (see page 180).

Research into the use of reinforcement principles has produced the following recommendations when considering extrinsic motivation:

- Positive reinforcement is 80–90 per cent more effective.
- Avoid the use of punishment, except when behaviour is intolerable or unwanted.
- In order to be effective, extrinsic feedback and reinforcement must meet the needs of the recipient (they must be important to or desired by the individual).
- Continuous reinforcement is desirable in the early stages of learning.
- Intermittent reinforcement is more effective with more advanced performers.
- Immediate reinforcement is generally more effective, particularly with beginners.
- Reward appropriate behaviour (cannot reward all behaviour):
    - reward successful approximations, particularly by beginners (shaping) – performance will not always be perfect (trial and error);
    - reward performance – do not just focus on the outcome (i.e. winning);
    - reward effort;
    - reward emotional and social skills.

**Table 8.2** Tangible and intangible extrinsic motivation

| Tangible | Intangible |
|---|---|
| • Trophies<br>• Medals<br>• Badges<br>• Certificates<br>• Money | • Social reinforcers<br>• Praise from teacher/coach/peers<br>• Smile<br>• Pat on the back<br>• Publicity/national recognition<br>• Winning/glory<br>• Social status<br>• Approval |

- Provide knowledge of results (information regarding accuracy and success of movement – see Feedback in Chapter 13).
- The use of punishment should be restricted or avoided, since although it can be effective in eliminating undesirable behaviour, it can also lead to bitterness, resentment, frustration and hostility. It can arouse a performer's fear of failure and thus hinder the learning of skills.

## Activity 5

Look at the list of strategies for the use of extrinsic rewards. Try to give practical examples of how a teacher or coach might implement them in real life.

## Activity 6

Consider top-level sports performers such as Johnny Wilkinson, Sir Steve Redgrave and Dame Kelly Holmes. In discussion with a partner, try to suggest what motivates them to carry on once they have reached the top.

### Combining intrinsic and extrinsic rewards

Both intrinsic and extrinsic motivation play important roles in the development of skilled performance and behavioural change (learning). Extrinsic rewards are used extensively in sporting situations. Most major sports have achievement performance incentives linked to some form of tangible reward system. At first glance it would appear that the additive effect of extrinsic rewards – money, cups and medals – and the high level of intrinsic motivation should result in performers showing a much greater level of overall motivation.

Intrinsic motivation can be affected by extrinsic rewards in two ways. The performer may perceive the reward as an attempt to control or manipulate their behaviour (the fun aspect becomes work). The performer may also perceive the reward as providing information about their level of performance. A reward could be perceived by a performer as increasing the individual importance of a particular achievement. In receiving the reward, that level of achievement is perceived as high. If they do achieve and gain the reward (positive information), this sign of high ability can help intrinsic motivation. If they fail to achieve the reward (negative information), however, they may perceive this as a sign of incompetence or low ability, thus lowering future intrinsic motivation.

If a person perceives extrinsic rewards as controlling their behaviour or providing information that they are competent, then intrinsic motivation will be reduced. To increase intrinsic motivation, the reward should provide information and positive feedback with regard to the performer's level of competence in performance.

Teachers and coaches should therefore try to involve the performer in decision making and planning with regard to their training programmes and performance goals. By becoming involved, the performer will feel a shared responsibility for any success or achievement, thus increasing their intrinsic motivation because they feel in control and competent. The now obvious link between competitive success and increased intrinsic motivation was shown by Weinberg (1978).

As success and failure in competitive situations provide high levels of information with regard to a person's level of competence or incompetence, it is important that a teacher or coach ensures that intrinsic motivation is not lost by a person who experiences defeat. This is done by emphasising performance or task goals and concentrating on more subjective outcomes (e.g. an action performed well). For instance: although you lost the tennis match it was to a better player; your number of successful serves increased and your tactical use of certain ground strokes also improved. By focusing on the subjective evaluation of success or performance outcomes (winning is not everything), teachers, coaches and parents can improve the performer's positive perceptions of themselves (self-image, self-confidence) and thus dramatically increase intrinsic motivation.

In conclusion, intrinsic motivation is highly satisfying because it gives the performer a sense of personal control over the situation in which they are performing. Being intrinsically motivated will ensure that an individual will train and practise enthusiastically, thus hopefully developing their acquisition of skill (learning) and overall performance.

Extrinsic rewards, however, do not inherently undermine intrinsic motivation. It is essential that physical education teachers and coaches use them effectively, in addition to other strategies. They must increase a learner's/performer's perceptions of success in order to develop intrinsic motivation within the overall educational and performance environment.

Successful strategies for the use of rewards to help develop intrinsic motivation should include:

- Manipulation of the environment to provide for successful experience.
- Ensuring that rewards are contingent on performance.
- Emphasising praise (verbal/non verbal).
- Providing variety in learning and practice situations.
- Allowing learners to participate in decision making.
- Setting realistic performance goals based on the learner's ability and present skill levels.

## EXAMINER'S TIP

Questions may focus on explaining different types of motivation with suitable practical examples. You should also be able to discuss the advantages and disadvantages of using different types of motivation.

### Activity 7

What happens when there are no further badges or trophies to obtain? How might a coach try to ensure that levels of motivation are maintained?

## Drive reduction theory

While drive reduction theory is primarily linked to motivation, it has strong links to learning and our understanding of S–R bonding (see the section on Theories of Learning page 179). C.L. Hull's (1943) theory suggested that continual repetition on its own may not serve to increase the strength of the S–R bond and thus shape the required performance. The strength of the S–R bond (learned behaviour) is affected by the:

- level of motivation or drive (desire to complete the task);
- intensity of the stimulus/problem;
- level of incentive or reward;
- amount of practice/reinforcements.

Hull believed that learning could only take place if drive reduction (acting as reinforcement) occurred, that is, the performer achieved the task they were driven to attempt, and all behaviour (learned performance) derived from a performer's need to satisfy their drives.

There have been many criticisms of Hull's work, but in relating it to physical education and sport we can see that once the S–R bond is strengthened and performance of the task has become a habit, the performer is no longer driven to keep working (drive reduction). In order to develop skills learning or performance levels further and prevent inhibition or lack of drive, a teacher or coach must set further goals or more complex tasks to ensure that drive is maintained. See Goal Setting page 190. Practices must be organised so that the learner is constantly motivated, preventing inhibition from occurring.

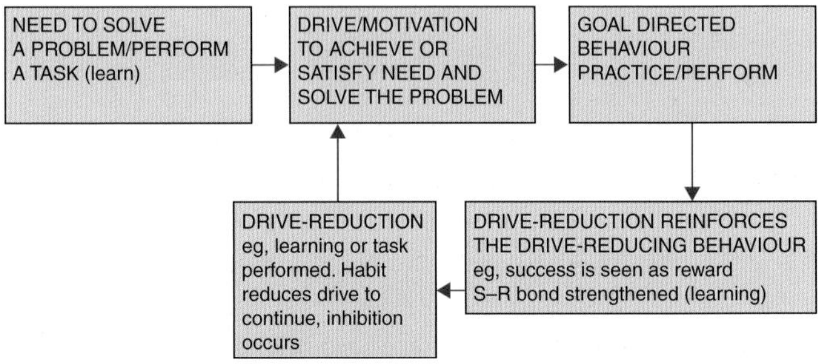


**Figure 8.12** Hull's drive reduction theory

It is also important that the teacher or coach ensures that only correct technique or good performance leads to the drive reduction, as it is *this* S–R bond that will be reinforced. Bad technique or habits must not be allowed to achieve drive reduction.

### Simplistic summary of drive theory

- We are all motivated or have desires to achieve or solve problems – these are known as drives.
- When faced with learning a new skill, we generally have a drive to achieve competent performance.
- Once we have practised and achieved this skill, our drive naturally reduces as we have accomplished what we wanted to do.
- This reduction in our drive acts as a form of reinforcement and strengthens the S–R bond.
- If we continue simply to do the same thing, inhibition occurs.
- At this point, more/new goals need to be set.

# Theories of learning

## Conditioning theories

In the early twentieth century, behaviourism was thought to provide a scientific basis for the explanation of human behaviour. This approach placed emphasis on the learning environment, where behaviour in response to specific stimuli could be observed and used to make predictions about future behaviour in relation to similar situations or stimuli. The early behaviourist approach was based on what became known as stimulus–response theories, or theories of association, where the outcome, or product, was more important than understanding the process.

Behaviourism has been referred to as a very mechanistic and generalised approach, implying that all learners can have their behaviour shaped or conditioned through regular association (i.e. practice) and manipulation of the learning practice environment by the teacher or coach. The performer learns to associate certain behaviour (response) with certain stimuli from within the environment. Once this connection between a particular stimulus and response occurs, the performer's behaviour becomes habitual, enabling predictions to be made about that person's future responses to the same or similar stimuli. Although dating from before the last century, stimulus (S) and response (R) theories as we know them owe much to the work carried out by Pavlov, Thorndike and Skinner. Although Pavlov (classical or respondent conditioning) and Skinner (operant conditioning) both represent the behaviouristic S–R approach to learning, there are some important distinctions we need to consider.

### Operant conditioning (Skinner 1904–1990)

In his later work on instrumental or operant conditioning, Skinner drew heavily on Thorndike's (1874–1949) three laws of learning. He saw the learner as being involved in the learning process. Behaviour was not seen as a reflex or as inevitable, with the learner having no choice or alternative, as is the case in classical conditioning. For Skinner, the learner's behaviour in the present situation was very much a result of the consequences of their previous actions.

The learner associates the consequences of their previous actions with the current situation (stimulus) and responds accordingly, taking into account whether those previous consequences were satisfactory, pleasing and successful, or unsatisfactory, unpleasant and unsuccessful. These consequences would serve either to strengthen the bond between a certain stimulus and response or to weaken it. Skinner suggested that these bonds could be further strengthened or weakened by the use of appropriate reinforcement, thus increasing or decreasing the probability of that behaviour happening again in the future. Both positive and negative reinforcement could be used to increase the probability of a certain behaviour happening again, and punishment could serve to weaken the bond and thus reduce the probability of certain unwanted behaviour or performance reoccurring.

**Key terms**

**Reinforcement:** Methods used to strengthen the stimulus–response bond and increase the likelihood of the action being repeated.
**Punishment:** Methods used to weaken the stimulus–response bond and decrease the likelihood of the action being repeated.

**EXAMINER'S TIP**

Take care not to confuse negative reinforcement with negative feedback or punishment. Develop an understanding of the role of reinforcement and give practical examples to support your answer.

**Activity 8**

Design a series of three progressive practices using operant conditioning for a sport of your choice.

### Thorndike's laws of learning

Skinner's studies in operant conditioning developed from considerable early research by Thorndike, who, in developing his own research on trial-and-error learning, linked to S–R bond theory, proposed many laws of learning, the most famous of which are outlined below.

**Law of readiness** In order for learning to be really effective, the performer has to be in the right frame of mind psychologically, as well as being physically prepared and capable of completing the task (i.e. appropriate maturational development, motivation and prerequisite learning).

**Law of exercise** In order for the bond between the stimulus and response to be strengthened, it is necessary for regular practice to take place under favourable conditions. Repetition of the correct technique is important, sometimes referred to as 'the law of use'. However, Thorndike suggests that failure to practise on a regular basis could also result in 'the law of disuse', when the bond is weakened. Appropriate or favourable conditions could be created by the use of reinforcement.

**Law of effect** The law of effect is central to understanding the essential differences between classical and operant conditioning. In his experiments to support this law, Thorndike placed a hungry cat in a 'puzzle box', from which it could escape to be fed by 'operating' the correct mechanism. Initially, although highly motivated, the cat struggled to get out, reacting in a very random way. Eventually, through a process of trial and error, when repeatedly placed in the box, the cat reduced its time in the box from 5 minutes to 5 seconds and was fed (pleasurable experience).

Thorndike concluded that:

1 What happens as a result of behaviour will influence that behaviour in the future.
2 Responses that bring satisfaction or pleasure are likely to be repeated.
3 Responses that bring discomfort are not likely to be repeated again.

This is not the same as classical conditioning, where the stimulus always produces the same response, whether it is good or bad. However, Thorndike's basic premise was that behaviour is shaped and maintained by its consequences.

Shaping is the gradual procedure/process for developing difficult/complex behaviour patterns in small stages. For example, if a badminton player receives a return which is only half-court and not too high, s/he will smash. If this proves to be successful, and therefore pleasurable, it will serve to strengthen the connection between the stimulus (half-court return) and the response (smash), thus making it more likely that this behaviour will be repeated the next time the same situation occurs. However, a problem sometimes associated with trial-and-error learning is that a beginner might learn a poor or wrong technique which may be effective in a limited way. This may result in having to relearn at a later date in order to weaken the S–R bond which has been developed.

Skinner went on to suggest that certain additional reinforcement or motivational techniques, such as praise or rewards, could serve to support even further his view of the law of effect.

The consequences of operants for behaviour (i.e. performance) can be:

1 positive reinforcement – strengthens behaviour;
2 negative reinforcement – strengthens behaviour;
3 punishment – weakens behaviour.

The above reinforcements or punishments can come in various guises.

**Definition of reinforcement** Reinforcement can be defined as any event, action or phenomenon which, by strengthening the S–R bond, increases the probability of a response occurring again. In other words, it is the system or process that is used to shape future behaviour.

Positive reinforcement usually follows when a learner has demonstrated a desirable performance (e.g. the basketball player has developed the correct set shot technique and receives praise from the coach). This will hopefully motivate and encourage the performer to repeat the correct set shot technique and try to improve.

Negative reinforcement also serves to increase the probability of a certain desirable behaviour happening again, but it is by the withdrawal of a possible aversive stimulus (e.g. a teacher or coach constantly shouting at their team from the sideline suddenly stops shouting). The team or players would assume that they were now behaving or performing in the correct way and thus would try to repeat the same actions or skills again.

Make sure that you do not confuse negative reinforcement with negative feedback or punishment.

## Activity 9

In discussion with a partner, try to think of other types of positive reinforcements that may increase the probability of a response being repeated.

**Definition of punishment** Punishment is an event or action, usually an aversive stimulus, used to try to reduce or eliminate undesirable behaviour (e.g. a penalty is given in football for a foul within the penalty area, or a red card is given to a player who repeatedly infringes the rules of the game). Punishment can be effective, but may result in frustration and bitterness, and is seen by many as a negative approach.

### Activity 10

1 In discussion with a partner, and using the table below, make a list of tangible and intangible reinforcers and punishments which could be used with a learner in the associative phase of learning.

| Reinforcers | | Punishments | |
|---|---|---|---|
| Tangible | Intangible | Tangible | Intangible |
| | | | |

2 Complete the same table for a professional sports performer.
3 Discuss the differences between the two tables.

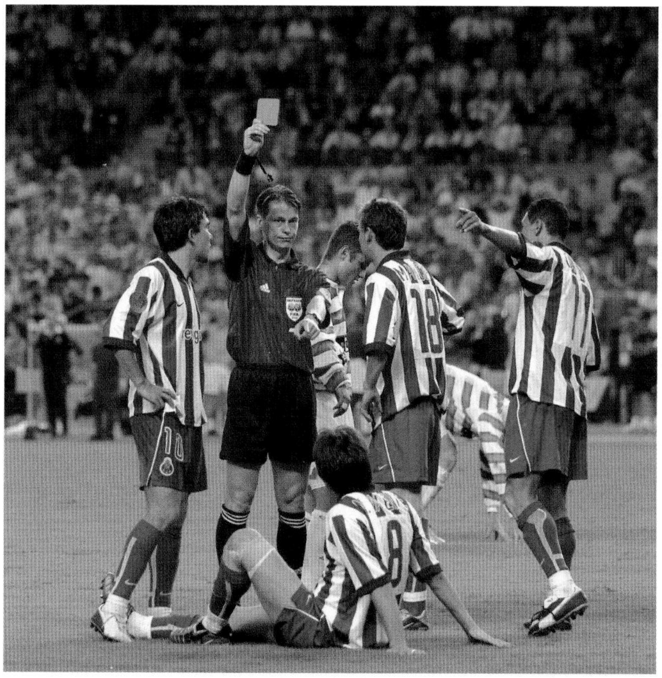

Figure 8.13 Punishment is used to eliminate undesirable behaviour; it tells us what not to do, rather than what we should do

**When and how to use reinforcers** In using reinforcement techniques, a teacher or coach needs to be aware of the effect that different reinforcers may have, and how and when to use them effectively to ensure the appropriate learning and performance of motor skills. Within operant conditioning, once the teacher or coach has decided on the desired level of performance or skill level, they will use their knowledge to employ reinforcers to condition the learner's behaviour in the appropriate way. It may be that the teacher plans lessons in order that success is gained quite easily in the first part of the session. Success itself can act as the reinforcer. As the skills become more demanding, praise for achieving aspects of the desired response may be given. The teacher or coach must ensure that the praise is given soon after the correct behaviour is performed in order that the beginner can link it to their actions and has no doubt what it is for (see Feedback on page 148).

In using reinforcers, a teacher or coach needs to consider the following:

1 How often to use them (too much or too little, partial or complete).
2 Ratio of positive to negative.
3 How soon after response.
4 What type to use.
5 Size and/or value of reinforcer.

All these points will be affected by the teacher's and beginner's interpretation and perception of the reinforcers used.

> **EXAMINER'S TIP**
> For each of the theories of learning, make sure you are able to explain the concept, discuss the advantages and disadvantages, and apply them to a practical situation in which they would be best suited to developing a skill or performance.

## Cognitive theories/insight theories

As research of human behaviour and performance developed further, many psychologists began to move away from the traditional behaviouristic approaches. Cognitive theorists saw the individual as being central to the process of learning, not merely reacting in a reflex manner (response) to outside influences (stimulus). Understanding of the total relationship between the many stimuli within the environment at any one time – and indeed their link to previous and future stimuli – was an essential part of cognitive theory.

Relationships between stimuli and certain responses were not learned in isolation, but were part of the learner's awareness of a variety of interrelated variables and experiences. It was argued that this would involve a whole host of cognitive processes, such as use of senses, perception/interpretation, problem solving and being able to relate the present situation to previous similar experiences, thus involving memory.

The main early supporters of this approach, whose views have become synonymous with the cognitive approach, were known as gestaltists. They believed that the whole is greater than the sum of its parts. They argued that in the learning situation, a beginner will continually organise and reorganise mentally, in relation to previous experiences, the various aspects they are faced with in order to solve a problem in the present situation, that is, they would 'figure it out'. The timescale involved, together with the strategies and methods used, were perceived as different for each individual.

This view of learning is known as insight learning: a learner suddenly discovers the relationship between the many stimuli they have been faced with and 'it all comes together' (e.g. a learner suddenly gets the timing of a serve right). Insight learning often results in the performer progressing very quickly after periods of apparently little progress. It is then important that further questions, problems or goals are set in order to motivate the learner to develop their performance further.

The association of S–R by trial-and-error learning (or chance, which is then reinforced when correct, thus gradually strengthening the bond) has no role to play in the cognitive perspective. Learning is not seen as a random process. What is learned within insight learning is therefore not a set of specific conditioned associations, but a real understanding (cognitive) of the relationship between the process and the means of achieving the end result. For instance, if it is explained to a defending hockey player why, when they are the last person in defence, they should not commit themselves, but should jockey their opponent, keeping goal-side, as this will enable other players to get in position to help or put pressure on the attacker, possibly forcing a mistake, the player is more likely to understand when and why to carry out the coach's instructions in future situations, and also to see the relevance of their role.

This, it is argued, is better in the long run than simply being told what to do, or possibly being punished if they do dive in and commit without thinking through their actions. In practice, following the cognitive approach, it would be important that the teacher or coach had an in-depth understanding and knowledge of both the individual learner and the various coaching strategies relevant to the skills being taught. It seems that a variety of experiences are essential for learners to develop insight of the present task or problem using knowledge gained from previous situations.

There is evidence to suggest that insight in the learner can be further developed by the teacher providing helpful hints or cues. This is particularly useful when considering transfers from previously learned activities or skills (see Transfer of learning on page 187). Gestaltists would suggest that a learner experiences the 'whole' skill or activity, learning individually to develop his/her own map of understanding, rather than making part or part-whole, step-to-step associations.

This whole learning approach allows learners to develop their own strategies and routes of understanding alongside general principles, thus enabling the quicker learners to progress at their own rate: this has obvious links to the promoting of motivation and the development of an individual's full potential.

## Socialisation

In global terms, socialisation is seen as the lifelong process of transmitting a culture by teaching and learning behaviours appropriate to the accepted norms, values and expectations of a society.

Socialisation, particularly within a sporting setting, is a dynamic process linked to the way in which people are influenced to conform to expected appropriate behaviour and to learn how to adopt a balanced and healthy lifestyle. Socialisation plays an important role in social integration.

General socialisation is heavily influenced by prime socialising agents. These are seen as:

- parents/family;
- teacher/school;
- peers/friendships;
- coach/club;
- media;
- role models.

Although the parents and family are seen as the most important agents of socialisation, all the others can exert a great influence in helping to create role models, real or imagined, that can be imitated. While socialisation can be considered in the global or national context of learning the norms, values and expectations of society, it can also be viewed in the more specific context of how:

- sport can act as an agent of socialisation for society in general;
- performers are socialised into specific sports'/teams' or groups' norms, values and expectations;
- through socialisation, individuals are able to learn the values associated with a healthy lifestyle. Active participation not only encourages positive behaviours and morals, it also promotes a better understanding of the benefits, leading to a positive attitude and regular participation.

### Sport as an agent of socialisation

Sport in its widest sense is seen by many as an important aspect of life in most societies, and therefore a fundamental component of the socialisation process experienced by the vast majority of young people. Research in this area, although often criticised, argues that performers, particularly young children, who take part in sport are being taught both physical (motor) and cognitive skills, which will enable them to participate fully and effectively within society as a whole (social learning).

The focus of this research has been on personality, moral behaviour, leadership roles, character building, cooperation, social roles, and so on. It has been claimed that games teach young performers to develop appropriate attitudes and values by providing specific learning experiences. It has been shown, however, that not all learning in these situations is positive. The specific type of experience is important and must be taken into account. The increasing professionalisation of sport can serve to promote the win-at-all-costs attitude, which may lead young performers to imitate deviant behaviour, such as cheating and aggression. It has also been suggested that the traditional values and roles portrayed by sport and performers have heavily influenced gender stereotyping, both within sport (e.g. females as weaker and less suited to sport) and outside. This influence is coming under increasing criticism from within society at present. It is felt that sport and physical education should be doing much more to influence the image of women positively, together with that of other equally under-represented groups in both sport and society in general.

## Social learning and observational learning

### Social learning

Social learning theory came about as an important alternative explanation to conditioning. It was Bandura who, in the 1960s and 1970s, carried out more extensive research in this area. Although he viewed learning and behaviour as being linked to reinforcements (as had conditioning theories), he viewed the reinforcements as being more closely related to vicarious reinforcement. He considered this vicarious reinforcement as the result of two elements, observation and imitation, particularly when related to the acquisition of social and moral behaviour. In introducing certain cognitive factors which can only be inferred from a person's social behaviour, social learning theorists, and Bandura in particular, emphasise the notion of learning through observation.

We discussed the concept of socialisation through sport above. The social learning perspective has been the traditional theme behind this notion. Learning is seen as taking place within a social setting in the presence of others, with the learner and the socialising agent involved in a two-way (reciprocal) interaction. An individual therefore observes other people's behaviour in various ways, not necessarily through direct interaction. The behaviour is observed, the consequences are assimilated and the behaviour is then copied in the appropriate situation at the appropriate time.

## Observational learning

In identifying observational learning, social learning theorists have emphasised a type of learning distinct from conditioning. New behaviour and attitudes are acquired by a performer in a sporting situation through watching and imitating the behaviour of others. The person who is being observed is referred to as the model, and modelling is a term used synonymously with observational learning.

Within physical education and sport, demonstrations are often used by teachers and coaches to give beginners a good technical model to work to. Very often this also serves to help a learner's specific confidence (self-efficacy). The degree of this effect will be enhanced if the person doing the demonstration is of similar ability (teammate) and/or is of high status (professional performer). In addition to showing a current technical model, observational learning, or modelling, can also influence a performer's attitudes and moral behaviour by inhibiting or encouraging certain behaviour/performance.

Teachers and coaches often hope that the consequences of disciplining a certain team member for unacceptable behaviour (e.g. substituting a player for fighting or arguing) will not only have an effect on the specific player, but will also affect the behaviour of other team members who are watching. The other players will internalise the consequences of their teammate's behaviour and are thus warned against copying it.

Modelling is not always carried out at a conscious or intentional level, either by the observer or the model. Very often the model does not intend their behaviour to be copied and is usually unaware that their behaviour is acting as a model for others. The behaviour of top professional sports performers can therefore have either positive or negative repercussions for the behaviour of beginners.

Although role models are an important factor within observational learning, they do not always have to be real or in direct contact with the observer. Remote sports stars, cartoon characters or fictional media-related models can prove equally influential. By identifying with the model, the performer will not only replicate existing behaviour, but may also reproduce certain behaviour in novel situations.

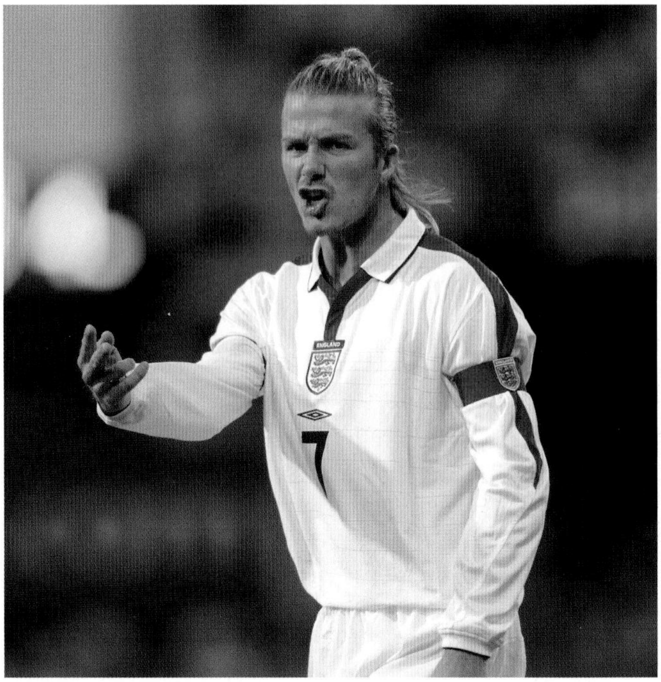

**Figure 8.14** Is David Beckham a positive role model for beginners?

People of influence in physical education and sport have to be aware that unacceptable models of behaviour or attitudes are often being presented and may influence the behaviour of others (e.g. gender stereotyping and aggression). Although for most learners and beginners the model is known directly by the observer and is usually a significant other (e.g. parent, teacher, coach, teammate or professional sportsperson), the degree of the effect or endurance of observational behaviour will depend on several factors.

Bandura's frequently cited Bobo doll experiments, in relation to children learning aggressive behaviour through the observation of others, led him to suggest that imitation is more than just copying a model's behaviour and depends very much on how appropriate, relevant, similar, nurturant, reinforced, powerful and consistent the behaviour is. Further research has shown that the learner not only imitates the behaviour, but also identifies with the role model.

## Important characteristics of models

### Appropriateness

If the behaviour of the model being observed is perceived by the observer as being appropriate in relation to accepted norms and values, it will increase the probability of the behaviour being imitated. For instance, in our society male aggressive behaviour appears more acceptable than female aggressive behaviour (accepted norm), and therefore young beginners/learners are more likely to copy male aggressive behaviour than female. This has obvious repercussions for male/female stereotyping in western culture.

### Relevance

In relation to the young performer's perceptions of the model, how relevant is the behaviour? Young males are more likely to imitate male models of aggression than are girls, as they have in general been socialised into seeing this as part of the accepted male role in society. The behaviour should also be realistic (i.e. a live performance is more likely to have an effect than a video).

### Similarity

Children as young as 3 years are already beginning to recognise their 'gender roles', and will identify more readily with similar models.

### Nurturant

Whether the model is warm and friendly will have an effect on the likelihood of their behaviour, attitudes and morals being imitated. A teacher presenting an activity in a friendly, unthreatening way is more likely to be taken notice of and is thus nurturing the appropriate behaviour.

### Reinforced

If a model's behaviour is reinforced or rewarded in any way, it is more likely to be imitated. Again, this has repercussions for the media, which very often, directly or indirectly, draw attention to certain behaviour, thus reinforcing it in the eyes of the beginner. The imitation of gender-appropriate behaviour is often reinforced by parents (significant others).

### Powerful

The more powerful the model, the more significant the effect is perceived to be (i.e. more likely to be copied if highly skilled).

### Consistency

The more consistent the model's behaviour is, the more likely it is to be imitated. Research has shown, however, that sometimes a role model's inconsistent behaviour can inadvertently have an effect on young performers' behaviour.

A performer will take into account the above factors and evaluate them in relation to the consequences of the behaviour. These consequences can be viewed in two ways, the second being more crucial than the first:

1. What were the consequences of the model's behaviour?
2. What are the perceived consequences of modelling the same behaviour for the observer (learner/beginner)?

The consequences may either be immediate or appear at a later stage.

If observers can imitate a certain behaviour at a later appropriate stage, they are said to have learned it socially. In physical education and sport, more long-term learning can also occur when young performers begin to think, feel and act as if they were the role model, rather than consciously copying technical motor skills. Over a longer period, young performers can assimilate the attitudes, values, views, philosophy and levels of motivation demonstrated by significant others (teacher or coach), to ensure that they become a 'model' professional themselves.

## Bandura's four-stage process model of observational learning

While social learning theory (and other learning theories) takes into account the effect of reinforcement, Bandura's original model referred to learning without any direct rewards or reinforcement. He argued that beginners/performers learn and behave by observing other performers or events (vicarious experience), not merely from the direct consequences of their own behaviour.

The practical application of Bandura's research to observational learning can be related to the four stages of the modelling process identified in Figure 8.15. This will help teachers and coaches to

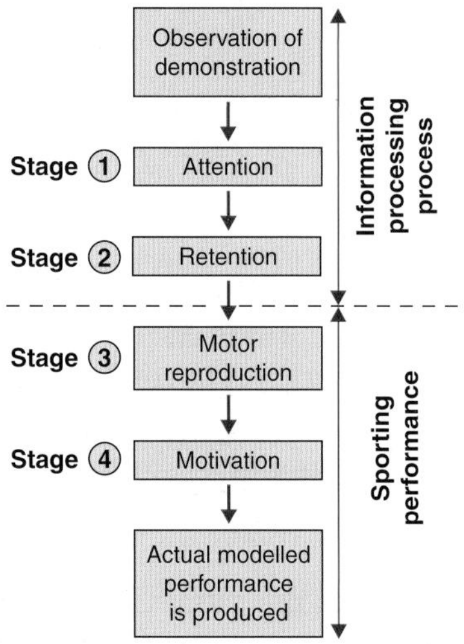


Figure 8.15 Adapted model of Bandura's observational learning process

ensure that learners are focused and maintain their attention, in order to produce a learned, competent performance.

## Stage 1: Attention

In order to ensure that a performer learns through observing, it is very important that they pay careful and specific attention to the model. The level of attention paid to a model will depend on the level of respect that the learner has for the perceived status and attractiveness of the model. A beginner, for instance, is much more likely to take notice of and try to emulate a highly skilled professional or a coach who has significant knowledge of the activity.

Attention is gained by models who are:

- attractive;
- successful;
- powerful;

  or by those whose behaviour is:
- functional.

Teachers and coaches must also be aware of the beginner's/learner's stage of learning, in order to ensure that they do not overload them with too much information. A good coach will ensure that a beginner focuses on the main points and that their attention is not distracted in any way from the task. It is important that the demonstration:

- can be seen and heard;
- is accurate;
- focuses attention on specific details and cues;
- maintains the level of motivation.

## Stage 2: Retention

In order that modelling is effective, the beginner must be able to retain the skill in their memory and recall it when appropriate. One way of achieving this is to use mental rehearsal. Another way is to ensure that the demonstration/practice is meaningful, relevant or realistic. By using symbolic coding in some form, a coach can help the performer retain the mental image of the skill. Thus retention often involves cognitive skills.

## Stage 3: Motor production

While a performer can pay attention and retain a clear picture of what is required of them, in general they will need time to practise the modelled technique if they are to be able to carry out the skill themselves. It is important, therefore, that the model is appropriate to the capability level of the learner/observer: the observer must be able to act out the task. If complex tasks are being developed, the methodology of teaching and practice must allow for general progression and provide opportunity for staged success.

## Stage 4: Motivation

If performance of the model is successful, this will provide the motivation for the learner to try to reproduce it at the appropriate time. Without motivation, a learner will not carry out the previous three stages (i.e. pay attention, remember and practise the task).

According to Bandura, the level of motivation is dependent on:

- the level of external reinforcement (praise, appropriate feedback);
- the level of vicarious reinforcement;
- the level of self-reinforcement (sense of pride or achievement);
- the perceived status of the model;
- the perceived importance of the task.

> **EXAMINER'S TIP**
>
> Practise drawing and labelling the model. It may help you to explain how the process works during an examination.

## Practical application of Bandura's model

In order to make demonstrations more effective, a teacher or coach should:

- make sure the learner is aware of the importance and relevance of the skill to the final performance;
- refer to a high-status model;
- get someone of similar ability to demonstrate to help self-efficacy;
- make sure the performer can see and hear well;
- show complex skills from various angles and at different speeds;
- highlight the main aspects of technique;
- focus attention on a few points, particularly for beginners and children;
- not allow too long a delay between instruction and demonstration;
- allow time for mental rehearsal;
- not allow too long a delay between demonstration and mental rehearsal;
- repeat the demonstration if necessary;
- reinforce successful performance.

# Schema theory

In the previous chapter we stated that motor programmes were traditionally considered to be a specific set of pre-organised muscle commands that control the full movement. This suggests that specific motor programmes for all possible types of action are stored in the long-term memory, awaiting selection and initiation. If we accept that motor programmes operate via continuously changing closed-loop and open-loop control (with or without the use of feedback), it is the stored motor programme which either directs all movements or is used as the point of reference for a movement to be compared against.

R.A. Schmidt presented his well-known schema theory as a way of dealing with the limitations, as he saw them, of Adams's closed-loop theory. Schmidt proposed that schemas, rather than the memory and perceptual traces suggested by Adams, explained recall of movement patterns. Instead of there being very specific traces for all learned or experienced movement, schemas as Schmidt saw them were 'a rule or set of rules that serve to provide the basis for a decision'.

**Key term**

**Schema:** A generalised series of movement patterns which are modified depending on the situation and the environment.

These generalised patterns or rules of movement solved the following dilemmas:

- How do we store possibly thousands, if not millions, of specific programmes of movement?
- How do we initiate and control fast and more complex movements?

In addition, if we can only initiate movement via memory traces developed through practice:

- How do we initiate movement in totally new situations that we have never faced before and have no memory trace of, or programme of movement for?

Schmidt suggested that we learn and control movements by developing generalised patterns of movement around certain types of movement experience (e.g. catching, throwing). A performer does not store all the many specific but different types of catching and throwing; rather they collate various items of information every time they experience either catching or throwing. This helps in building up their knowledge of catching or throwing in general. Performers thus construct schemas which enable them at some future time to successfully carry out a variety of movements.

**EXAMINER'S TIP**

Learn the different sources of information used in the schema theory which are required to control movement. Explain your understanding with a practical example. Do not confuse schema theory with transfer of learning.

A schema for throwing can be adapted:

- returning a cricket ball to the wicketkeeper;
- a long pass in basketball/netball;
- a goalkeeper in football setting up an attack;
- throwing a javelin;
- playing darts.

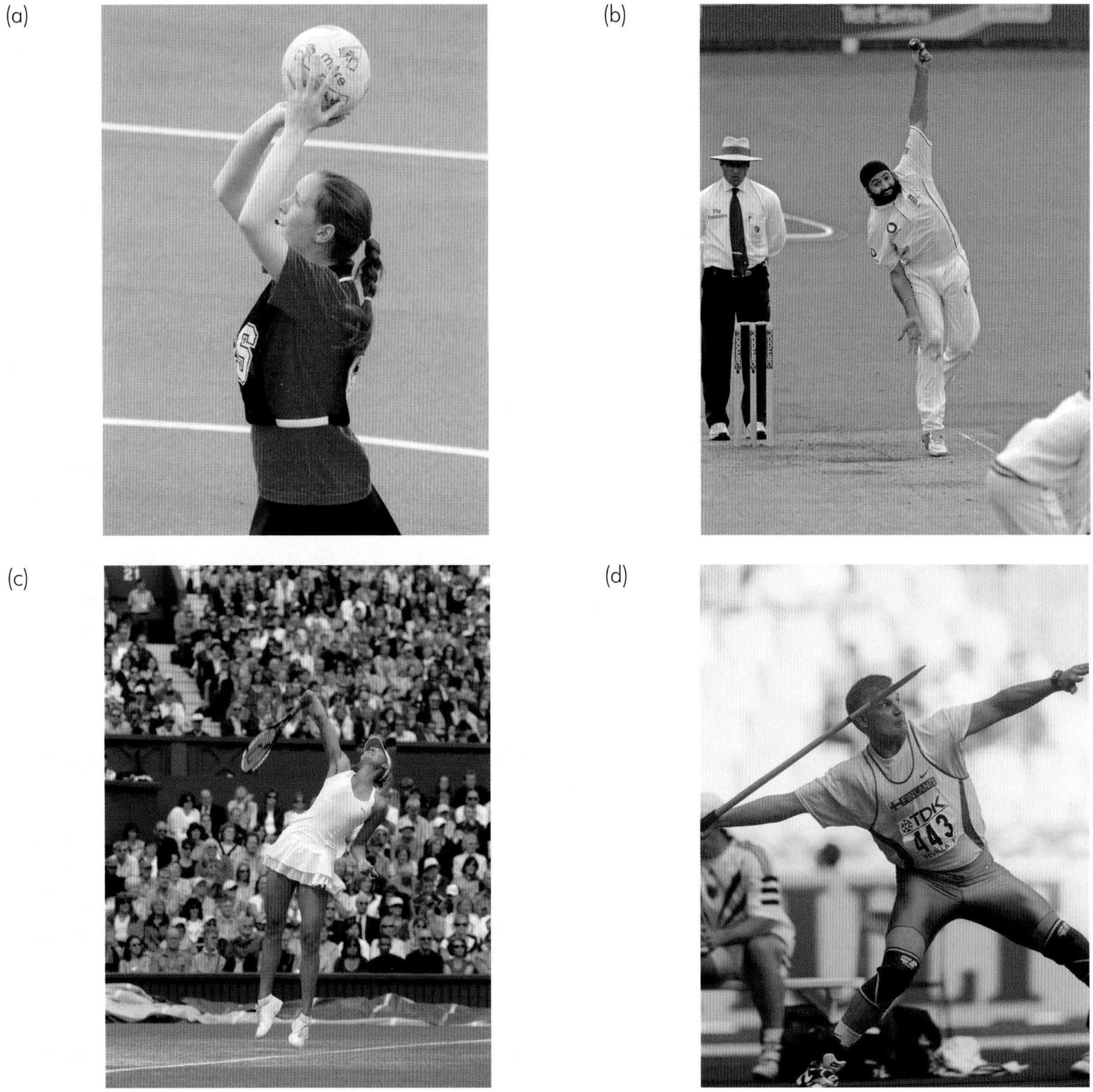


**Figure 8.16** All the throwing actions are based on a similar schema, which is adapted to suit the different skills

By collating as much movement information as possible with regard to throwing, we can adapt to new situations because we know the general rules associated with throwing long, short, high, low, and so on. Variety of practice is essential. In order for schemas to be constructed and developed, the performer has to collate information from four areas of the movement (see Table 8.3).

Whenever a performer takes part in an activity, s/he will collate these four areas of information to form schemas of movement and store them in the long-term memory. The fact that these are abstract rules of response will enable the performer to cope in unfamiliar surroundings. In order to increase the possibility of the performer making the correct decision and being able to carry it out effectively, variety of practice is essential. It is important that the teacher or coach not only ensures repetition, but that practice is organised in order to take into account the various demands that the skill places on the performer in the real-life situation.

Table 8.3 Recall and recognition schemas

| | | |
|---|---|---|
| **Recall schemas**<br>Information is stored about determining and producing the desired movement (similar to memory trace). | 1 Initial conditions (where we are) | • Knowledge of environment<br>• Position of body<br>• Position of limbs |
| | 2 Response specification (what we have to do) | • Specific demands of the situation<br>• Direction<br>• Speed<br>• Force |
| **Recognition schemas**<br>Information is stored enabling evaluation of movement. | 3 Sensory consequences (what movement feels like) | • Information based on sensory feedback<br>• During and after movement<br>• Involves all sensory systems |
| | 4 Response outcomes (what has happened) | • Comparisons are made between actual outcome and intended outcome<br>• KR is important |

### Strategies/methods to enable schema to develop

- Varied practice conditions.
- Avoid blocked or massed practice.
- Practice relevant to the game (e.g. opposition).
- Include plenty of feedback – continuous and terminal.
- Realistic practice.
- Tasks should be challenging/gradually more difficult.
- Slow-motion practice.
- Include transferable elements.

## Transfer of learning

Having considered the complexity, organisation and classification of a skill/task, a teacher needs to consider structuring the learning environment in order to take into account the concept of transfer. The instructional approaches used to introduce and teach skills/tasks to performers often depend on the relationship between various skills that have either been taught previously or are going to be taught in the future. The transfer of performance and learning from one situation to another has been an essential element of organisational and instructional approaches for many years.

There is evidence to support the following general points:

1 That different types of transfer possibilities exist.
2 That certain practice conditions can either help or hinder the actual effect or degree of transfer.
3 That the amount and direction of transfer can be affected by many factors.
4 That teachers need to be aware of the principles associated with transfer.
5 That teachers need to be able to apply these principles in order to structure effective teaching or coaching situations.

### Types of transfer

The following are types of transfer:

- proactive;
- retroactive;
- positive;
- negative;
- bilateral.

#### Proactive transfer

When a skill/task presently being learned has an effect on future skills/tasks, this effect is said to be proactive. A teacher ultimately aiming to teach basketball may start off by introducing beginners to throwing, catching, passing, moving and dribbling, thus building up skills to be transferred into the future game situation. Simplified forms of more complex activities are introduced.

### Retroactive

When a skill/task presently being learned has an effect on previously learned skills/tasks, this effect is said to be retroactive. This transfer is seen as working backwards in time.

### Positive transfer

Positive transfer, as the term suggests, is when skills/tasks that have been learned/experienced help or facilitate the learning of other skills. This can be positive retroactive or positive proactive. Similarities in both skill components and information-processing characteristics will help increase the possibilities of positive transfer. If these similarities are pointed out, particularly to beginners in the associative phase of learning, the effect of transfer can be enhanced further.

It is suggested that transfer possibilities are greater between tasks that have common elements. If the S–R bond expected in one task were the same as earlier learned S–R bonds, the effect of transfer would be greater. For example, a diver wishing to improve their coordination of turning and twisting might take part in trampolining practice in order to develop more control and possibly increase their understanding of rotation and twisting. The components in the practice situation (trampolining) are very similar to the main task and are realistic, thus improving the likelihood of positive transfer occurring.

It is important, therefore, if we accept this basic principle, that a teacher or coach must ensure that practice situations are as realistic as possible. Research on similarities between stimulus and response has shown that maximum positive transfer is produced when the stimulus and response characteristics of the new skill are identical to those of the old skill. Other theories have supported the idea that it is general principles of understanding and movement that are transferred as well as the specific elements of a skill. Thus, when the information-processing requirements (cognitive components) are similar, the effect of transfer is greater.

A player involved in a team game, such as football or hockey, would be able to transfer their spatial awareness, and their tactical understanding of passing, moving and tackling, from one game to another. Having learned to throw a cricket ball, the

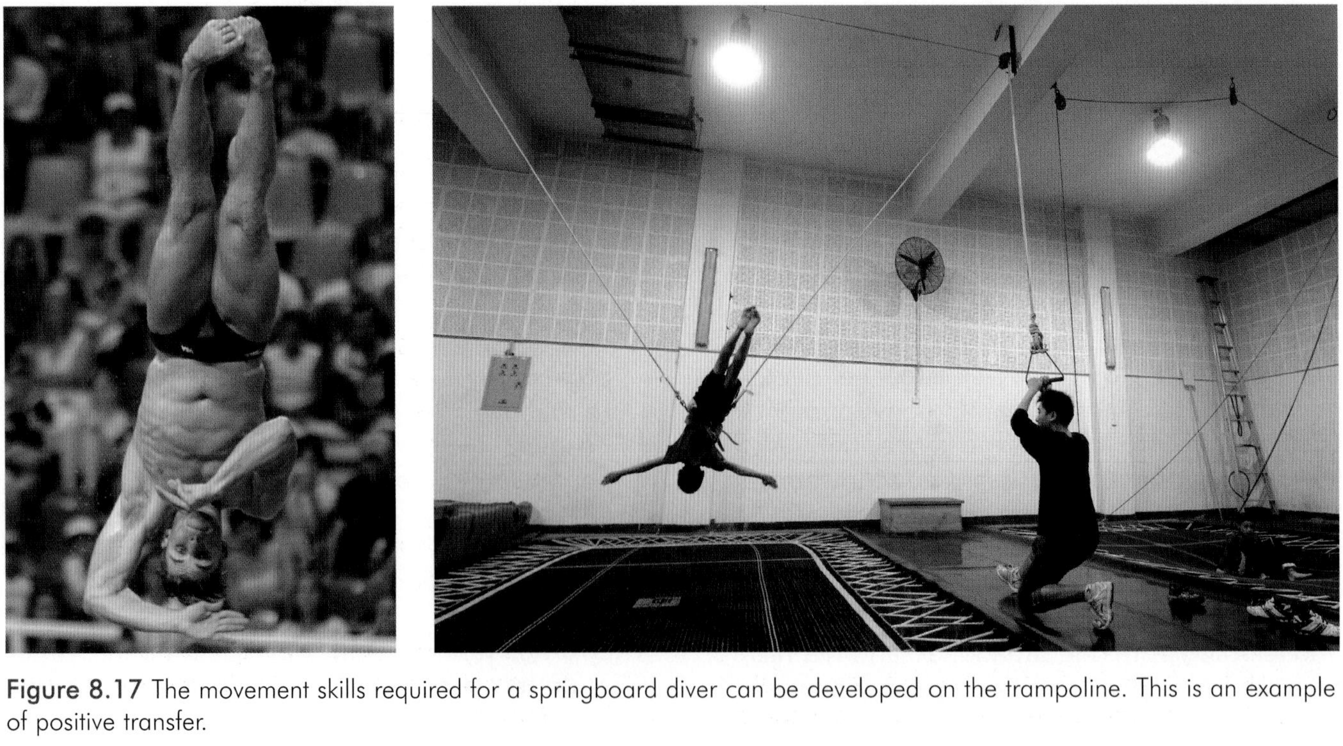

**Figure 8.17** The movement skills required for a springboard diver can be developed on the trampoline. This is an example of positive transfer.

basic principles of the movement can be transferred to throwing a javelin (see Schema theory on page 185). This view of positive transfer being more likely between activities with similar cognitive elements (information-processing conditions) has been termed transfer-appropriate processing.

## Negative transfer

When one skill/task hinders or inhibits the learning or performance of another skill/task, this is known as negative transfer. Sports performers and coaches tend to believe that this happens on a regular basis. Thankfully, the effects of negative transfer are thought to be limited and certainly temporary. It is thought to occur when a performer is required to produce a new response in a well-known situation (familiar stimulus). Stimuli are identical or similar, but the response requirements are different. Initial confusion is thought to be created more as a result of the performer having to readjust their cognitive processes than because of problems associated with the motor control of the movement. The familiar example of tennis having a negative effect on badminton is often quoted, but although the two games have similar aspects (tactics, use of space, court, net, racket, hand–eye coordination, etc.), the wrist and arm action are very different.

When a basketball or hockey coach changes tactics at set plays, any initial negative transfer is thought to be a result of the players having to readjust cognitive processes, rather than an inability to complete the movement required of them. For example, a rugby player has always been taught to fall to the ground when tackled in order to set up a ruck for his teammates. If the coach changes tactics and decides to develop a mauling game, it will be difficult for the player to stay on his feet in the tackle in order to set up a maul.

In order to overcome or limit the effects of negative transfer, teachers and coaches should be aware of areas that may cause initial confusion. Practices need to be planned accordingly, ensuring that the players are aware (direct attention) of possible difficulties they might experience. At the same time, the teacher or coach needs to be aware of possible positive effects and try to ensure that these outweigh the negative possibilities. In addition, the psychological habits of positive attitude, sustained motivation and a conscientious approach to training and practice can also be transferred positively in order to limit any negative effect, as can an understanding of how to deal with new problems.

## Bilateral transfer

In our earlier discussion of transfer we considered transfer from one skill/task to another. Bilateral transfer, however, occurs when learning is transferred from limb to limb (e.g. from the right leg to the left leg). When a basketball coach tries to develop their player's weaker dribbling hand by relating it to earlier learned skills with the strong hand, they are using bilateral transfer. This involves the player in transferring both motor proficiency and levels of cognitive involvement. The performer is thought to adjust and transfer the parameters of stored motor programmes linked to one limb action to the other (schema theory). Thus, with the appropriate practice, the levels of learning developed with the performer's stronger or preferred hand or side can be transferred to the weaker hand or side.

### Activity 11

Select a skill (e.g. a badminton serve or basketball lay-up) and attempt to execute the skill with your non-dominant hand. Discuss your experiences with a partner and explain how you modified your technique in an attempt to improve.

## Strategies a coach/teacher could employ to promote positive transfer

- Ensure that the movement and cognitive requirements of the skills are similar.
- Ensure that the performer understands the principles of transfer.
- Ensure that the performer is involved in the analysis of the skills.
- Ensure that the original skill is well learned before starting the new skill.
- Ensure that the performer practises the skill in a closed situation before trying it in a game.
- Ensure that practice is realistic.
- Ensure a variety of practice once the basics are mastered.
- Ensure that the principles of games are understood (e.g. width in attack, depth in defence).

# Goal setting

> 'A goal is what an individual is trying to accomplish. It is the object or aim of an action.'
>
> (Lock, 1981)

Goal setting is generally seen as an extremely powerful technique for enhancing performance. However, it must be carried out correctly. When used effectively, goal setting can help focus a performer's attention, help self-confidence, enhance both the intensity and persistence dimensions of motivation, and ultimately have a positive effect on performance. As can be understood from the previous section, goal setting can be used to help performers feel in control of relatively stress-provoking situations and thus help them to cope with their anxieties. However, if you refer back to intrinsic and extrinsic motivation, you will understand that when used improperly, the setting of goals, particularly wrong or unrealistic goals, not only has a negative effect on motivation but can also be a significant source of stress and anxiety in the immediate performance situation. This can lead in turn to impairment, not enhancement, of performance in the long term. Goal setting should be used with caution by coaches and teachers.

According to industrial research carried out by Lock et al. (1985) goals are seen as direct motivational strategies setting standards a performer is psychologically motivated to try to achieve, usually within a specific time.

In these discrete terms goal setting is generally thought to affect performance in the following way:

1 *Attention* – goal setting helps to direct a performer's attention (focus) to the important aspects of the task.
2 *Effort* – goal setting helps to mobilise or increase the appropriate degree of effort a performer needs to make in relation to a specific task.
3 *Persistence* – goal setting helps a performer maintain their efforts over time.
4 *New strategies* – goal setting helps a performer to develop new and various strategies in order to achieve their goals, e.g., learning (problem solving).

## Goal orientation

In considering all the factors that can affect the effectiveness of goal setting, the personality of the performer is important. The level or style of the performer's goal orientation has a differential influence (Lambert Moore Dixon 1999). High achievers (see achievement motivation) with high n.ach and low n.af motivational levels prefer challenging but realistic goals. In comparison, low achievers (low n.ach/high n.af) avoid challenging goals and usually adopt either very easy or incredibly hard goals. In addition children in the 'social comparison' stage usually focus on competitive and outcome goals. Task-orientated performers prefer performance and process goals.

Goal orientation could be:

- performance-orientated
- success-orientated (outcome)
- failure-orientated.

Most coaches and performers in sport, and people throughout their lives in general, set goals for themselves: the secret is to set the right goals and use them in the right context. Generally, in order to be effective, goals need to provide direction and enhance motivation. Goals are also seen as playing an important role in stress management. They are the standards against which perceived success or failure are measured and thus link to present attributions of success or failure.

## Types of goals

The types of goals a performer adopts or are set by the coach (goal orientation) can have a significant effect on the performer and ultimately the performance. In addition to subjective goals, e.g., having fun and enjoyment, and objective goals, e.g., reaching a particular standard, two further goals have been identified: **outcome** goals and **performance** goals.

### Outcome goals

Outcome goals generally focus on the end product. Successful competitive results, that is, winning a match or gaining some tangible reward, are usually the standard or goal set. Performers who continually make social comparisons of themselves against other performers are said to be outcome-goal-orientated. Winning and being successful enables this type of performer to maintain a positive self-image as they perceive themselves as having high personal ability (see intrinsic and extrinsic motivation and attribution.) However, a performer may produce the best game or time in their lives and still lose, as their level of achievement depends on the performance of others. If others play better, you do not achieve your outcome goal, i.e. failure.

## Performance and process goals

These generally focus on a performer's present standard of performance compared with their own previous performance, that is, they are self-referent. Levels of success are judged in terms of mastering new skills or beating a personal best. Developing a performance goal orientation has been shown to reduce anxiety in competitive situations as the performers are not worrying about social comparisons and demonstrating their competence. They can concentrate on the process of developing their performance further, i.e. process goals. Process goals focus on what can be done in order to achieve the improvement in performance required, for example, keeping your head down and following through more in order to improve your effective strike rate off the tee in golf. Performance-orientated individuals tend to attribute success to internal and controllable factors, e.g., effort, and therefore are able to experience and maintain higher levels of pride and self-satisfaction. A performer adopting performance goals (goal-orientated approach) is able to maintain motivation for longer and more consistently as competition for social comparisons is not the be all and end all of their lives. What matters for them is raising their levels of perceived ability by learning new skills.

Sports psychologists have suggested that performers who adopt different goal setting styles (outcome or performance) set different types of practice and competitive goals that will affect future cognitions and ultimately performance.

Although it is difficult for performers in modern sport not to consider winning and losing, by continually emphasising and focusing on performance goals the coach should ensure that ultimately outcome goals are achieved. For every outcome goal that is set there should be several performance and process goals.

## Principles of goal setting

In order for goals to be effective and have a positive impact on performance there are some simple principles which should be applied. Unrealistic goals can lead to a decrease in motivation, the possible development of a negative attitude and a change in behaviour, which may result in the performer becoming disillusioned as they feel unable to meet their targets.

A commonly used acronym to remember the basic principles is SMARTER:

S – Specific

M – Measureable

A – Accepted

R – Realistic

T – Time phased

E – Exciting

R – Recorded

Each of the above points are discussed in detail below.

### Specificity

Very often when teachers or coaches set goals for performers they are far too general. Telling a performer to 'try hard' or 'do your best' have been shown to be less effective than more specific objective goals. It is important that goals are specific, clear and unambiguous. This helps when evaluating goals as improvements can be assessed more easily.

### Measureable

In setting short- and long-term goals in order to chart progression, it is important that the goals can be measured in order that evaluation can take place. Setting goals without evaluation is generally a waste of time – evaluation should be accurate and happen on a regular basis. However, if evaluation becomes excessive it could possibly lead to an outcome orientated approach rather than a performance process approach.

It may be that, in the light of progress, new short-term goals can be negotiated and set. A performer may be finding the training too easy or may have achieved certain levels of success earlier than expected. New variables not thought of at first may also need to be taken into account. However, goals should not be continually changed as this may lead to a performer's uncertainty. It may also prove difficult to lower goals as performers may perceive this as some form of failure. It is important to emphasise their temporary nature and inform the performer of possible setbacks.

This point links closely with the fact that a coach must take on the following responsibilities.

**Develop goal achievement strategies** – there is no point in goals being set if a performer is not given strategies for reaching those goals. These strategies can actually also be the short-term goals. This is where the teachers or coaches sporting specific knowledge comes into play. Running, training or skills schedules can be put into operation, e.g., a performer may have to cover so many miles per week or train for longer than 20 minutes, three times per week, etc.

**Provide goal support** – in order to achieve certain goals the performer will need to make a certain commitment in terms of time and possibly even financially. This may need the regular support and understanding of their families. Facilities will be needed along with possible physiotherapy and rehabilitation support. Financial backing, motivation or an occasional shoulder to cry on may be needed.

### Accepted

It is important that the performer is involved in the goal setting process rather than having them set from some external source. The performer is more able to perceive the targets as fair and achievable and therefore more likely to accept them. They are also far more likely to be prepared to work towards them if they have been responsible for setting the goals in the first place. By understanding the needs and personality of the performer a coach is more aware of how much time is available for training etc, and through negotiation they can endeavour to foster goal acceptance and commitment.

### Realistic

In general, psychological research supports the view that difficult but realistic goals are the most effective type of goals to set. Setting easy goals has been shown to be of little value as this can result in lack of real effort and therefore motivation. Goals that are very difficult have not been shown to significantly impair performance in the long run, particularly for performance-orientated athletes. However, unrealistic goals have been shown to be stressful leading to heightened arousal, high A-state anxiety, possibly frustration, reduced future confidence and ultimately poor performance. It is obviously important, therefore, that teachers and coaches have a good understanding of the performer's or group's level of experience, ability and skill in order that appropriate goals can be set. For example, a performer with a high need to avoid failure (n.A.f) may set inappropriate goals which ensure either easy success or definite failure.

## Time Phased

### Long- and short-term goals

Individual research into whether short- or long-term goals are best is somewhat equivocal. It has generally supported the view that both need to be set. A performer needs to have an overview of where they are heading. At the same time they need to have sub-goals to enhance and reinforce development towards the main long-term goal. Short-term goals can be used to give the performer levels of progress and achievement. Interim success can serve to develop confidence, reduce anxiety, and maintain levels of motivation. Developing psychological training goals in order to reduce aspects of anxiety, such as learning relaxation techniques, can be seen as short-term goals within the context of overall performance, so set both short- and long-term goals.

### Exciting

In order to motivate the performer the goals should be viewed as a challenge. Remember in an earlier chapter we discussed the concept of the Drive Reduction Theory. If the individual or team are given a challenge which they feel is not only realistic but one that will stretch them and provide a great deal of satisfaction if are successful, their motivation levels will be higher.

### Recorded

The coach and/or the performer should always make a written record of the agreed goals. By committing the goals to paper there is no chance of their being forgotten or misinterpreted. It can be seen as a kind of unofficial contract between performer and coach/teacher. It also allows the performer to refer back to them in the future, allowing comparisons and modifications of training programmes to be made.

## What you need to know

* Learning is relatively permanent.
* Learning is due to practice or experience.
* Learning is inferred.
* There are different types of learning (cognitive, affective, effective).
* There are different phases of learning (cognitive, associative, autonomous).
* Learning develops along a continuum.
* There are different types of performance curves.
* Plateaus are to be avoided.
* Learning is affected by many variables.
* Teachers or coaches can adapt a variety of guidance techniques appropriate to the individual needs of the learner. Visual, verbal and mechanical/physical are the main types of guidance.
* Practice over an extended period, with short practice periods and limited rest periods, is generally found to be most effective.
* The effectiveness of massed or distributed practice depends on the type of task, the level of the learner and the situation.
* Sticking rigidly to one method of either whole or part practice is generally not advised. A combination is often more effective.
* Research studies have shown that learners can benefit greatly from mental practice. The effectiveness of mental practice is increased considerably if used in conjunction with, rather than instead of, physical practice.
* It is important that learners are taught how to use mental practice effectively.
* Schema are seen as generalised sets of movement patterns stored in the long-term memory, allowing performers to tailor movements to the specific demands of the situation they are faced with.
* Schema are built up through practice and experience.
* Schema theory works on the basis that there are four sources of information which are used and stored in order to modify the programme of movement.
* Variability of practice helps to develop schemas by the performer experiencing different situations.
* Schema theory suggests that every variation of a particular task/skill does not require the learning of a new motor programme.
* The principle of transfer between tasks/skills is supported by schema theory.

* Motivation is seen as energised, goal-directed, purposeful behaviour.
* Motivation is closely linked to inner drives and arousal.
* Motivation can affect the direction and intensity of behaviour.
* Motivation can be intrinsic or extrinsic.
* Extrinsic motivation is behaviour motivated by external rewards – tangible and intangible – or punishment.
* Intrinsic motivation develops as a result of internal drives to achieve feelings of personal satisfaction and fulfilment (the flow experience).
* Rewards should be monitored carefully and linked to giving information regarding a performer's level of competence.
* The key components of the behaviouristic perspective are stimulus (S) and response (R). The S–R theory is based on the concept that learning involves the development of connections or bonds between specific stimuli and responses.
* In operant conditioning, reinforcement is central to shaping behaviour.
* The teacher or coach must try to produce feelings of satisfaction to give strong reinforcements (law of effect).
* Hull's drive theory links motivation to the strengthening of the S–R bond.
* Cognitive theories suggest that performers must be able to understand events. The concept of insight is a major aspect of cognitive theories.
* When the skill/performance (response) achieved relates closely to the desired action (response) the teacher can:
  - give knowledge of results;
  - give praise/positive feedback/positive reinforcement.

  This will strengthen the S–R bond and promote success.
* If the required skill/performance is not produced, the teacher can weaken the bond between the stimulus and the inappropriate response (S–R) by:
  - giving negative feedback;
  - using punishment.
* Most behaviour in sport takes place within a social setting.
* Socialisation is the general continuous process of transmitting a culture to people and teaching them behaviour appropriate to the accepted norms, values and expectations of society.

* As a member of a sports group/team, a performer can be socialised into the 'modelled' norms of that subculture. These may be carried over and influence behaviour outside the sporting situation.
* The family is the most important prime socialising agent. However, teachers, coaches and high-status models and peers can also heavily influence a performer's behaviour.
* Social learning theory advocates that we learn and acquire new behaviours and attitudes, both acceptable and unacceptable, as a result of vicarious reinforcement through observation and imitation.
* The person being observed is the model.
* The effect of observational learning is dependent on the model having certain characteristics.
* Observational learning can take place without intention.
* The effect and level of social learning through observation is increased if the model is of a high status and their behaviour is reinforced.
* Demonstrations are an important aspect of observational learning.
* The process of observational learning involves four stages: attention, retention, motor production and motivation.
* Transfer refers to the influence of one activity/skill on another. There are a variety of types of transfer and transfer can be effective forwards or backwards in time.
* Transfer between tasks that are very similar is greater than transfer between dissimilar skills.
* The relationships between skills/concepts and cognitive processes need to be pointed out and explained to learners in order to increase the probability of positive transfer taking place.
* Teachers should try to minimise the possibility of negative transfer occurring.
* Goals will not be effective unless they are linked to specific and realistic strategies for achieving them.
* The effectiveness of goals is dependent on the interaction between individuals, i.e. coach/performer and the situation.
* Goals can be subjective or objective and can be focused on performance process or outcome.
* Performance goals should adhere to the 'SMARTER' principles.

## Review questions

1 Explain the difference between performance and learning.
2 Why can we only infer if learning has or has not taken place?
3 What are the characteristics associated with the three stages of Fitts and Posner's model of learning?
4 In what ways does a performer in the autonomous phase differ from a performer in the cognitive phase?
5 How is the notion of a continuum related to learning development?
6 Why is the term 'performance curve' used rather than 'learning curve'?
7 What is a plateau in a performance curve? What do you think it would feel like to experience it?
8 Should we infer that plateaus in performance mean learning is not taking place?
9 How might you learn from performing wrongly?
10 What factors may cause plateaus in performance?
11 Consider an ogive-shaped curve of performance for a beginner and explain the reasons behind the shape.
12 What is a schema?
13 Explain the function of recall schemas and recognition schemas.
14 What four sources of information are used to modify schemas?
15 Why is variability of practice important for the development of schemas?
16 What are the main strategies a coach can adopt in order to develop quality schemas?
17 Explain the different types of extrinsic and intrinsic motivation and provide examples of each.
18 Why is intrinsic motivation thought to be more effective than extrinsic motivation?
19 What factors should a teacher or coach be aware of when using extrinsic rewards?
20 Identify three disadvantages of extrinsic motivation.
21 If a performer is intrinsically motivated, will the introduction of extrinsic rewards enhance motivation? Explain your answer.
22 Explain three ways to develop intrinsic motivation.
23 In what ways can a teacher try to reduce the effect of negative transfer?
24 Give two practical examples of negative transfer.
25 What are the main effects of goal setting?
26 Explain outcome goals and performance goals.
27 Why are social comparisons important for outcome-goal-orientated athletes?
28 Explain the many important factors that have to be taken into account when setting goals.
29 What are goal achievement strategies?

# Opportunities for participation

SECTION

C

CHAPTER 9

# Concepts of physical activity

## Learning outcomes

**By the end of this chapter you should be able to understand the characteristics and objectives of:**

- play
- leisure, recreation and active leisure
- physical education
- outdoor and adventurous activities within educational [outdoor education] and recreational [outdoor recreation] settings
- sport
- the relationships between these concepts and be able to compare and contrast one concept with another
- the benefits of each concept, to the individual and to society

## Chapter Introduction

Society is a dynamic concept as it is constantly changing and adapting, sometimes gradually evolving over centuries, and in other instances revolutionary changes are experienced almost overnight. Sport will reflect and influence the society of which it forms an integral part.

The following chapters will hopefully highlight to you the impact society has on sport and vice versa, how this process is ongoing, continuing to affect **your** personal experiences of participating in sporting activities. Imagine a situation where you have no facilities to train, no clubs to belong to, and where the system of coaching is so underdeveloped athletes cannot improve. Imagine living in Victorian times, how different your experiences in terms of leisure, recreation, sport and education would have been. In comparison to the Victorian era:

- there is now more equality of opportunity for different social groups;
- sport has enhanced international communication;
- sport as big business has created questions about ethics and the politics of sport;
- perhaps more importantly, experiencing the human emotions connected to participation in sporting activities is what makes it a valuable subject of study.

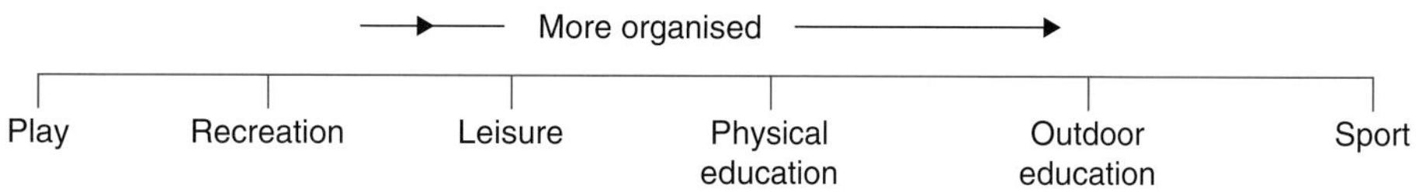


Figure 9.1 The physical activity continuum

# Factors affecting sport in society

Several factors can influence and be influenced by the system of sport and they are outlined in the diagram on the previous page. The arrows suggest the symbiotic relationship.

### Activity 1

Consider each factor and try and extend them into sub categories. For example, Education could include:

- state and private schools
- facilities
- government policies
- National Curriculum
- physical education and so on.

It is useful at this stage to choose one factor that interests you and research what influence it may have had on sport or vice versa in the past or present day.

This should give you some understanding of the type of issues that will be covered in later chapters.

Physical activity is an umbrella term for a variety of activities participated in with different motivations, for example as a:

- recreational activity;
- form of compulsory education;
- sport.

Now we need to discover exactly what we mean by these terms.

## Play

Play is something which children and adults do. It takes different forms and has different motives and benefits for each, but it can assume a great significance and importance to people's lives. A quick look in the dictionary to investigate what we mean by the word 'play' reveals that it conjures up many different meanings; e.g. 'to occupy or amuse oneself in a sport; to fulfil a particular role – he played defence; a dramatic production; play fair'. It is very difficult to extract one meaning alone, but we must attempt to tease out the common characteristics which are relevant to our field of study.

### Huizinga

The contribution of Huizinga, a Dutch cultural historian, lies in the detailed way he describes play; he provides observations but does not attempt an explanation of play. His descriptions include the following:

- Play is creative; it is repeated, alternated, transmitted; it becomes tradition.
- Play is a stepping out of real life.
- Play is uncertain. The end result cannot be determined.
- All play has rules, and as soon as the rules are transgressed, the whole play world collapses.
- Play is social. A play community generally tends to become permanent, encouraging the feeling of being together in an exceptional situation, of mutually withdrawing from the rest of the world.

> 'Play is a voluntary activity or occupation exercised within certain fixed rules of time and place, according to rules freely accepted but absolutely binding, having its aim in itself and accompanied by a feeling of tension, joy, and the consciousness that this is different from ordinary life'
>
> *(Huizinga, 1964)*

### Piaget

Piaget, a Swiss psychologist, claimed that play is:

- an end in itself;
- distinguished by the spontaneity of play as opposed to the compulsion of work;
- an activity for pleasure;
- devoid of organised structure.

Piaget believed that play was the most effective aspect of early learning. Much educational thinking has been influenced by this thought. Play is crucial for development and intelligence: the child uses its intelligence in play and is manipulative; s/he adapts to the environment by modifying feelings and thoughts.

The following definition is a useful amalgamation of the different theories of play.

'Play is activity – mental, passive or active. Play is undertaken freely and is usually spontaneous. It is fun, purposeless, self initiated and often extremely serious. Play is indulged in for its own sake; it has intrinsic value; there is innate satisfaction in the doing. Play transports the player, as it were, to a world outside his or her normal world. It can heighten arousal. It can be vivid, colourful, creative and innovative. Because the player shrugs off inhibitions and is lost in the play, it seems to be much harder for adults, with social and personal inhibitions to really play.'

(Adults play but children just play more *G. Torkildsen*)

## Implications of play

### Education

The importance given to play in terms of children's ability to learn more effectively has been taken seriously by many educationalists. Certainly in the early years there is a focus on play activities through which children will learn.

Exploratory learning led to a more **heuristic** teaching style (a device or strategy that serves to stimulate investigation). The teacher's role changed from being purely instructional to one of initiating a guidance form of learning.

**Key term**

**Heuristic:** Comes from the Greek word 'eurisko' meaning 'serves to discover or reaches understanding of'. Through heuristic play children are satisfying their natural need to explore, and are discovering for themselves the properties and behaviour of different objects and materials. The play eliminates any sense of failure as it has open-ended possibilities rather than pre-determined goals set by adults.

### Physical education lessons

There are aspects of physical education which do not match the concept of play. For example: it is compulsory; the content is chosen by the teacher; the teacher is in authority over the group; the group does not initiate the activity spontaneously.

### Recreation

Recreation managers should also take note of the positive experiences which play can generate in everyone's lives, not only children's.

### Central government

Children's play is in receipt of central government funding, which highlights the importance placed upon it. The Children's Secretary Ed Balls recently announced 'the largest government investment in children's play in this government's history' in the Children's Plan.

The Children's Plan states:

> Parents and children told us that they wanted safe places to play outside, and we know that play has real benefits for children. We will spend £225 million over the next three years to: allow up to 3,500 playgrounds nationally to be rebuilt or renewed and made accessible to children with disabilities; create 30 new adventure playgrounds for 8- to 13-year-olds in disadvantaged areas, supervised by trained staff; and a play strategy

# Leisure

The Ancient Greeks regarded 'leisure' as important for the development of the 'whole' man, his mind and body. This, however, was a state reserved only for the wealthy members of society. The growth of Christianity had a negative effect on leisure time, believing it to have little value in the preparation of the soul for the later life. The Puritan work ethic is a concept developed in the sixteenth and seventeenth centuries which valued the benefits of labour as opposed to the temptations of idleness. It has had far-reaching effects on how we view leisure; even today, work is given a much higher status than leisure activities.

## Theories of leisure

There are four major approaches to looking at leisure.

### Leisure as time

This refers to surplus time, i.e. time left over when practical necessities have been attended to. These necessities were referred to by the Countryside Recreation Research Advisory Group in 1970 as 'work, sleep, and other needs' (including family and social duties). C. Brightbill claims that people need the time, opportunity and choice to enjoy true leisure. He contrasts true leisure with enforced leisure, such as illness, unemployment or forced retirement.

## Activity 2

- Fill in a weekly timetable with all the 'necessities' mentioned on the previous page, including sleep, paid work, college/school work, domestic responsibilities, etc. Then try to approximate the amount of time you have left as leisure.
- Fill in the activities you consider to be part of your leisure time.

### Leisure as activity

Leisure activities can be subdivided into different categories of interest: sport; home entertainment; hobbies and pastimes; reading; public entertainment; holiday activities such as sightseeing.

J. Nash believes that leisure activities occur on four levels:

| | |
|---|---|
| 1 creative involvement | 2 active |
| 3 emotional | 4 passive |

Each is attributed a value; those at the apex are considered more worthy as leisure than those at the base.

Other theories claim that it is the meaning the activities have for the individuals participating which is more important than the activities themselves.

J. Dumazadier believes that leisure must be freely chosen and should benefit the individual in terms of relaxation, diversion or broadening of horizons. He uses the term 'semi-leisure' to include such activities as DIY which can be pleasurable as well as being functional.

### Leisure as an end in itself

This contradicts the idea of free time being leisure. The state of mind with which a person approaches this free time is crucial. In its ideal state, leisure should be an opportunity for self expression (J. Pieper; C. Brightbill; S. de Grazia).

### The holistic approach

J. Dumazadier believes leisure has three main functions:

1 relaxation
2 entertainment
3 self fulfilment.

In other words, leisure holds a meaning for people and this is what is most important. It can relieve stress, be an antidote to boredom and allow freer movement than is allowed in many work places.

The concept of leisure is still undergoing changes. Many people are now motivated to work, not for the sake of work but to allow them the opportunity to enjoy their leisure status. Many feel their true identity is not that which occurs at work, but that which emerges during leisure.

## Leisure and work

- Leisure is generally something people do not have to do, whereas most people have to work to earn a living.
- Work and leisure can both create a sense of self worth, creativity and personal development within a person.
- The common belief that people have more free time for leisure in the modern world, can be challenged by the fact that economic circumstances can force people to take on extra work.

In modern industrial societies, work can determine:

- how much time a person has for leisure;
- how much energy they can bring to their leisure;
- whether leisure can be pursued through work.

## Growth and change in leisure time

There are many reasons for the growth and change in leisure time in the UK:

- working hours have been reduced by the application of technology;
- labour-saving gadgets enable people to spend much less time on domestic chores in the home;
- increase in life expectancy;
- increase in disposable incomes;
- decline in the role of traditional social structures like the church and family;
- education for everyone;
- mobility of a large section of the population;
- public provision of leisure facilities including the ability to hire equipment which would otherwise be out of reach of the majority of the population;
- early retirement;
- high unemployment.

## Popular (low) culture

Individuals choose their own leisure within the context of their own culture, values and identity; the majority of the population will also be exposed to marketing forces of leisure. Popular culture is therefore defined by what is available and what represents social development.

Popular culture can also create change and trends, e.g. skateboarding, public marathons. Different aspects are given prominence at different times but generally there is less of a tendency to maintain traditional established practices. The far-reaching effects of the mass media as it transmits Western popular culture across the world can, however, result in a uniformity of cultures, rather than the richness and variety of cultures which characterise different countries.

## High culture

This traditionally refers to the cultural pursuits of the higher social classes and they usually reflect the privileged lifestyles of wealth, education and more free time. Activities pursued by this group of people are often not made easily accessible to the lower social classes, and there is a sense of cultural separation. These activities are often considered to operate on a more intellectual and refined manner to those of popular culture.

# Integrating play, recreation and leisure

Each concept has its own distinct nature, but they also have similarities; they are multidimensional and link together.

**Similarities**

- freedom
- self expression
- satisfaction
- quality
- self initiated
- no pressure or obligation to take part
- range of activities
- experiential

**Differences**

- emphasis, e.g. play has a strong emphasis on childlike spontaneity and unreality
- functions, e.g. for learning, refreshing, recreating or just being!

## Interrelationships

Leisure can be the pivot upon which the other two concepts can be embraced.

> 'leisure can conceptually embrace the freedom of play, the recreation process and the recreation institution. Leisure can be presented as the opportunity and the means for play and recreation to occur.'
>
> (*Torkildsen*)

A recreation programme combines planning, scheduling, timetabling and implementation, using resources, facilities (e.g. swimming pools, parks, natural resources, etc.) and staff to offer a wide range of services and activities. The activities will range from allowing spontaneity to being completely structured.

### Activity 3

Discuss the following philosophical viewpoints with a partner or as a class:

- All participants, regardless of athletic ability, should have equal amounts of playing time on the school curriculum.
- Physical educators should be role models and practise on the playing fields what they preach in the classroom!
- Physical education is only useful in that it provides a break from academic lessons.
- Physical education should be compulsory.

# Physical education

## What is physical education?

Physical education is an academic discipline (an organised, formal body of knowledge), which has as its primary focus the study of human movement. It may be viewed as a field of knowledge, drawing on the physical and human sciences and philosophy, with its main emphasis on physical activity. As this field of knowledge has broadened, the subject-specific areas have increased. Sub-disciplines have emerged which have diversified the subject and related it to career opportunities. Examples of such sub-disciplines are: sport sociology, biomechanics, sports medicine, exercise physiology, sport philosophy, history of sport, sports psychology and sports management. You will probably recognise some of these from your own AS level physical education course.

Physical education at this level may seem a far cry from what you have experienced during your time at school. At this stage, it is necessary to know what is meant by the term 'physical education', and to appreciate that over the last century a philosophy has developed (and will continue to develop), sometimes changing radically the practice of this subject.

Physical education is an educational process which aims to enhance total human development and performance, through movement and the experience of a range of physical activities within an educational setting. Total development means acquiring activity-specific skills and knowledge, as well as fostering positive attitudes and values which will be useful in later life. Physical education can help us to achieve a quality of life and a vitality which can be lacking in sedentary lifestyles.

**Key term**

**Sedentary:** A tendency to sit about, without taking much exercise.

### Activity 4

Consider the key words below and provide an example for each one (e.g. Knowledge: the learning of rules).

- Range of physical activities;
- Movement;
- Activity-specific skills;
- Knowledge;
- Values;
- Educational setting.

## Aims and objectives

Physical activity involves doing, thinking and feeling. Children need to know *how* to perform or express themselves; to know *about* physical activities; and to benefit from the enriching experience of knowing how it *feels* to perform.

Already we have given physical education some very difficult challenges. We are assuming that all the outcomes are positive, but this is clearly not the case. Among your peers there will be those who enjoy their physical education experiences, but

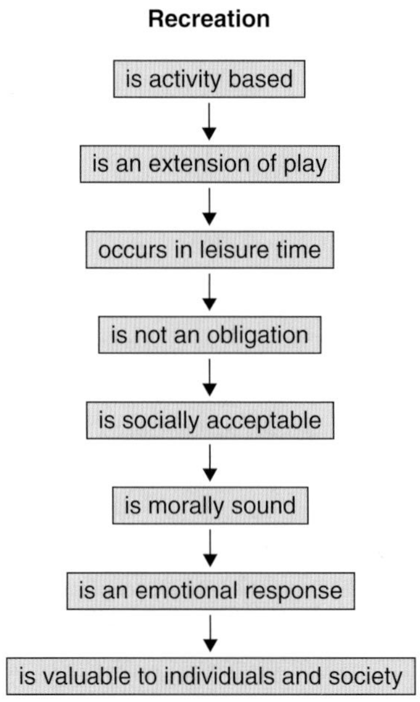
Recreation
is activity based
is an extension of play
occurs in leisure time
is not an obligation
is socially acceptable
is morally sound
is an emotional response
is valuable to individuals and society

**Figure 9.2** Values of recreation

there will also be some who definitely do not! Before we can hope to achieve the positive benefits, we must clarify the aims, objectives and desired outcomes of the physical education curriculum.

### Aims

Physical education aims to:

- develop a range of psycho-motor skills;
- maintain and increase physical mobility and flexibility, stamina and strength;
- develop understanding and appreciation of a range of physical activities;
- develop positive values and attitudes, such as sportsmanship, competition and abiding by the rules;
- help children to acquire self-esteem and confidence through the acquisition of skills, knowledge and values [**OPE**];
- develop an understanding of the importance of exercise in maintaining a healthy lifestyle.

### Objectives

Physical education can affect different areas of development. For example:

- The children will be able to complete a 20-minute run – physical development.
- The children will execute the correct technique for a gymnastic vault – motor development.
- The children will be able to explain the scoring system in badminton – cognitive development.

- The children will display enthusiasm and enjoyment and participate in extracurricular activities – affective or emotional development.

## A balanced physical education programme

A balanced programme should attempt to offer a variety of activities selected from each group in Table 9.1 (below), in order to maximise fully the opportunities to be gained from the different activities. There should be a balance of activities which are:

- team-orientated;
- individual;
- competitive;
- non-competitive movement-based.

**Table 9.1** What a child receives from quality physical education

| **Physical skills** | **Physical fitness** | **Knowledge & understanding** | **Social skills** | **Attitudes & appreciations** |
|---|---|---|---|---|
| ↓ | ↓ | ↓ | ↓ | ↓ |
| in: | such as: | of: | such as: | such as: |
| • games;<br>• gymnastics;<br>• dance;<br>• swimming;<br>• track and field;<br>• outdoor and adventurous activities;<br>• fitness programme. | • functional fitness capacities essential to health and well-being;<br>• cardiorespiratory efficiency;<br>• muscular strength;<br>• muscular endurance;<br>• flexibility;<br>• motor ability capacities: speed, balance, agility, coordination and reaction time. | • safety;<br>• physical skills;<br>• physical fitness;<br>• body systems;<br>• learning processes;<br>• social skills;<br>• scientific principles of movement;<br>• environmental concerns;<br>• rules;<br>• strategies;<br>• community recreational opportunities. | • fair play;<br>• cooperation, teamwork and sharing;<br>• responsibility;<br>• leadership and citizenship;<br>• competition;<br>• communication: listening, speaking, performance and demonstrating;<br>• operating with rules;<br>• self-control: work under pressure;<br>• following directions;<br>• resourcefulness;<br>• self-direction;<br>• consideration of others. | • desire to participate in physical activities;<br>• desire to be physically active;<br>• interest in health and responsibility for personal care;<br>• appreciation of fair play operating within the rules;<br>• respect for team-mates, opponents and officials;<br>• appreciation of own abilities and the abilities of others;<br>• appreciation of the relationship between exercise and health;<br>• appreciation of the quality effort in the work of others;<br>• feelings of pride and loyalty in the accomplishments of self, school and others;<br>• interest in a positive self-concept. |

Source: *The British Journal of Teaching Physical Education*, Autumn 2002

## Activity 5

Think of a couple of activities you regularly participate in but possibly at different levels with different attitudes. List the reasons why you may participate in both.

## Activity 6

Ask a group of your peers about their experiences of physical education (including the types of activities, and what they enjoyed most or least). You can ask general or more specific questions.

## Activity 7

1 Study the aims of physical education and see how you might link these to the activities shown in Table 9.2.
2 Tick the activities which you have experienced during your secondary education. Do you think you received a balanced physical education programme?
3 Conduct a survey of approximately six schools in your local area. Try to find out what they offer their pupils. Can you find parallels or many variations? Does what is on offer reflect the different nature of the schools?

**Table 9.2** A balanced physical education programme

| Games | | | | Movement |
|---|---|---|---|---|
| **Invasion** | **Net** | **Striking/field** | **Rebounding** | |
| football | tennis | cricket | squash | gymnastics |
| netball | volleyball | rounders | | dance |
| hockey | table tennis | softball | | trampolining |
| rugby | | | | athletics |
| | | | | swimming |

## Who chooses the physical education programme?

In the UK there is a decentralised system, by which the teacher and the individual school have the power to produce their own programme, though they are increasingly bound by government guidelines. The national curriculum now sets out which subjects are to be taught at each key stage of a pupil's schooling. Physical education is compulsory from Key Stage 1 (ages 5 to 7) through to Key Stage 4 (up to age 16).

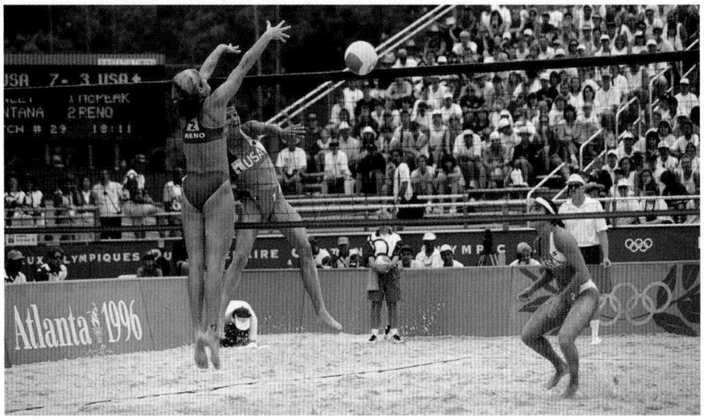


**Figure 9.3** Play, recreation, leisure or sport?

**National curriculum** The national curriculum attempts to raise standards in education and make schools more accountable for what they teach. Physical education continues to be one of only five subjects which pupils of all abilities must pursue, from their entry to school at age 5, until the end of compulsory schooling at age 16.

Attainment targets and programmes of study have been written for physical education. Children are required to demonstrate the knowledge, skills and understanding involved in areas of various physical activities, including dance, athletics, gymnastics, outdoor and adventurous activities, and swimming. There are four key stages.

**Key Stage 1**

During key stage 1 pupils build on their natural enthusiasm for movement, using it to explore and learn about their world. They start to work and play with other pupils in pairs and small groups. By watching, listening and experimenting, they develop their skills in movement and coordination, and enjoy expressing and testing themselves in a variety of situations.

*Breadth of study*
During the key stage, pupils should be taught the knowledge, skills and understanding through dance activities, games activities and gymnastic activities.

**Figure 9.4** Key Stage 1 – programme of study

**Key Stage 2**

During key stage 2 pupils enjoy being active and using their creativity and imagination in physical activity. They learn new skills, find out how to use them in different ways, and link them to make actions, phrases and sequences of movement. They enjoy communicating, collaborating and competing with each other. They develop an understanding of how to succeed in different activities and learn how to evaluate and recognise their own success.

*Breadth of study*
During the key stage, pupils should be taught the knowledge, skills and understanding through five areas of activity:

a) dance activities
b) games activities
c) gymnastic activities

and two activity areas from:

d) swimming activities and water safety
e) athletic activities
f) outdoor and adventurous activities.

**Figure 9.5** Key Stage 2 – programme of study

**Key Stage 3**

During key stage 3 pupils become more expert in their skills and techniques, and how to apply them in different activities. They start to understand what makes a performance effective and how to apply these principles to their own and others' work. They learn to take the initiative and make decisions for themselves about what to do to improve performance. They start to identify the types of activity they prefer to be involved with, and to take a variety of roles such as leader and official.

*Breadth of study*
During the key stage, pupils should be taught the knowledge, skills and understanding through four areas of activity. These should include:

a) games activities

and three of the following, at least one of which must be dance or gymnastic activities:

b) dance activities
c) gymnastic activities
d) swimming activities and water safety
e) athletic activities
f) outdoor and adventurous activities.

**Figure 9.6** Key Stage 3 – programme of study

**Key Stage 4**

During key stage 4 pupils tackle complex and demanding activities applying their knowledge of skills, techniques and effective performance. They decide whether to get involved in physical activity that is mainly focused on competing or performing, promoting health and well-being, or developing personal fitness. They also decide on roles that suit them best including performer, coach, choreographer, leader and official. The view they have of their skilfulness and physical competence gives them the confidence to get involved in exercise and activity out of school and in later life.

*Breadth of study*
During the key stage, pupils should be taught the knowledge, skills and understanding through two of the six activity areas.

**Figure 9.7** Key Stage 4 – programme of study

## Activity 8

Beach Volleyball (Figure 9.3) has grown significantly in the last decade. How can it meet the needs of the individual in terms of recreation and sport?

## Activity 9

1 Summarise the general requirements for each key stage of the national curriculum.
2 What factors may a teacher have to take into account when devising a syllabus?

## The importance of physical education

Physical education develops pupils' physical competence and confidence, and their ability to use these to perform in a range of activities. It promotes physical skilfulness, physical development and a knowledge of the body in action. Physical education provides opportunities for students to be creative, competitive and to face up to different challenges, as individuals and in groups and teams. It promotes positive attitudes towards active and healthy lifestyles.

Students learn how to think in different ways, to suit a wide variety of creative, competitive and challenging activities. They learn how to plan, perform and evaluate actions, ideas and performances, to improve their quality and effectiveness. Through this process, pupils discover their aptitudes, abilities and preferences, and make choices about how to become involved in lifelong physical activity.

**IN CONTEXT**

**Figure 9.8 shows data from a survey published by the European Union of Physical Education Associations. The survey shows the amount of time spent per week on physical education in schools in the USA and Europe. At primary level, the UK is ninth out of ten, and at secondary level, the UK ranks bottom.**

The DfES also conducted a survey in the 1990s, which showed that many schools are still not devoting two hours a week to physical education, as recommended.

### Activity 10

Suggest reasons why one-third of secondary schools in the UK do not manage to provide the recommended two hours of physical education per week.

### Physical education as preparation for leisure

As young people approach the end of their compulsory years of schooling, it is necessary to foster an awareness of the opportunities available in the community. As a result of the philosophy of educating children for their leisure time, schools began to offer options in the later years of schooling, where a wider variety of activities could be experienced, sometimes using community facilities. This was made possible by smaller groups, guided by additional non-specialist staff. Students should be informed about and put in contact with local clubs and sports centres.

This is an area of weakness in the UK, as there are traditionally poor links between schools and community sport, as a result of trying to maintain a distance between sport and physical education.

## Developments in school sport

The term 'sport' refers to the 'physical activities with established rules engaged in by individuals attempting to outperform their competitors' (Wuest and Bucher 1991). Sport provides different opportunities for physical activity while at school. Its main focus is on improving performance standards, rather than the educational process, and it takes place mainly outside the formal curriculum. It is usually viewed as an opportunity for children to extend their interest or ability in physical activities.

The changes which have taken place in society and education since the mid 1980s (e.g. extracurricular opportunities) have affected school sport, with a reduction in emphasis on the sporting elite, which sometimes required a disproportionate amount of resources for a small number of children. Extracurricular clubs, open to all, became more acceptable. However, extracurricular activities were affected by some of the following factors:

1 The teachers' strikes in the early 1980s – the contractual hours and lack of monetary incentives tended to diminish teachers' goodwill, and clubs were disbanded.
2 Financial cuts were felt in terms of transport.
3 The local management of schools allowed schools to supplement their funds by selling off school fields.
4 The increasing amount of leisure and employment opportunities for children meant they were less attracted to competing for their school team.
5 The anticompetitive lobby became more vocal – they espoused the theory that competition in sport was not good for children's development.

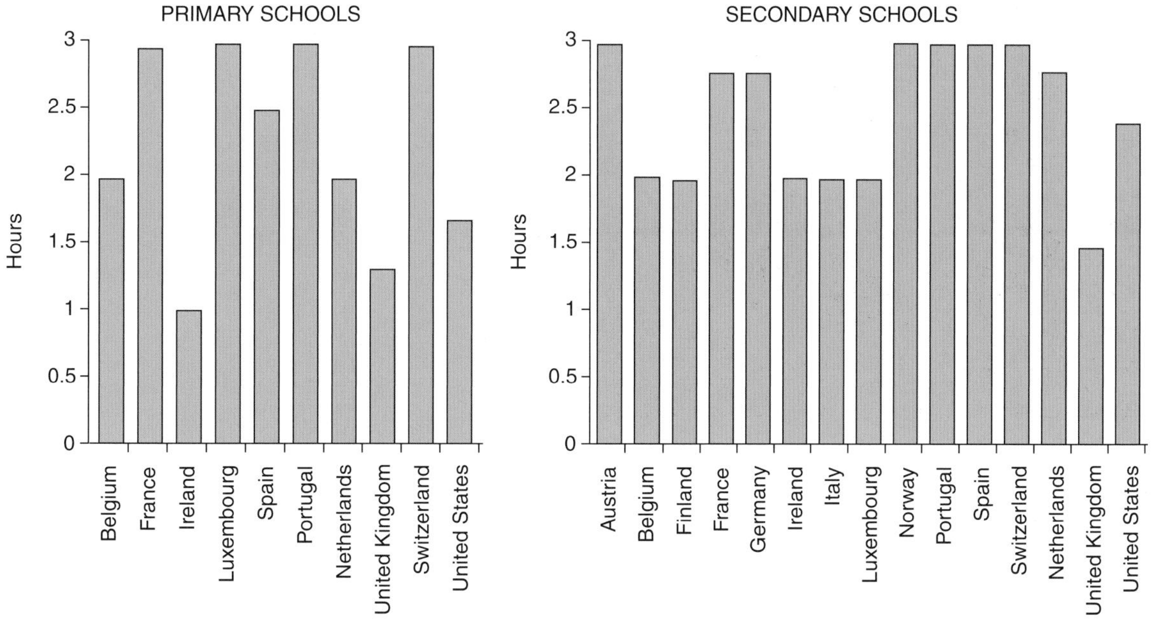


**Figure 9.8** The amount of time devoted to PE in schools in the UK compared to the rest of Europe and the USA
*Source*: European Union of Physical Education Associations

Through its Department for Children, Schools and Families, the government has put forward a number of initiatives to increase the range and amount of school sport available to young people aged 5–16 years:

- By 2008, they hope to engage 75 per cent of children in each school partnership in two hours of high-quality PE and school sport per week, within and beyond the curriculum.
- By 2010 the ambition is to offer all children at least four hours of sport, made up of at least two hours of high-quality PE within the curriculum, and at least an additional two to three hours out of school, delivered by a range of school, community and club providers.

Some of the initiatives in operation are set out below:

1 Club Links – This programme links schools with local sports clubs and is being delivered through the national governing bodies of 22 sports.
2 Competition Managers – The government's Department for Culture, Media and Sport is appointing Competition Managers to develop a programme of inter-school competitions in a number of pilot areas. The Department aims to have a Competition Manager in all School Sport Partnerships by 2010.
3 Step into Sport – This is a joint initiative with the Department for Children, Schools and Families, and is one of the eight strands in the national School Sports Strategy. Step into Sport provides sports leadership and volunteering opportunities for young people aged 14–19 years.
4 Sport kitemarks for schools – Following consultation on proposals to introduce changes to sport kitemarks, two key changes have been agreed:
    1 Kitemarks will reward delivery of the national PE, School Sports and Club Links strategy. They will therefore only be open to schools which are in a School Sport Partnership.
    2 Kitemarks will be awarded annually, and this will happen automatically through the national school sport survey, so there will be no need to complete a separate application form.

A high-quality physical education for all children is central to the Government's new PE School Sport and Club Links Strategy (PESSCL).

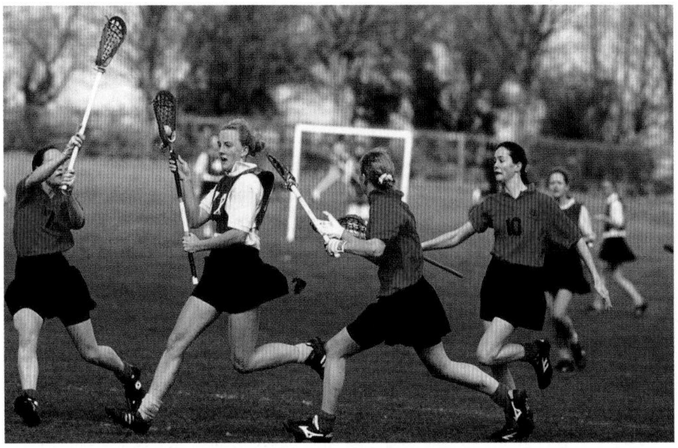

Figure 9.9 School sport encourages teamwork

Table 9.3 Advantages and disadvantages of competitive sport

| Advantages | Disadvantages |
|---|---|
| Children have a natural competitive instinct, and as they are more motivated to practise, enjoyment of sport increases | Continued feelings of failure can cause stress and anxiety |
| Can raise self-esteem and help children learn how to cope with failure and success | The need to win can encourage unsporting behaviour |

## Physical education or sport?

This is an ongoing debate, which resurfaced in the 1995 document *Sport: Raising the Game*, with the government's decision to give competitive sport a higher status. The terms 'physical education' and 'sport' are complex. There is an overlap between them, but the central focus of each one is different. The aim of physical education is to educate the individual, while sport has other purposes, such as achieving excellence, fitness and earning an income. A good physical education programme can be the foundation on which extracurricular opportunities can be extended and enhanced. However, physical education teachers should not necessarily feel pressured into allowing a 'sport' ethos to creep into the curriculum.

## Sport education

'Sport education' is a term used to describe a pupil-centred rather than teacher-centred approach. Children are encouraged to be continually involved in the learning process. This gives every child an opportunity to have some form of success within school physical education, even if they are not particularly physically gifted. Children are given responsibility for organising aspects of lessons, such as equipment management, practice drills and working constructively in teams to include each member. Inclusion of all children is therefore a key factor.

# Outdoor and adventurous activities

Outdoor and adventurous activities take place in the natural environment, including situations which are dangerous and challenging, suggesting conquest of natural obstacles or terrain. Examples of such activities are rock climbing, skiing and skydiving. New activities continue to develop, mostly as a result of technological advances, such as jet-skiing and windsurfing.

It is possible to participate in these activities through a recreational and/or an educational approach:

- Outdoor education: participation in outdoor and adventurous activities in the natural environment, developing educational values. For example, a school may offer orienteering within the school grounds, or arrange a visit to a national park or other area where adventurous activities may be undertaken.
- Outdoor recreation: participation in outdoor and adventurous activities within the natural environment in an individual's free time.

When individuals participate in a *recreational* capacity there are no rules as such, no winners or losers and therefore no officials. There is usually a code of etiquette, however, concerning safety and the conservation of the natural environment.

### Activity 11

1. List as many activities as you can which take place in the natural environments of water, mountains, air and countryside.
2. Where people do not have easy access to these areas, how could you adapt the urban environment for them to learn the basic skills of some of these sports?

Recently, many of these activities have become *sports*, involving scoring systems and officials, for example, white-water slalom races and speed climbing. These activities can place the individual in situations which are dangerous and challenging, and which induce exhilaration, fear and excitement. They can be competitive, but more often the competition is against the elements or the human body rather than against another person. When an individual is facing the elements, the main challenge they face is differentiating between real and perceived risk.

The personal qualities required for and enhanced by these activities include:

- self-reliance;
- decision-making skills;
- leadership;
- the ability to trust others;
- trustworthiness.

Such activities are not usually done alone, and the ability to work with others to overcome obstacles is often important.

**Key terms**

**Risk:** The possibility of incurring injury or loss; being exposed to danger or a hazard. Outdoor and adventurous activities pose situations of real and perceived risk.

**Real risk:** Risk from the natural environment, such as a rock fall. Leaders need to be aware of the potential risks when planning routes and so on.

**Perceived risk:** This is where the sense of adventure comes from, and leaders need to be aware of this. If the perceived risk is too great for the ability level of the performer, however, feelings of anxiety could become overwhelming.

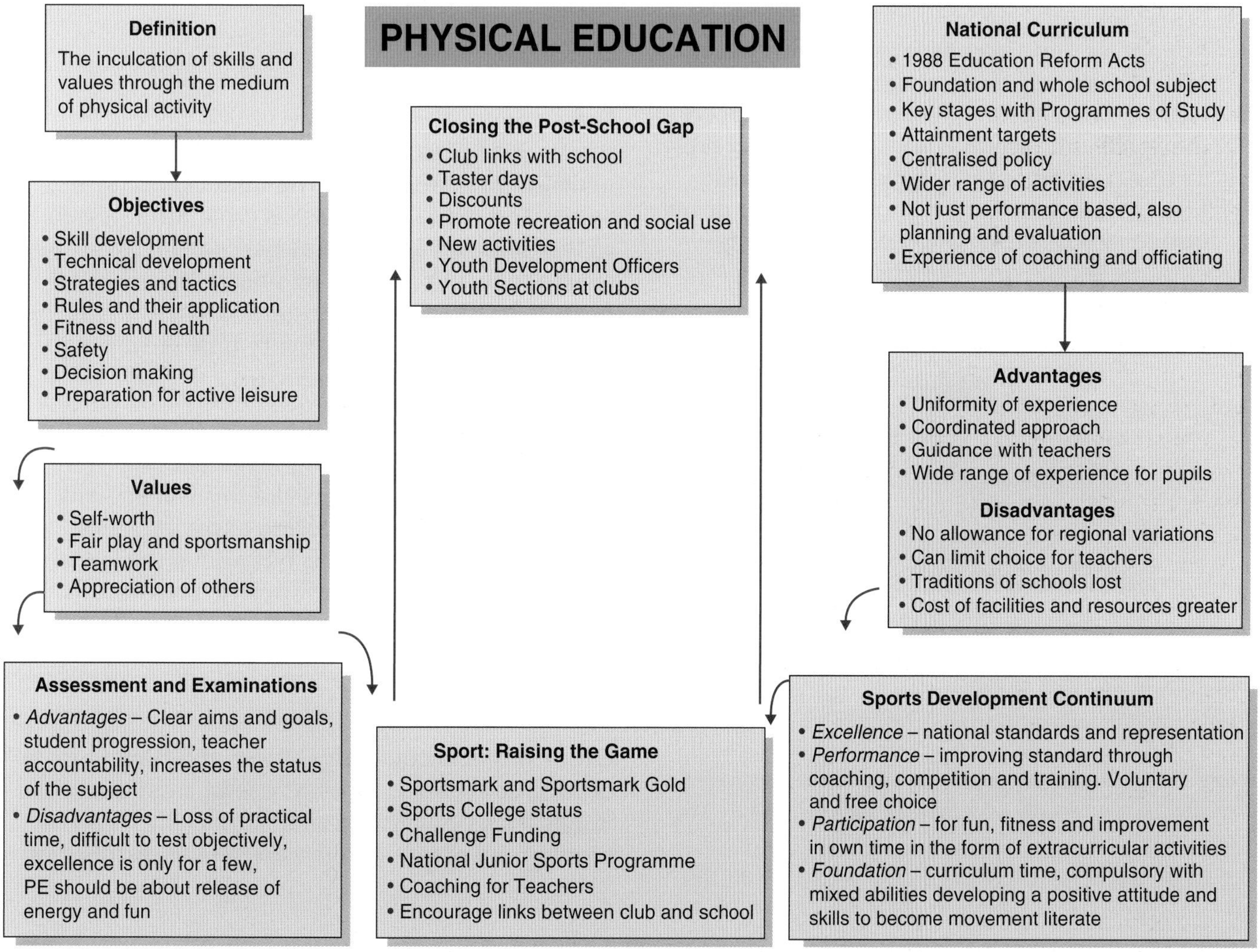


**Figure 9.10** Physical education

## Growth of outdoor and adventurous activities

There has been considerable growth in both traditional (e.g. canoeing, rock climbing, abseiling, climbing) and 'new' (e.g. jet-skiing, snowboarding, mountain biking) adventure sports. The reasons for this growth can be explained by:

- increasingly sedentary lifestyles, which make some people seek more active and exciting leisure time;
- increased leisure time and standards of living, which make these activities more accessible;
- the development of new and exciting sports technology;
- the appreciation of the natural environment, particularly as a release from urban pressures.

According to Mortlock, there are four broad stages of adventure:

- Play – little challenge in developing skills/ boredom could set in.
- Adventure – more challenging environment/ skills developed under safe conditions.
- Frontier adventure – the individual is placed in more difficult terrain where well-learned skills can be put to the test/challenge/conquest.
- Misadventure – where things go wrong, either due to lack of preparation or due to more extreme terrain and climatic conditions.

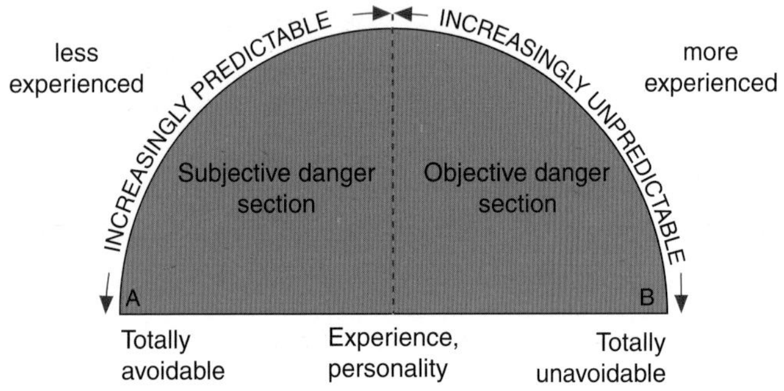


**Figure 9.11** Mortlock diagram
*Source*: C. Mortlock (1984) *The Adventure Alternative*, Cicerone Press

**Note:** Beginners will work at the left end of the base line AB. Experienced climbers will work from the right end of the base line.

### Activity 12

1 If you were a leader of a mixed ability group, which stages of adventure would you aim to achieve for your group, and which factors would you aim to avoid?
2 Plan an activity which could come under the outdoor education umbrella. Note the pitfalls which could arise.

### Danger

Danger is the state of being vulnerable to injury. In the sporting arena this risk is heightened in outdoor and adventurous activities. Two types of danger are outlined by Mortlock. Subjective danger is that which is under the control of the individual, such as the choice of safe and appropriate equipment, and the choice of route. There is no such control over objective danger, however, such as an avalanche.

## Risk assessment

Fears about liability are preventing people from teaching and learning about risk. Outdoor activities *are* dangerous. The freedom to face, assess and manage the risk is what attracts people to these sports. Society has become increasingly averse to facing risk and all efforts are made to protect children from dangerous situations. Is this really a healthy attitude? Every time we cross the road we make a risk assessment.

'Risk assessment' is becoming a familiar term to anyone involved in leading other people. There is a danger that precautions like this will actually prevent schools from offering experiences of outdoor activities. Sport is not above the law and the changing attitudes of society have had an impact in this area, as elsewhere.

## Cross-curricular issues

Other subjects could also utilise and benefit from outdoor education as it has useful cross-curricular implications; environmental issues which can be highlighted are inequalities in wealth distribution, land use, forestation and deforestation, energy sources and the problems caused by people and pollution. However, it must not lose its own unique contribution in its own right. The United Kingdom lags far behind many other countries in its provision, and many outdoor education residential centres have been threatened with closure.

## Outdoor education and the school curriculum

There are strong reasons why outdoor education should be included in the school curriculum: namely, the benefit to the personal and social education of children, through experiential learning. Other subjects could also utilise and benefit from outdoor education, which has useful cross-curricular implications.

The national curriculum does not require that outdoor education is taught, though schools can arrange for it to be included. The skills which can be experienced and learned directly are an intrinsic element of Key Stages 3 and 4 of the adventurous activity option in physical education.

In an already constricted timetable, few schools have the commitment to the subject to support and sustain outdoor education:

- The Education Reform Act 1988 increased the problems schools experienced in offering these activities.
- The fundamental changes to the way in which schools are funded have also seriously affected the opportunities for teachers to gain valuable in-service training in order to achieve the appropriate qualifications.
- Local education authorities may no longer have access to sufficient funds to provide for this training.
- The law regarding charging pupils for out-of-school activities may cause schools to limit or abandon such activities, as voluntary contributions may not be sufficient. This could mean that only the wealthier schools are able to participate, so these activities would retain their elite image.
- The increasing concern over safety issues presents another problem for schools.

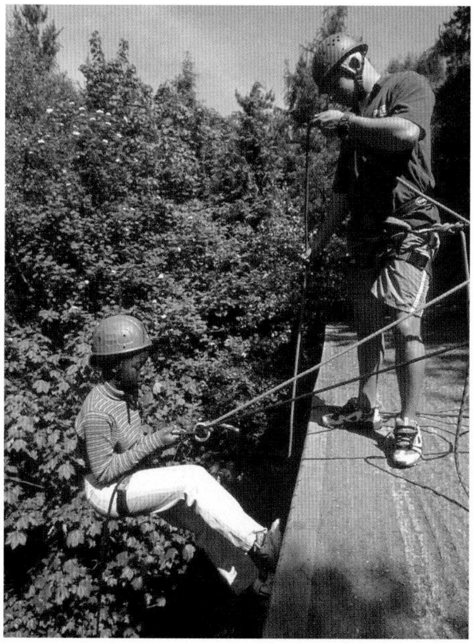

Figure 9.12 Outdoor activities should be available to everyone

## Tourism and environmental safeguards

Outdoor pursuits are growth sports, but there are also some problems which need to be addressed. The UK lags far behind many other countries in its provision of outdoor activities, and many outdoor education residential centres have been threatened with closure.

The areas in which these activities often take place are country parks, nature reserves, green belt areas, areas of outstanding natural beauty and national parks. Conflicts can emerge between the sport participants, landowners and the environment. The UK is a relatively small island, with high-density population. Problems caused by the growth in tourism and outdoor activities will be felt here more keenly than in much larger countries such as the USA and France, which have lower population density.

Some of the problems caused are:

- erosion of land and river banks;
- pollution caused by motor sports;
- the increase in the number of vehicles disturbing wildlife and local residents.

The most radical solution would be to ban the activities, but it might be more viable to plan for these activities in order to minimise the damage inflicted on the environment. The agencies concerned need to liaise with each other to produce effective strategies. These agencies

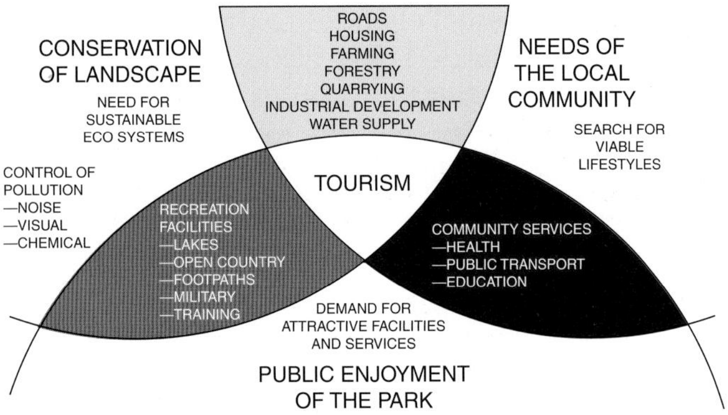


**Figure 9.13** Causes of conflict in a national park

include the home country sports council, the CCPR, the governing bodies of the individual sports, local authorities, the Countryside Commission and the Association of National Park Authorities.

**IN CONTEXT**

**The Outward Bound Trust began to pioneer outdoor activities in the 1940s. It has five centres in Britain, including Aberdovey in Wales, Ullswater in the Lake District and Loch Eil in Scotland. It is now a worldwide organisation. Outward Bound works in partnership with the Duke of Edinburgh's Award Scheme. Its main aim is to promote personal development training for young people, placing them in challenging situations, such as physical expeditions, skills courses and the city challenge (an urban alternative). The challenging and often rugged activities include living in the wilderness, mountain climbing, canoeing, skiing and touring on bicycles.**

## Exam-style questions

**1** The following activities are examples of outdoor education activities:

Abseiling Orienteering Canoeing Hill Walking

What can young people gain from outdoor education and why do our children not have the opportunity to experience regular or varied outdoor education?

# Sport

What is sport? We know that Sport England refers to numerous activities as sport; we have sports clubs; hunting is called a sport; a person can be referred to as 'a good sport', and so on. In general we use the term loosely in normal conversation, but when we are relating important sociological concepts to sport (such as discrimination, funding and its relationship to physical education), it is necessary to focus quite specifically on what we mean by the term.

A definition of sport would be useful, to examine the key elements. Sport can be defined as:

> 'institutionalised competitive activities that involve vigorous physical exertion or the use of relatively complex physical skills by individuals whose participation is motivated by a combination of intrinsic and extrinsic factors'
>
> *(Coakley, 1993)*

What do we mean by some of these terms?

### Institutionalised

- A standardised set of behaviour recurs in different situations;
- Rules are standardised;
- Officials regulate the activity;
- Rationalised activities involve strategies, training schedules and technological advances;
- Skills are formally learned.

### Physical activities

- skills, prowess, exertion;
- balance, coordination;
- accuracy;
- strength, endurance.

The extent of the physical nature of the activity can vary and can lead us to question whether an activity such as darts is a sport. Darts is referred to as a sport via the media, but the fact that it does not require much physical exertion can place it lower down on the sport continuum, even though it meets other criteria for inclusion as a sport. Any activity which does not meet all the criteria listed above would have less status as a sport.

## Activity 13

Using a variety of equipment, devise a game within a group.

- What characterised the development of this game?
- What would you have to do to change it into a PE lesson?
- What would you have to do to turn this game into an Olympic activity?

**Key terms**

**Physical Endeavour:** Where the body is working very hard and expending a considerable amount of energy.
**Physical Prowess:** Outstanding or superior physical skill.

## Motivation for participation in sport

| Intrinsic | Extrinsic |
|---|---|
| • self satisfaction | • money |
| • fun | • medals |
| • enjoyment | • fame |
| • own choice | • obligation |
| • 'play spirit'. | • praise. |

Most people will combine both of these motivations in the approaches they adopt towards sport participation. Colin Montgomerie says:

> 'I used to get tense about the money angle of it, the financial situation you found yourself in when suddenly you had to putt for a prize the size of someone's salary. Now it's not the financial side, it's trying to beat my peers. I don't need to be paid. Don't tell the sponsors that. But when I finish a tournament and I've beaten my peers, I don't need to be paid. The feeling I have is terrific, of success and freedom, if you like. That's what I do it for.'
>
> (*The Daily Telegraph* Sat. Oct. 16, 1999)

**IN CONTEXT**

**Progression from recreation → sport**

**The following situation may help clarify this complex concept as we have developed the argument so far:**

**Two friends who kick a football in the street are involved in an informal, social occasion. Physical exertion is present and skills are developing, but the people are involved in recreation rather than sport. If they challenged two other friends to a competition, this has moved to a situation called a contest or match. It is competitive but still under informal conditions. Only when they follow formalised rules and confront each other under standardised conditions can their situation be called sport.**

**Merely playing a recognised physical activity is not enough to allow us to call it sport. The situation under which it is operating is also important and needs consideration.**

**EXAMINER'S TIP**

Though you may not be directly examined on the historical development of sport it is worth remembering that the present day is the culmination of many centuries, and to truly understand the values and judgements we make about sport we need to be able to analyse it in the context of the past.

## Benefits of sport

Sport can:

- act as an emotional release;
- offer individuals an opportunity to express their own individuality;
- help in the socialisation of people, i.e. encourage a collective spirit and persuade people away from social unrest;
- provide people with values which are positively viewed by society such as fair play and sportsmanship;
- help people achieve success when other avenues of achievement are not available to them;
- help highlight issues which can be changed;
- help achieve health and fitness;
- have economic benefits to individuals (income) and nations' economies;
- create a challenge and provide enjoyment.

## Problematic areas

- Sport can help to retain and reinforce discrimination.
- Too much emphasis can be placed on winning, and financial rewards intensify this. Gamesmanship has become more acceptable in the modern day sports world.
- Competition, if not handled well, can be damaging to an individual.
- Excessive behaviour can be encouraged through sport, such as deviancy.
- Spectator sport can begin to outweigh active participation.
- Media coverage can dominate sports and their type of coverage can determine the wealth of a sport.

## Summary


- You should have a clearer picture of differences between the concepts of play, physical and outdoor recreation/education and sport; their unique features and also features which complement and relate to each other.
- People become involved in sport for various reasons and at various levels; each activity provides different challenges and experiences.
- Each of the concepts has implications for the individual and for society.
- It is useful to understand how they have developed over a period of time in order to fully appreciate the present situation
- Very often the physical activities used are the same – it is the attitude with which they are undertaken which makes the difference.


### Activity 14

Using an A3 sheet of paper, list as many key words as you can under recreation, leisure, physical education, outdoor recreation and sport.

## What you need to know

* Physical activity is an umbrella term for a variety of energetic pursuits from games to athletic, gymnastic and outdoor and adventurous activities.
* Physical activities can be participated in either recreationally or on a more formalised and structured level.
* Regular participation in physical activities provides benefits to the individual and society.
* The benefits of regular participation to the individual occur on a:
  - physiological level, such as improved cardiovascular endurance;
  - psychological level, as in releasing aggressive tendencies;
  - emotional level, such as making an individual feel a worthwhile person with a sense of achievement.
* Many factors (for example, the growth in electronic games) are responsible for people adopting a more sedentary lifestyle.
* Young people in particular are at risk from future health problems.
* The government needs to develop policies to try and counteract the problem, but first needs to understand some of the barriers that face young people in their level of participation.
* Physical recreation offers participation opportunities to all members of the community for them to enjoy in their own leisure time and voluntarily. It operates on a relaxed and more informal level. Opportunities can be provided by social agencies, such as a local Authority, and must have a positive effect on an individual's life.
* Outdoor recreation is the participation in outdoor and adventurous activities in the natural environment in an individual's free time. An example would be a skiing trip with friends.
* Physical education is the instilling of knowledge, skills and values through the medium of physical activity in an educational setting.
* Outdoor education is participation in outdoor and adventurous activities in the natural environment within an educational setting. An example would be a school ski trip.
* Sport is the most formalised of all the concepts. It is institutionalised and competitive and requires a more highly developed level of skill.

## Review Questions

1 Give five characteristics of the concept of Play.

2 What word does the term 'recreation' derive from and what does it mean?

3 What is the implication of the words 'activity' and 'experience' when applied to the term recreation?

4 How can work affect people's leisure time?

5 What factors have led to the growth in leisure time?

6 What are the key terms that characterise the term Physical Education?

7 Name five aims of Physical Education.

8 What is the main difference between Outdoor Education and Outdoor Recreation?

9 What constraints determine the level of Outdoor Education whilst at school in the United Kingdom?

10 What are some of the benefits and problems associated with participating in sporting activities?

# CHAPTER 10

# Current provision for active leisure

## Learning outcomes

**By the end of this chapter you should understand the following:**

- the characteristics and goals of the public, private and voluntary sectors;
- the advantages and disadvantages for the public, private and voluntary sectors;
- the concept of Best Value in relation to public sector provision.

## CHAPTER INTRODUCTION

This chapter explores the role that sport assumes in the political and social arena. It examines the organisation, administration and policymaking process of sport, helping you to reflect on major sporting and social issues. The importance with which the government in power views sport makes a huge difference to the opportunities available, from the grass roots of sport to sporting excellence.

Before we study the provision for sport at varying levels of participation, we are going to look at a summary of participation trends outlined by the DCMS, which will highlight the significance of this chapter.

## Participation

### A summary of participation trends

- The quality and quantity of participation in sport and physical activity in the UK is lower than it could be, and levels have not changed significantly over recent years:
  - for sport: only 46 per cent of the population participate in sport more than 12 times a year, compared to 70 per cent in Sweden and almost 80 per cent in Finland;
  - for physical activity: only 32 per cent of adults in England take 30 minutes of moderate exercise five times a week, compared to 57 per cent of Australians and 70 per cent of Finns.
- Young white males are most likely to take part in sport and physical activity, and the most disadvantaged groups are least likely to do so. Participation falls dramatically after leaving school, and continues to drop with age. But the more active you are in sport and physical activity at a young age, the more likely you are to continue to participate throughout your life.
- The UK's performance in international sport is better than we might think. UK Sport's index of success places us third in the world. However, we are not as successful in the sports we care most about as a nation.
- The UK successfully hosts major sporting events each year (such as Wimbledon and the London Marathon), with little government

involvement. Problems have arisen with the so-called 'mega events' (Olympics, FIFA World Cup, UEFA European Championships, World Athletics Championships and Commonwealth Games), which require significant infrastructure investment. Historically, there has been poor investment appraisal, management and coordination for some of these events.

- Total government and lottery expenditure on sport and physical activity in England is estimated to be roughly £2.2 billion per year. A significant proportion of this is distributed via local authorities. The funding of sport and physical activity is fragmented, and some strands of funding may not be sustainable, as money from the National Lottery and TV rights is decreasing and local government budgets are being squeezed. In contrast, there is major public investment planned for school sports facilities.
- Broadly speaking, sport and physical activity are delivered through four sectors:
  1. local government (e.g. your local council);
  2. education (schools, FE and HE);
  3. voluntary sector (clubs and national governing bodies of sport);
  4. private sector (e.g. privately owned golf clubs). The role of the health sector in physical activity is also important. However, government's interaction with these sectors is through a complex set of organisations, with overlapping responsibilities and unclear accountability. The situation is further complicated at the international level, because some sports compete as United Kingdom/Great Britain, some as home countries, and some as both.

## Participation pyramid

As part of our study we need to investigate the various levels of participation in sporting activities. This will range from:

- the broad base of the pyramid, where the main emphasis is on participation; to the
- apex of the pyramid, where the focus is on the standard of performance.

For ease of study, society will be categorised into distinct groups based on age, disability, gender, socio-economics, culture and race, and we will consider each one in relation to the opportunities for sporting participation provided.

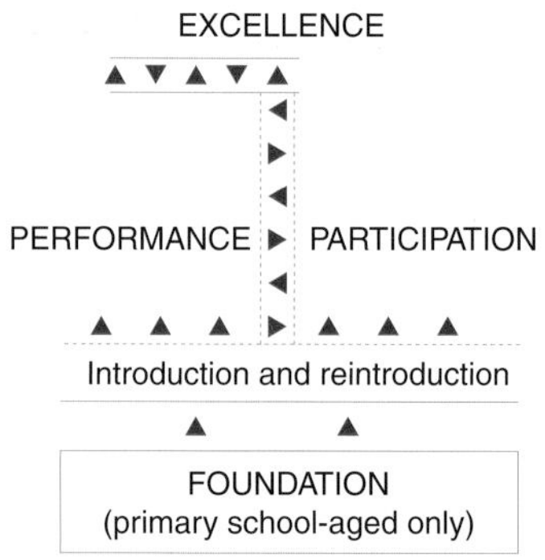


**Figure 10.1** Sports development continuum model

The need for a more coordinated and fair approach to the provision of sporting activities addresses two main areas:

1. sports development: enabling people to learn basic sports skills, with the possibility of reaching a standard of sporting excellence;
2. sports equity: redressing the balance of inequalities in sport, that is, equality of access for everyone, regardless of race, age, gender or level of ability.

Sport England has a sport development continuum:

- Foundation – learning basic movement skills, knowledge and understanding; developing a positive attitude to physical activity.
- Participation – exercising one's leisure option for a variety of reasons – health, fitness, social.
- Performance – improving standards through coaching, competition and training.
- Excellence – reaching national and publicly recognised standards of performance.

Sport England is required to widen the base of the participation pyramid by ensuring equality of opportunity through the provision of facilities and sporting programmes in order that people from all sections of society are able to feel the benefit from participating in a variety of activities. Many of the organisations and policies are outlined below

**Key term**

**Participation:** The active involvement of people in recreational and sporting activities.

# The organisation of sport in the UK

The organisation of sport and physical education has a dynamic aspect, so it is important (and more interesting!) if you try to keep up to date with changes as they occur. The web addresses for some of the major organisations are provided below (these are correct at the time of writing).

The main focus of this section is to appreciate that opportunities for participation and excellence should not be the result of luck or coincidence, but the culmination of specific aims and policies of organisations with a remit to develop sport at these levels. The opportunities people have to initiate and further develop their interest in sporting activities are dependent on many factors, including:

- provision within their country/community;
- personal factors, such as race, gender, age and socio-economics.

We need to understand how sport and politics interact. It will be useful to begin with a definition of politics:

> the science and art of government; dealing with the form, organisation and administration of a state or part of one, and of the regulation of its relations with other states... Political [means] belonging to or pertaining to the state, its government and policy. (Oxford English Dictionary)

We will look at some of the key words that make up this definition and consider their possible meaning in relation to sport.

**EXAMINER'S TIP**

You may not be examined directly on the aspect of sport and politics, but it can help you to understand and appreciate in more depth the issues we will discuss during this section of the book.

## Administration

The administration of sport can be seen as developing from the community. For example, a local sports club forms the base of the pyramid, with its regional, national and international counterparts above. The international governing bodies of sport (the International Olympic Committee, the Commonwealth Games Federation and the European sports bodies) are political bodies and their dealings must reflect the political climate in which they operate. They are concerned with:

- governing sport;
- making decisions;
- creating and distributing finances and resources.

## IN DEPTH: Relations with other states

The relationships between states with regard to sport began as soon as worldwide travel and unified rules of competition developed. Sport can have a positive and a negative influence within and between societies.

| Positive | Negative |
|---|---|
| • International goodwill<br>• Promotes cultural empathy and understanding between nations<br>• Athletes are seen as ambassadors of their country<br>• The Olympic Charter sets out the view that sport promotes world peace by improving international understanding and respect<br>• The sense of belonging to a country encourages patriotism and nationalism | • Patriotism and nationalism are more powerful when conflict is prevalent<br>• Reinforces conflict<br>• Results in winners and losers: winners can be viewed as superior and powerful, whereas losers are inferior and powerless<br>• Success is attributed to countries as much as to the athletes themselves<br>• Other nations can be seen as 'the enemy' |

## Policy

Policy suggests decision making based on the ideology (set of ideas) or philosophy of those in power. This is relevant from local to international situations. Numerous indicators can be used to determine the importance a government places on sport:

- the expenditure for sport;
- the position or status of sports ministers within a government;
- the type and amount of sport legislation produced.

Politics reflects the power systems within a culture – who has the power and how do they use it? Sport and physical activities have sometimes been used by various governments, individuals and administrators for political reasons.

The commercial world plays an extremely important role in sports decision making, at local, national and international levels. The cost of staging sports events such as the Olympic Games, for example, is extraordinarily high:

- The construction of stadiums requires capital which often only governments can raise.
- The running of events increasingly involves those who pay international television fees.
- Revenue for major events requires huge commitment from governments.

## IN DEPTH: Political uses of sport

### Social factors

Sport can be used to introduce or reinforce social harmony. Government inquiries into inner-city riots usually refer to the need to provide better sporting facilities. This can be taken to have various meanings:

- Boredom creates dysfunctional activity. By providing the highest standard of sporting facilities and educating people to use them constructively in their leisure time, we can help to improve people's quality and enjoyment of life, giving them less reason to become involved in antisocial activities.
- The 'bread and circuses' theory – this is more controversial, and claims that sport can be used to divert the attention and energy of the masses away from the problems of the political and social system in which they live.

**IN CONTEXT**

**In the film *Gladiator*, the emperor stages a festival of games to keep the population happy and has bread thrown to the crowds to make him popular.**

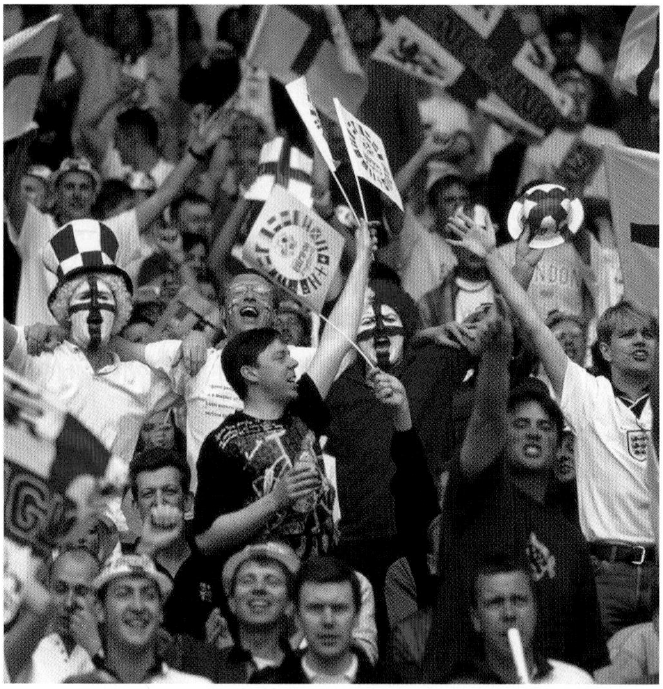

**Figure 10.2** Does sport divert people's attention away from political and social problems?

### Sport as 'character-building'

Sport would also seem to have socialising qualities, which can be used as a political tool. For example, involvement in team games helps develop the ability to work in a team, as well as qualities of cooperation, leadership, obeying rules and respecting authority; team games have always been popular with governments when they emphasise the value of a population participating in sporting activities.

### Propaganda

Sport can be used as political propaganda. For example, in the 1930s, the Nazi youth groups aimed to indoctrinate young people in the values of Nazi Germany.

### Defence and work

Sport has also been used to raise the fitness level of populations in order to better prepare them for defending their country, make them more productive in the workplace and decrease health costs.

So we can see that there are various reasons why national governments become involved in sport. Figure 10.3 summarises these points.

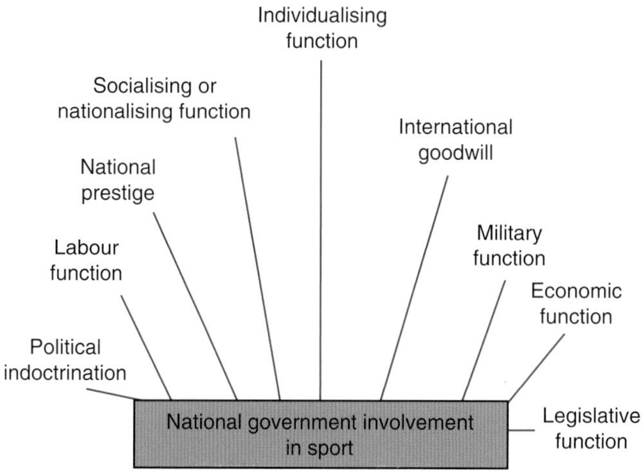


Figure 10.3 National government involvement in sport

## Activity 1

1 Choose four functions of sport from Figure 10.3. Explain in detail how each one operates.
2 Consider the stance of the Department for Culture, Media and Sport. Which of these functions is the British government most concerned with?

# Sport and government in the UK

We have been suggesting that sport cannot be seen as an activity which only has relevance to those who practise it; it also serves various functions of a society. In the current climate, the government policies for participation and excellence in sport have become crucial to all the other sports organisations, such as Sport England and UK Sport. It is therefore necessary at this stage to determine exactly why the national government would become more involved in sports policy.

## Government policies

In recent years, both Conservative and Labour governments in the UK have sought increasingly to assume more control over physical education and sport. Why should the government wish to spend money on sport and leisure? The stance taken is that sport can make a valuable contribution to delivering the four key outcomes of:

1 lower long-term unemployment;
2 less crime;
3 better health;
4 better qualifications.

It can also develop:

- individual pride;
- community spirit to enable communities to run regeneration programmes themselves;
- neighbourhood regeneration.

**Key terms**

**Function:** The special activity, purpose or role of an organisation or person. An example of the function of a school would be to educate young people.
**Funding:** Income that is generated, internally or externally, and expenditure incurred to meet the function of the organisation.

## The role of central government

### Minister for Sport

- The role of the minister is to advise and consult, not to direct.
- S/he coordinates sport rather than controls it.
- S/he now comes under the DCMS, which also has competing responsibilities.

However, these limitations should not be overstated, for the minister can exert considerable influence on policy, when required. This would mainly depend on:

- the prominence of sporting issues to the government;
- the quality, ambition and style of the minister in office.

Make sure you know who the current Minister for Sport is and try to keep track of any initiatives, opinions or events with which s/he becomes involved.

**Executive summary**

**Findings**

Arts and sport, cultural and recreational activity, can contribute to neighbourhood renewal and make a real difference to health, crime, unemployment and education in deprived communities.

1. This is because they:
   a appeal directly to individuals' interests and develop their potential and self-confidence
   b relate to community identity and encourage collective effort
   c help build positive links with the wider community
   d are associated with rapidly growing industries.
2. Barriers to be overcome are:
   a projects being tailored to programme/policy criteria, rather than to community needs
   b short-term perspectives
   c promoting arts/sport in communities being seen as peripheral, both to culture/leisure organisations and in regeneration programmes
   d lack of hard information on the regeneration impact of arts/sport
   e poor links between arts/sport bodies and major 'players', including schools.
3. Principles which help to exploit the potential of arts/sport in regenerating communities are:
   a valuing diversity
   b embedding local control
   c supporting local commitment
   d promoting equitable partnerships
   e defining common objectives in relation to actual needs
   f working flexibly with charge
   g securing sustainability
   h pursuing quality across the spectrum: and
   i connecting with the mainstream of art and sport activities.
4. Social exclusion issues arise with various groups irrespective of their geographic location. This is particularly the case with ethnic minority groups and disabled people where special and systematic arrangements need to be made:
   a to invest in people and capacity within these groups and to build an information base against which future progress can be measured
   b to cater specifically for their needs in general regeneration programmes and culture/leisure policies
   c to engage directly with people within these groups, and actively to value and recognise diversity
   d to develop, monitor and deliver action plans to promote their access and involvement and to meet their needs.

**Figure 10.4** Executive summary – policy action team 10
*Source*: Department for Culture, Media and Sport

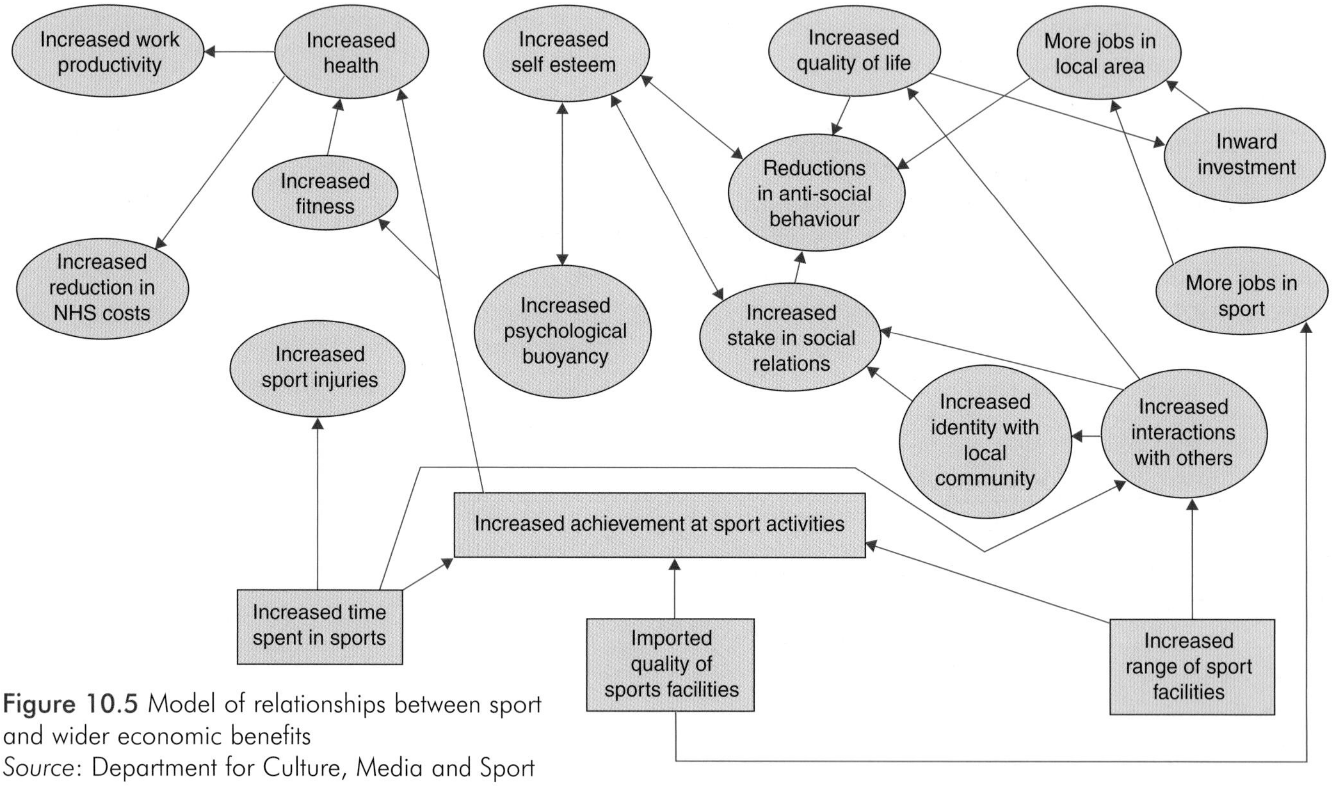


**Figure 10.5** Model of relationships between sport and wider economic benefits
*Source*: Department for Culture, Media and Sport

Table 10.1 The benefits of sport

| Nature of benefit | Experienced by excluded | Strength of evidence | Nature of evidence | | | |
|---|---|---|---|---|---|---|
| | | | Lab/ experi-mental | National/ large survey | Case study | Meta analysis/ study review |
| *National* | | | | | | |
| Identity | – | + | | | | |
| Prestige | ++ | + | | | * | |
| Reduced health | – – | + + | | * | * | * |
| Costs | | | | | | |
| Trade | | + + | | * | | |
| *Communal* | | | | | | |
| Community/ family coherence | – – | | | | * | * |
| Lower law and order costs (especially for youth) | – – – | + | | | * | * |
| Job creation | + / – | + | | | * | * |
| Environmental (created/ renewed) | | | | | | |
| *Personal* | | | | | | |
| Physical health (heart, lungs, joints, bones, muscles) | | | | | | |
| Better mental health (coping, depression) | – – – | + + + + | * | * | * | * |
| Better self-esteem/ image/ competence | + / – | + + | * | | * | * |
| Socialisation/ integration/ tolerance | + + + | + + + | * | | * | * |
| General quality of life | + + | + + | * | | * | * |

*Source*: Department for Culture, Media and Sport

**Note**: The strength of positive and negative experience in column 2 and of evidence in column 3 is shown by the number of + and – signs. * indicates where the particular form of evidence is available.

## Department for Culture, Media and Sport (DCMS)

www.culture.gov.uk

Following restructuring, this department assumed control of sport, becoming the central government department responsible for government policy on areas including the arts, sport and recreation, the National Lottery, libraries, museums and galleries, broadcasting and films. Sport therefore has to compete alongside these other areas.

| Policies for participation | Policies for excellence |
|---|---|
| • Sport: Raising the Game (1995)<br>• A Sporting Future for All (2000)<br>• Game Plan (2002)<br>• Best Value through Sport<br>• Step into Sport: Leadership and Volunteering | • Sport: Raising the Game<br>• A Sporting Future for All<br>• Game Plan<br>• Best Value through Sport<br>• Step into Sport: Leadership and Volunteering<br>• PE School Sport and Club Links Strategy (PESSCL) |

## Game Plan: A strategy for delivering government sport and physical activity objectives (December 2002)

Game Plan provides a broad context and research evidence for sports policy. It covers broad issues:

- Grass-roots participation could be improved.
- International success is better than perceived.
- The hosting of mega events has not always been successful.
- There are problems of funding in sport.
- There are complex structures responsible for delivering sport policy.

In less than a decade, numerous government policies for sport highlight government's belief in the importance sport is beginning to have in the UK. The following organisations must try to address many of these issues. In some cases their responsibilities overlap.

## Sport England

www.sportengland.org

Sport England began its role in January 1997 and is accountable to Parliament through the Secretary of State for Culture, Media and Sport, who operates under the DCMS. Sport England also operates ten regional offices in England, providing partnerships across public and private sectors.

Local authorities and Sport England have worked in partnership to improve the cause of sport through facility development, raising standards of management, sports development initiatives, events and campaigns. It is a relationship that balances national objectives and priorities with those at a local level.

### Objectives

The objectives of Sport England are to lead the development of sport in England by influencing and serving the public. Its aims are:

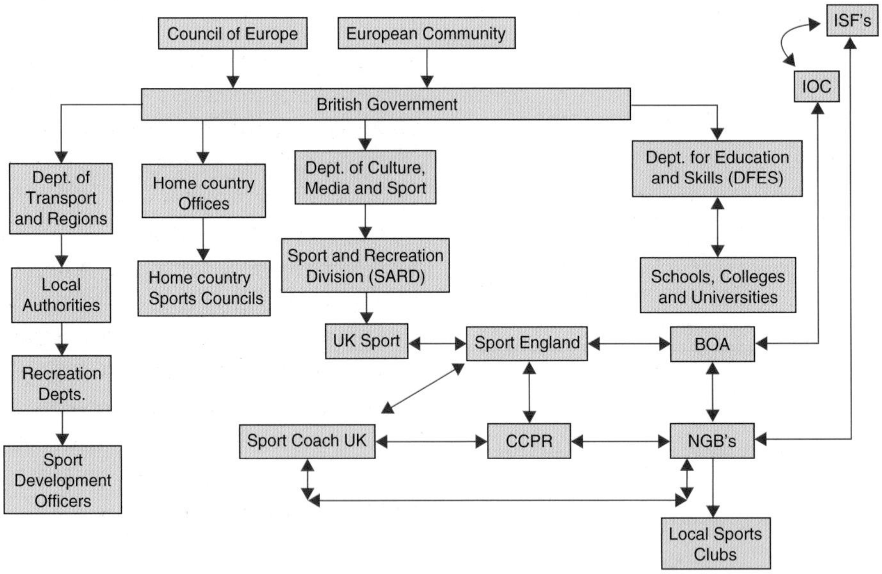


**Figure 10.6** Organisation of sport in the UK

- start – get people to participate;
- stay – retain people once they have started;
- succeed – achieve higher levels of performance.

Members of the Council are appointed by the Secretary of State for Culture, Media and Sport. Their responsibilities include:

- approving all policy matters and operational and corporate plans for Sport England;
- bringing independent judgement to issues such as strategy and resources;
- ensuring all financial matters are regulated and operate efficiently.

A series of advisory panels guide Sport England in the following areas:

- lottery;
- local authorities;
- women and sport;
- disability;
- racial equality;
- government body investment.

### Funding

The work of Sport England is jointly funded by:

- the Exchequer, for maintaining England's sports infrastructure;
- the National Lottery via the Sport England Lottery Fund, which is earmarked for the development of sport in England;
- sport as part of the overall social inclusion policy and neighbourhood regeneration work.

| **Policies for participation** | **Policies for elite/ excellence** |
|---|---|
| • Active programme<br>• Sportsmark/ Activemark<br>• National Junior Sports<br>• Sport Action Zones<br>• Step into Sport | • World-class programme<br>• Academies Scheme<br>• Sportsearch Programme (TOP) |

## Youth Sports Trust

The Youth Sports Trust is a registered charity, set up in 1994 to improve sporting provision for young people in the UK. Its mission is to develop and implement a linked series of quality sports programmes, known under the umbrella term, the National Junior Sports Programme. The Trust also works alongside the Department for Children, Families and Schools to support maintained secondary schools that are applying for Specialist Sports College status. The organisation is becoming increasingly influential in the coordination and provision of sport, both in schools and in the local community.

| **Policies for participation** |
|---|
| • National Junior Sports Programme<br>• Step into Sport<br>• School Sports Coordinators<br>• Sports Colleges |

## Local provision for leisure

Local leisure provision has traditionally come from three main sectors:

1. private
2. public
3. voluntary.

### Private provision

Private provision for leisure has existed ever since wealthy people have been able to belong to exclusive clubs and where individuals/ entrepreneurs have seen the opportunities for making a profit from providing a service to those who can afford to pay. Private leisure facilities increased dramatically during the late twentieth century and are a reflection of the growing wealth amongst the masses. These facilities range from private golf clubs to fitness clubs. Their primary aim is to make a profit. The attraction for many of their clients is the exclusive or elitist ethos. However, the proliferation of such facilities could take away trade from local authority-run facilities which in turn could lead to a decrease in public (local authority) provision.

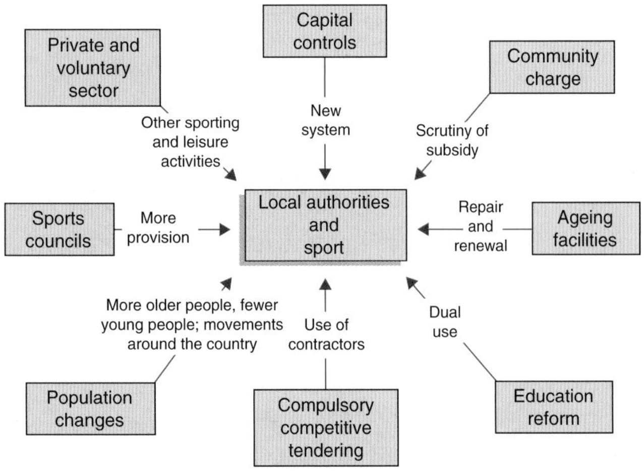


**Figure 10.7** Pressures on local authority sports policy

## Activity 2

What are the advantages and disadvantages of the growing number of private fitness clubs?

## Public provision (local authorities)

Public provision began as far back as the late nineteenth century with facilities such as town parks and baths. The motives behind this movement were:

- social control – the middle classes wanted to control the behaviour of the working classes by providing socially acceptable recreational activities;
- to reduce crime rates;
- to instil a sense of morality;
- to improve the health and fitness of the working classes;
- to respond to a growing social conscience to improve the lot of the poor – the development of philanthropy and social justice.

Have things really changed over the last 150 years? Today local authorities bear a heavy burden to provide leisure facilities, so why should they spend huge sums of money on this public service?

- Leisure is a popular demand from local residents – they expect sporting facilities in the same way that they expect hospitals and libraries and they are the ones who elect the local councils.
- Leisure provision can help reduce crime and improve people's health.
- Leisure can provide an economic boost in terms of tourism to an area as well as employment.
- Leisure can help integrate a society and provide people with skills which could be transferred into other areas of life.
- Leisure can improve the morale and feelgood factor for a local population.
- Some people would not be able to afford the membership fees to some of the more exclusive facilities. Local authorities are supposed to provide a social need.

## Voluntary provision

This is the area in which most sporting activity occurs. Individuals come together to form clubs and associations which are run to benefit the participants. They are generally self-financing. Annual subscriptions and match fees provide the bulk of the revenue and indicate the grass roots development of sport in the UK.

## Activity 3

Research a local sports club in your area, possibly one you belong to, and investigate how it is run, who runs it and the general financing of the club.

**Table 10.2** Various leisure activities

| Sport | Education | Tourism | Social | Cultural |
|---|---|---|---|---|
| Sports centres | Libraries | Museums | Youth clubs | Theatres |
| Playing fields | Swimming pools | Conservation | Community centres | Art galleries |
| Ski slopes | | Country parks | | |

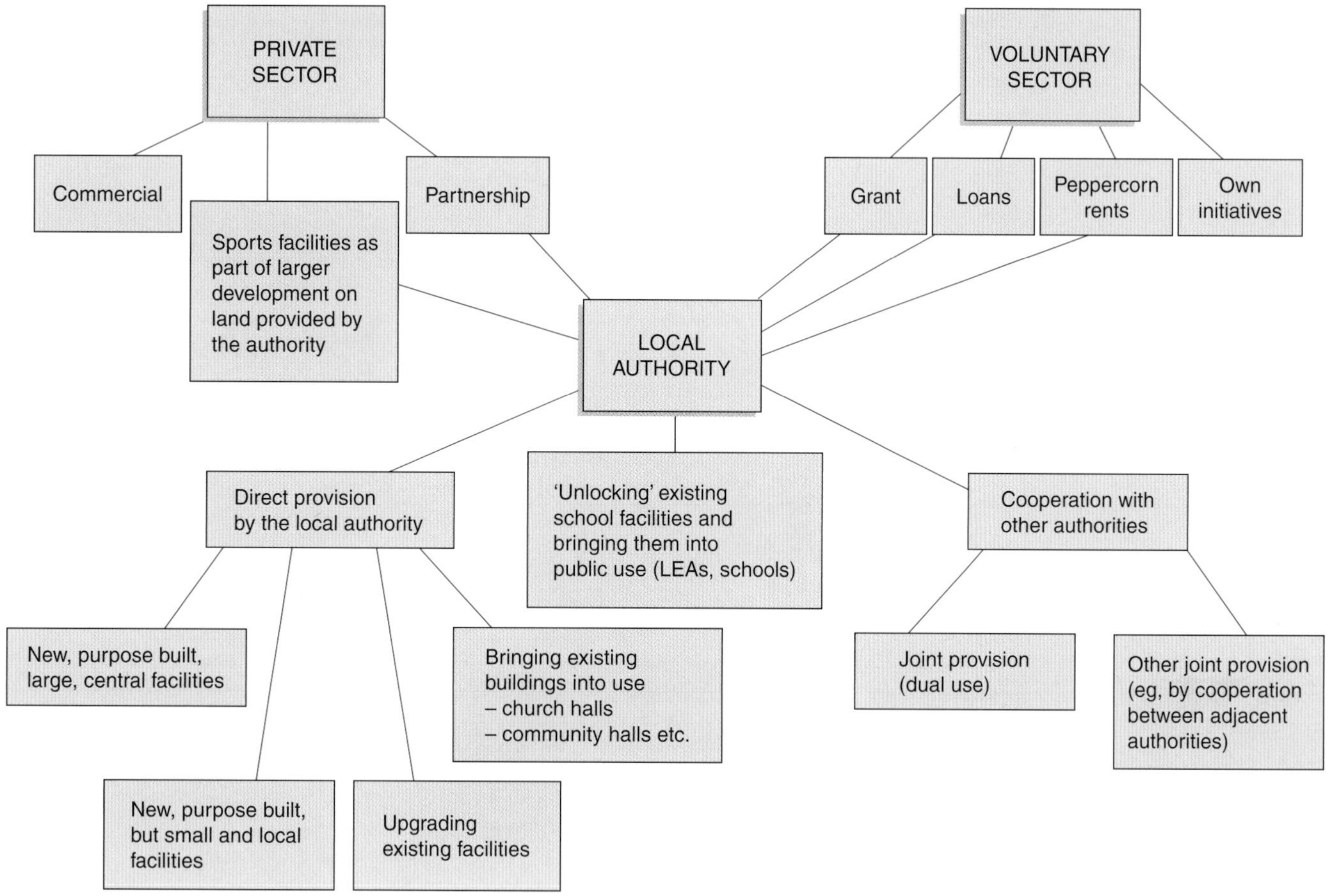


Figure 10.8 Provision of leisure services

| Private sector | Public sector | Voluntary sector |
|---|---|---|
| • Privately owned/registered companies<br>• Trading on normal profit and loss/self-financed<br>• Membership entrance fees<br>• Managed by owners/their employees<br>• Must operate and survive in open market/make a profit/compete | • Business operations run by local authority departments<br>• Trading on set prices/charges, etc.<br>• According to a pre-set budget<br>• May involve subsidies as a matter of policy/Council tax or equivalent<br>• Managed by local authority employees | • Business operations owned by 'members'<br>• Possibly on trust/charity basis<br>• Trading on normal profit and loss/break even<br>• Managed through a members' committee<br>• May employ staff<br>• Financed by membership fees/fund-raising/ sponsorship |

## Best Value

The government has a major policy called Best Value which local authorities and sport organisations such as Sport England are expected to deliver.

Best Value was a part of New Labour's wider modernisation programme aimed at bringing councils closer to their communities and promoting the role of councils in community leadership and governance. There was a statutory duty upon all

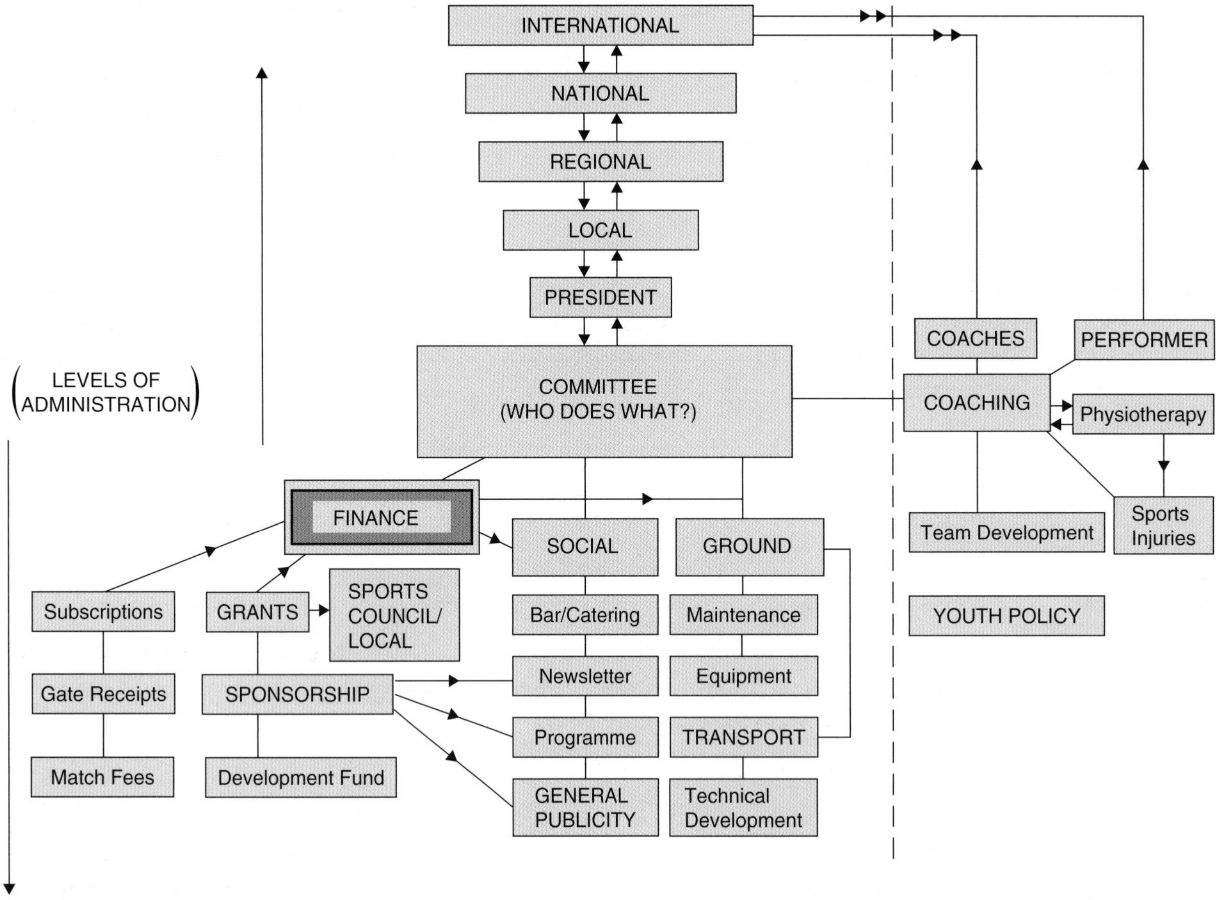


**Figure 10.9** Administrative framework of a large athletic club

local authorities to meet the requirements of Best Value as set out in the Local Government Bill published on 30 September 1998. Best Value applied to all local authorities as from 1 April 2000.

> A modern council – or authority – which puts people first will seek to provide services which bear comparison with the best ... Continuous improvements in both the quality and cost of services will therefore be the hallmark of a modern council and the test of Best Value.
>
> (Department of the Environment, Transport and the Regions 1998)

The document 'The Value of Sport' responds to the challenge: Why invest in sport? It demonstrates that sport can make a difference to people's lives and to the communities in which they live. It emphasises that for every pound spent on sport there are multiple returns in improved health, reduced crime, economic regeneration and improved employment opportunities.

> We can all appreciate the many benefits that sport can provide for individuals and society, but sport needs to demonstrate tangible benefits to individuals, communities and the nation as a whole, if it is to compete with many other worthy causes for a share of limited public resources'.
>
> (Trevor Brooking)

- *Best Value through Sport: Case studies* has been designed to illustrate examples of progressive practice within local government, to complement The Value of Sport and to provide guidance on how to enhance sports services within a Best Value context.
- *Performance Indicators* is an inter-centre comparison framework on key performance indicators developed through a combination of secondary data analysis of the use of management of sport halls and swimming pools in England 1997–1999 and primary research.

- *Model Survey Package 5* is a series of 'standard' questionnaires to be used as part of the consultation process for both user and non-user surveys.
- *Quest: Facilities* is the UK Quality Scheme for Sport and Leisure that has now been operational in facility management for three years. Over 90 sites have achieved external accreditation. Quest provides standards of good practice and a framework for continuous improvement that are endorsed by the Local Government Association and the sport and leisure industry.
- *Quest: Sports Development* is being extended to the sports development sector following a successful feasibility study. The work has reached its piloting stage and will take account of the demands of Best Value.

## Activity 4

Research a local authority website (preferably your local one) to discover how it delivers Best Value in the field of sport and recreation.

## What you need to know

* Local provision of leisure is the responsibility of three main sectors:
  - rivate sector – where the primary aim is for an owner to make a profit by providing an exclusive service which requires customers to pay a premium membership fee;
  - public sector – or local authority provision where a service is provided to a local population and has developed since the nineteenth century;
  - voluntary sector – where interested individuals come together to organise and participate in a recreational and sporting activity. They need to break even but profit is not the aim.
* Best Value is a government policy which local authorities and organisations such as Sport England must adhere to in providing good quality services for the best money possible.
* There is heavy reliance on local government to provide opportunities and facilities for sport and recreation.

## Review questions

1. Draw the sport participation pyramid or sport development continuum and briefly explain each stage.
2. What do the terms 'private', public' and 'voluntary' mean in relation to provision for leisure?
3. What are the advantages and disadvantages of public provision for leisure?
4. Outline some major participation trends in the UK.
5. Who is the current Minister for Sport?
6. What are the objectives of Sport England?
7. Outline the major features of the 'Best Value' policy.

CHAPTER 11

# Creating opportunities to increase participation

## Learning outcomes

**By the end of this chapter you should understand the following:**

- the legacy of the public schools in the nineteenth century, especially the terms:
  - technical development of activities, particularly games
  - athleticism
  - concept of fair play
- the state school system of education from 1870, linking up to the present day, with an emphasis on:
  - the transition from:
    - drill (military style) 1870–1902, to
    - physical training, through the syllabuses of physical training (1904–1933), to
    - physical education including Moving and Growing (1950s)
- present-day National Curriculum
- the characteristics of each Key Stage of the National Curriculum
- how the Key Stages can help increase participation.
- the changing level of government control over education
- current initiatives to increase participation of young people in school sport such as PESSCLS (Physical Education and School Sport Club Links Strategy), sports colleges and school sport coordinators and whole sport plans of national governing bodies; Sports Leaders UK and the TOPS programme

### EXAMINER'S TIP

Although for ease of study we will deal with the state and private sector separately, it is important to remember that the private or public schools that operated for the gentry or upper classes were already well established by the nineteenth century. The state schools were established much later following the Forster Education Act 1870, educating different people for very different purposes.

## Victorian Britain

Victoria became queen in 1837. Her reign was a period of dramatic social change reflected in the development of games and sport during the nineteenth century.

The United Kingdom became the birthplace of modern sport, with many sports becoming rationalised, that is, rule-bound with codes of behaviour or etiquette. The middle and upper classes through their public schools were to be one of the most influential social factors in this development.

## Nineteenth-century public schools

The sons of the gentry were educated at the public schools, characteristically being sophisticated, prestigious, fee-paying boarding schools. There were originally nine elite institutions, which were called 'Barbarian' schools as they maintained the gentry tradition: Eton, Harrow, Rugby, Shrewsbury, Charterhouse, Westminster, Winchester, St Paul's and Merchant Taylor's.

The emergence of the middle classes resulted in them building their own proprietary colleges, which were based on the elite schools. Examples of these 'Philistine' schools are Cheltenham College, Marlborough and Clifton.

**Key terms**

**Rationalisation**
Popular recreations were changed by the addition of both written and unwritten rules.

## Technical/formal development of activities

The development of sport in the public schools radically changed previous concepts of sport. The boys brought to their schools their experiences of games like cricket and mob football and country pursuits such as fishing and coursing. Before the formalisation of team games, the boys would leave the school grounds and participate in rowdy behaviour; this often involved poaching, fighting and trespassing, drinking alcohol and generally bringing the school's name into disrepute, causing conflict with local landowners and gamekeepers.

However, during this stage they began the process of organising their own activities and devising new ways of playing. These were often associated with individual architectural features of the different schools, such as cloisters for fives and the Eton wall game, an old form of football which survives to this day. It developed from the unique architectural feature of a long, red brick wall which separates the school playing fields from the Slough road. The wall was built in 1717, but the game became popular in the nineteenth century. Ten players per side work the small ball along a narrow strip, 4–5 yards wide and 118 yards long. The players are assigned their playing position and specialised role according to their physique.

Thomas Arnold, the head of Rugby School, encouraged the boys to develop activities which could be played on the school grounds and which would also highlight the more moral features of teamwork, such as self-discipline, loyalty, courage -- character-building qualities suitable for the prospective leaders of society.

Cricket was already a fairly well-established game in society and as such was considered suitable for the boys. Mob football, however, was played by the lower classes and was not so acceptable, until the boys devised a more organised format. The game of rugby supposedly began at Rugby School, when William Webb Ellis picked up the ball during a game of football and ran with it.

The boys were in charge of organising the games, and senior bands of boys (normally called prefects) would be in control. Games committees were formed, e.g. the Harrow Philathletic Club. The masters actively discouraged some activities (poaching and gambling) while others were allowed to exist on an informal recreational basis among the boys (fives and fighting). They actively encouraged the boys to organise team games. Boys who excelled in games were admired by the other pupils, becoming the 'games elite'.

**Table 11.1** Cricket, football and society

| Cricket | Football |
|---|---|
| Earliest established game in English society, accepted by boys' families | Still a 'mob' game in the nineteenth century |
| Differing positional roles made it acceptable for both social classes to play | Played by the lower classes in society |
| Reflected the ideals of athleticism: teamwork/honour/etiquette; team before individual | Not popular with the gentry until boys devised rules within the schools |
| | 'Contact' nature of the game meant that the social classes would play separately for a long time |

Initially, inter-school fixtures were not feasible as no two schools had the same rules. However, by the mid-nineteenth century, headmasters and staff started to organise sports. Games were seen as a medium for achieving educational aims with a moral social sense; they could also help combat idleness and as such were a form of social control.

Technical development of games led to the following:

- boys brought local variations to the schools from their villages;
- played regularly in free time;
- developed individual school rules/skills/boundaries, etc.;
- played competitively, i.e. house matches;
- self-government meant boys organised activities initially;
- later codified rules allowed inter-school fixtures;
- development of games elite.

## Athleticism

The cult of athleticism stressed the physical and social benefits of sports:

- The physical benefits were seen to counteract the effects of a sedentary lifestyle. Sport was viewed as therapeutic, invigorating and cathartic. It was also seen as a break from work.
- Sport would take place within a competitive situation which would help the boys learn how to cope with winning and losing in a dignified manner. It helped to develop leadership qualities, and being captain was a high-status office to hold.

The house system was fundamental to the competitive sport events, in which the manner of the performance was considered more important than the result.

Athleticism also met middle-class values of respectability and order, for example values such as sportsmanship, leadership and abiding by rules. The middle classes were to become the organisers and administrators of society, particularly highlighted in their role within governing bodies of sports clubs.

The public schools instituted the idea of the sports day, which operated as a public relations exercise for the old boys, parents and governors of the school. School funds could benefit from generous donations and valuable publicity could be gained.

**Key terms**

**Athleticism**
Physical endeavour with moral integrity.

The moral development of games encompassed:

- teamwork and group loyalty;
- playing to the written and unwritten rules of the sport;
- fair play and sportsmanship;
- courage and bravery;
- character building and leadership skills.

**Key terms**

**Fair play**
More than playing to the written rules, fair play incorporates the concepts of friendship, respect for others and always playing in the right spirit. Often referred to as 'sportsmanship'.

**EXAMINER'S TIP**

Make sure you understand the difference between the terms 'technical' and 'moral'.

**IN CONTEXT**

**Influential headmaster: Thomas Arnold**

**Thomas Arnold became headmaster in 1828 of Rugby School where he directed a crusade against personal sin, e.g. bullying, lying, swearing, cheating, running wild. Pupils were to remain on the school grounds, he forbade shooting and beagling as these activities encouraged poaching, and fights should occur only within his presence and be supervised by the prefects who enforced his authority.**

**Arnold is known for his contribution to Muscular Christianity, but he valued games only for what they could contribute towards the social control of the boys. The development of athleticism followed the cooperation of the boys in maintaining discipline and achieving Arnold's reforms.**

***Tom Brown's Schooldays* by Thomas Hughes was published in 1860 and highlighted the Victorian ideal of the physical side of the Christian gentleman.**

**EXAMINER'S TIP**

Understand that questions asking 'how' and 'why' games were rationalised would require very different answers.

Athleticism spread nationally and worldwide via the following means:

- old boys'/girls' network;
- universities codified rules, developed activities technically, improved and devised new ways of playing;
- sports clubs and governing bodies became significant administrative features;
- officers in army and navy were influential on troops;
- clergy influenced parishioners;
- teachers went back into schools;
- employers encouraged games in their workforce;
- the British Empire enabled these developments to be spread around the world.

## IN DEPTH: Muscular Christianity

Running parallel to the development of athleticism in the public schools was the Muscular Christian movement. Muscular Christianity was an evangelical movement, of which Charles Kingsley was one of the most influential exponents. Kingsley helped to combine the Christian and the chivalric ideal of manliness. It was the return of the Platonic concept, the 'whole man'. It improved one's ability to be gentle and courteous, brave and enterprising, reverent and truthful, selfless and devoted.

Kingsley believed healthy bodies were needed alongside healthy minds. Neglect of health was as lazy as a neglected mind. He also led the hygienic movement which was to have a deep effect on the working conditions of the poor.

There was little or no support for sport for its own sake at this time; sport should increase physical health and military valour, and create Christian soldiers. It was a fusion of physical with moral training.

Evangelical developments were directly linked with two philosophies:

- Muscular Christians regarded cricket, boating and football as positive recreation.
- The Church was attempting to attract workers from the pubs by forming alternative social clubs.

Eventually there was a strong link with the club development of working-class sport, particularly football.

**Activity 1**

Consider the similarities and differences between the status and characteristics of team games in the nineteenth century and in schools today.

### Summary

Nineteenth-century public schools:

- provided an education for the social elite;
- developed many traditional activities and games;
- gave rise to the cult of athleticism parallel with the Muscular Christian movement;
- allowed games associated with character-building qualities, for example courage and loyalty;
- influenced the development of sport nationally and worldwide through their positions of leadership in society.

## State education

Prior to 1870, the education of the masses had been the responsibility of the parish and was very inconsistent. The Forster Education Act 1870 was a great milestone in social welfare, as it created a state system of education. There was a developing initiative to build more schools and the Act was the result of some radical changes in social thinking among philanthropists and social reformers.

From the time that the first Board Schools were built in 1870, teachers in the poorest districts were faced with the extreme poverty of many of their pupils – as many as 3–4 million children were living below the poverty line.

## Characteristics of state schools

Experiences of children at state schools were very different from those of their gentry counterparts. Small buildings with little space and no recreational facilities allied with a philosophy which denied any recreational rights to the working class, and placed its own constraints on the physical activities available to the state school system.

Gymnastics formed the bedrock of early state school physical exercise. Foreign influence, in the form of Swedish gymnastics, was important. The School Board tended to favour the Swedish system for its free-flowing, freestanding exercises, possibly due to the employment of Swedish inspectors.

### Swedish gymnastics

This was suitable for state schools as it aimed to:

- suit the diverse objectives of physical exercise for the working classes;
- promote health and fitness based on scientific principles, gaining approval with the School Board;
- encourage military preparedness through its drill style of instruction;
- improve industrial efficiency/work productivity;
- foster social order/social control/discipline of large numbers of children;
- promote the harmonious development of the whole body;
- be safe and cheap;
- be easy to learn and instruct.

The lack of fitness and discipline and the poor general health of the working classes had been noted in the Boer War (1899–1902) and blamed for the heavy loss of life. Swedish gymnastics also came under threat as not being effective enough in improving the fitness of the working classes sufficiently for the hardships of war.

## The Model Course

A policy of drill and physical training was initiated but had little recreational value. In 1902 the Model Course was instituted by Colonel Fox of the War Office. The main aim of the course was to:

- improve the fitness of the working classes for military preparation;
- increase their familiarity with combat and weapons;
- improve discipline and obedience amongst the working classes.

Drill was characterised by commands issued by the teacher or NCOs (non-commissioned officers) to the children, who would be standing in uniform, military-style rows and obeying the commands in unison. Large numbers could be catered for in a small space and as the movements were freestanding and required no apparatus, they were cheap. After 1873 boys and girls received drill.

The problems with this approach were that they were essentially adult exercises for children, they did not take children's needs and physical and mental development into account, there was no educative content and individualism was submerged within a group response. The use of NCOs also reduced the status of the subject as it did not use qualified teachers.

> **Key terms**
>
> **Model Course**
> A form of military drill, instigated by Colonel Fox of the War Office between 1902 and 1904.

Owing to the problems and concerns over the Model Course, the Board of Education established a syllabus of physical training in 1904, 1909, 1919, 1927 and 1933. It stressed the physical and educative effect of sport:

- The physical content would have been very much influenced by the Board's primary concern for the medical and physiological base from which it approached the subject. As such the therapeutic effect, the correction of posture faults, and exercises to improve the circulatory systems would have been foremost in its aims.
- The educational aims would try to develop alertness and decision making. [BL: end]

The 1919 syllabus took into consideration the loss of life in the First World War and the flu epidemic which hit the country shortly afterwards. Sir George Newman had recognised the beneficial effects of recreational activities in helping to rehabilitate injured soldiers.

By 1933 there were fewer tables , there was more freedom of movement and a more decentralised lesson. This was recognition of the increasing rights of the working classes and the educational value of group work.

**EXAMINER'S TIP**

You need to be able to contrast the early syllabuses with the later syllabuses and also with the present-day National Curriculum.

**Activity 2**

Why were Swedish gymnastics and military drill suitable for state schools?

## First World War

The First World War, also known as the Great War, was fought from 1914 to 1918, mainly in Europe and the Middle East. The allies (France, Russia, Britain, Italy and the United States after 1917) defeated the central powers (Germany, Austria, Hungary and Turkey). Millions died in static trench warfare.

Nationalism revealed itself in war. Public schoolmen with their ideals of service were enthusiastic about the conflict. It was glorified like a football match and the football match between British and German soldiers at Christmas 1914 set the tone for how sport was to be perceived during wartime. Football grounds were used extensively for recruiting and eventually the Football League bowed to moral pressure to stop fixtures for the duration of the war. Following the war there were hopes of a more equal society due to the massive loss of life sustained from all echelons of society.

**EXAMINER'S TIP**

You will not be directly examined on the two World Wars but you need to understand how they would have influenced the thinking and policies of people and organisations in those times.

## Post-Second World War developments

The Butler Education Act 1944 planned to reform education in Britain. It was a major social reform, with the aim of removing special privileges and ensuring equality of opportunity for all. Its main provisions were as follows:

- There were to be 146 local education authorities to replace the previous 300. They were required to provide recreational facilities to specific sizes.
- The school leaving age was to be raised to 15 from 1947.
- All education in state-maintained grammar schools was to be free. To attend grammar schools children now needed to pass the eleven-plus exam, rather than pay.
- All children would leave the elementary school at 11 and move to a secondary school – either grammar or secondary modern. This was a complete separation of the primary from secondary education and meant that new schools had to be built.
- More mature forms of physical education were required to suit the higher ages of the children.

The Second World War had the following effects:

- destruction of schools/deterioration of equipment;
- evacuation of children to rural areas;
- male physical education teachers enlisted;
- work taken over by older men and women;
- more mobile style of fighting;
- apparatus for schools from commando training;
- movement away from therapeutic and medical value of physical education;
- more emphasis on heuristic/guidance style of teaching.

After the war there was an extensive rebuilding programme and facilities were more sophisticated than before. The therapeutic effect of recreational activities was again valued. The commando training during the war had developed the use of obstacle training and this was how the first apparatus began to appear in schools – scramble nets, rope ladders, mats and frames, hoops, wooden tables and benches.

The 'movement' approach began in physical education lessons – children were required to use their initiative and learn by discovery. This also demanded new teaching methods and there was the development of a more heuristic style, which placed the teacher in the role of guiding the children rather than being purely instructional.

The form of dance favoured by Isadora Duncan and Laban, using the body as an expressive medium, was taken up by women teachers. Modern Educational Dance 1948 gave 16 basic movement themes and rudiments of free dance technique and space orientation. The word 'movement' came to reflect the 1940s and 1950s as 'posture' had reflected the 1930s.

## *Moving and Growing* and *Planning the Programme*

These two publications were issued by the Ministry of Education in 1952 and 1953 respectively. They replaced the old syllabuses and were to be implemented in primary schools. They combined the two influences of:

- obstacle training from the army;
- movement training from centres of dance.

Running parallel to these changes were:

- circuit training (devised by G.T. Adamson and R.E. Morgan at the University of Leeds);
- weight training – progressive resistance exercises;
- outward bound schools promoting adventurous activities to develop the personality within the natural environment in challenging conditions.

These publications developed as a result of changes in educational thinking which was to make learning stem from a more child-centred approach. The physical education teacher was now more autonomous, with personal control over the physical education syllabus. The activities included agility, playground and more major game skills, dance and movement to music, national dances and swimming. The key words which separate them from earlier forms of physical activity in state schools are:

- exploratory
- creative
- individual
- fun.

**Key terms**

**Child centred**
Devising a programme which takes into account the physiological, psychological and emotional development of children at different ages.

## Educational gymnastics

From the 1950s to the 1970s there was a significant rise in the uses of modern educational gymnastics. In this type of activity children were encouraged to respond with movement to a stimulus, or movement problem. For example, a teacher might set a task of finding as many different ways to travel across, along or over a bench. The child would be required to use a certain amount of imagination and creativity to solve the task.

However, there would be no right or wrong solution. The child was not forced to perform cartwheels but they could respond to the task with movements within their capabilities and therefore would develop confidence as they achieved a level of success.

This was very much a heuristic style of teaching as opposed to the more didactic and prescribed approach of the early twentieth century.

### Summary

- Physical activity in state schools at the end of the nineteenth century concentrated on military drill and Swedish gymnastics.
- Emphasis was placed on activities suitable for the poor conditions in state schools and discipline of the working classes.
- Disenchantment with these systems led to:
  - the Board of Education producing syllabuses in the first three decades of the twentieth century which schools were required to follow;
  - the syllabuses laid out the content and style of teaching as a guideline for teachers to follow;
  - strong emphasis was placed on teacher authority;

  - there was still very limited major games teaching.
- Syllabuses became defunct with the improvements in teacher training.
- The publications *Planning the Programme* and *Moving and Growing* reflected the change in emphasis from purely physical and organic developments to a focus on the development of the 'whole' child through the movement approach.
- The use of different terms over the years (drill, physical training and then physical education) reflect the gradual development of certain ideas. Changes occurred in content as well as in the relationship between the teacher and the class.

# Present-day physical education

## National Curriculum for England

### New Secondary Curriculum

The new Secondary Curriculum for England has been launched and will be implemented in schools from September 2008–2011.

The Government believes that two hours of physical activity a week, including the National Curriculum for physical education and extra-curricular activities, should be an aspiration for all schools.

| | Key stage I | Key stage 3 |
|---|---|---|
| **Acquiring and developing skills** | 1) Pupils should be taught to:<br>a. explore basic skills, actions and ideas with increasing understanding<br>b. remember and repeat simple skills and actions with increasing control and coordination. | 1) Pupils should be taught to:<br>a. refine and adapt existing skills<br>b. develop them into specific techniques that suit different activities and perform these with consistent control. |
| **Selecting and applying skills, tactics and compositional ideas** | 2) Pupils should be taught to:<br>a. explore how to choose and apply skills and actions in sequence and in combination<br>b. vary the way they perform skills by using simple tactics and movement phrases<br>c. apply rules and conventions for different activities. | 2) Pupils should be taught to:<br>a. use principles to plan and implement strategies, compositional and organisational ideas in individual, pair, group and team activities<br>b. modify and develop their plans<br>c. apply rules and conventions for different activities. |
| **Evaluating and improving performance** | 3) Pupils should be taught to:<br>a. describe what they have done<br>b. observe, describe and copy what others have done<br>c. use what they have learnt to improve the quality and control of their work | 3) Pupils should be taught to:<br>a. be clear about what they want to achieve in their own work, and what they have actually achieved<br>b. take the initiative to analyse their own and others' work, using this information to improve its quality. |

| | Key stage 1 | Key stage 3 |
|---|---|---|
| **Knowledge and understanding of fitness and health** | 4) Pupils should be taught:<br>a. how important it is to be active<br>b. to recognise and describe how their bodies feel during different activities | 4) Pupils should be taught::<br>a. how to prepare for and recover from specific activities<br>b. how different types of activity affect specific aspects of their fitness<br>c. the benefits of regular exercise and good hygiene<br>d. how to go about getting involved in activities that are good for their personal and social health and well-being |
| **Breadth of study** | 5) During the key stage, pupils should be taught the knowledge, skills and understanding through dance activities, games activities and gymnastic activities. | 5) During the key stage, pupils should be taught the knowledge, skills and understanding through four areas of activity. These should include:<br>a. games activities and three of the following, *at least one of which must be dance or gymnastic activities*:<br>b. dance activities<br>c. gymnastic activities<br>d. swimming activities and water safety<br>e. athletic activities<br>f. outdoor and adventurous activities |

## Summary

**During key stage 1** pupils build on their natural enthusiasm for movement, using it to explore and learn about their world. They start to work and play with other pupils in pairs and small groups. By watching, listening and experimenting, they develop their skills in movement and coordination, and enjoy expressing and testing themselves in a variety of situations.

**During key stage 3** pupils become more expert in their skills and techniques, and how to apply them in different activities. They start to understand what makes a performance effective and how to apply these principles to their own and others' work. They learn to take the initiative and make decisions for themselves about what to do to improve performance. They start to identify the types of activity they prefer to be involved with, and to take a variety of roles such as leader and official.

Competitive game activites are compulsory at key stage 3.

# Physical Education and School Sport (PESS)

## Achieving high quality PE

PE is the programme of study that schools offer in PE lessons. This section provides guidance on how your school can improve the quality of its PE.

## Achieving high quality school sport

School sport is physical activity, dance and sport that takes place outside PE lessons but is still organised by the school.

## Increasing participation in PESS

All of the schools involved in QCA's PESS investigation have succeeded in meeting the Government's target for 85% of pupils aged 5 to 16 to take part in a minumum of two hours of high quality PESS each week, both within and beyond the curriculum. In primary schools in the investigation 100% of pupils are involved in PESS for more than two hours each week. Most secondary schools in the investigation have two hours of PE timetabled for all pupils in key stage 4, and many more pupils have additional time for GCSE PE and related qualifications. In some schools in the investigation, this totals more than five hours of curriculum time.

The schools involved in the PESS investigation have achieved this by focusing on helping all pupils to:

- become fully involved in PE, school and community sport, making the most of the opportunities on offer
- enjoy PESS more, so that they want to take part
- have the confidence to get involved in different activities.

Schools involved in the investigation have worked hard to raise the participation of pupils of both sexes, whatever their culture, ethnicity, ability or disability.

## Ten Ways of increasing Physical Education and School Sport at Key Stages 3 and 4

1 Change the way PE is timetabled, e.g. more frequent and longer lessons/blocking activities
2 Change teaching approaches, e.g. sport education with differing roles such as official, manager, etc; use ITC – some pupils find this motivating; group pupils appropriately
3 Offer a wider range of qualifications, e.g. GCSE; JSLA; vocational and NGB awards
4 Develop Curriculum Pathways – offer a range of options
5 Ask pupils what they want – through surveys, school councils
6 Give pupils recognition – as mentors, class representatives and awards ceremonies
7 Make the most of Young Leaders – they can help teachers; become play leaders at playtime
8 Activities at lunchtimes – through informal recreational opportunities with equipment made available
9 Use local coaches and clubs – ensure they understand the ethos of the school; they can develop all aspects from skill development to NGB awards and encourage pupils to join clubs
10 Link with Heathly Lifestyles

For more information: visit qca.org.uk

### Activity 3

What are the similarities and differences between Key Stages 1 and 3 in terms of content, delivery and objectives?

Research information on Key Stages 2 and 4.

## Summary

The following points should be noted. In 1988 the government introduced the National Curriculum which was a return to a centralised approach towards education. The government wanted more control over education and to set national standards for which teachers would be accountable, through the attainment targets.

A wide range of physical activities is emphasised, with teachers being able to select activities from a set of guidelines. There are six sport classifications:

- games;
- gymnastics;
- dance;
- swimming;
- athletics;
- outdoor and adventurous activities.

This is to try to ensure all children receive a high-quality physical education.

As well as learning to perform a range of sports and activities, the National Curriculum encourages children to adopt other roles such as organiser/manager, informed spectator and critical performer, and advocates analysis and evaluation skills and coaching. Physical education should include physical, psychological and social benefits for the child which in turn should benefit society.

The 'movement' approach (educational gymnastics and dance), begun in the 1940s and 1950s, and the 'child-centred' and guidance discovery approach towards teaching and learning continue to be strong influences. The teaching of games has also to some extent adopted some of these ideas, such as encouraging children to create their own games and make up their own rules.

The tradition of keeping physical education and school sport (extra-curricular activities) separate has remained. The government is emphasising the benefits of physical education by increasing the number of hours it *suggests* schools should offer.

There is a variety of factors which affects the experiences children are offered during their physical education at primary and secondary school. These include:

- government guidelines/requirements;
- facilities available;
- wealth of the school;
- traditions of the school/local community;
- head teacher/physical education teacher preferences;
- type of school, e.g. private, public or state.

The government is also stressing the important role school sport has to play by introducing numerous policies, such as Physical Education and School Club Links Strategy [PESSCLS], but nevertheless it remains an optional activity for teachers and children.

Physical education and school sport are recognised as the foundation upon which children can develop active participation in physical recreation and sport. In the UK the 'drop-out rate' from active participation in sporting activities on leaving full-time education is one of the worst in Europe. Factors such as school finances, lack of teachers' goodwill, competing leisure interests for young people, poor physical education experiences alongside traditionally poor school club links help to account for this situation.

**Activity 4**

What are the advantages and disadvantages of keeping competitive school sport optional?

## Sport for young people

First of all we must recognise that not all young people share common lifestyles: they may have different socio-economic backgrounds, parental attitudes, social experiences, and so on. Youth is often seen as a transition from school and childhood to work and adulthood. Individuals who struggle with this transition often become isolated from the main community and 'drop out'; some may become deviant and when considered in larger numbers can form an underclass. This group will experience exclusion from society. Sport participation is mostly a result of early positive experiences in physical education curricula and recreational activities.

**Key terms**

**Post-school gap:** The drop in sport participation when people leave full-time education.

As early as 1960, the Wolfenden Report was concerned that the provision of sport in the UK was poorer than in other European states, leading to the post school gap, which results in a drop in participation on leaving school.

Some constraining factors are:

- the concentration in clubs on the talented youngsters;
- the tradition of single sport clubs in the UK, compared to more multi-sport clubs in Europe.

Physical activities are promoted by a wide range of individuals and agencies, such as:

- the education system, in particular the physical education programme;
- sports clubs and governing bodies;
- play workers;
- the youth service;
- local authorities.

It is necessary for these agencies to coordinate their efforts. For example, national governing bodies and schools associations need to plan programmes jointly which will support a common youth sport policy.

In previous years, the Sports Council targeted the age band 13–24 years. However, recent research (General Household Survey) suggested that low participation was not the problem, but that young people do not play as many sports as children. However, young females still participate less than their male counterparts. On leaving school, more casual sports are enjoyed, alongside adventure sports and health-related activities.

### Obesity and young children

The British Heart Foundation report *Couch Kids – the growing epidemic*, published in 2000, says that:

> Tackling overweight and obesity must start in childhood for two reasons:
> - because it is much easier to prevent becoming overweight than to correct it;
> - because it is easier to adopt healthy eating patterns when children are young.

The report contains some alarming statistics:

- Nearly 70 per cent of 2–12 year olds eat biscuits, sweets or chocolate at least once a day, while less than 20 per cent eat fruit and vegetables more than once a day.
- More than a third of children are not meeting the recommended activity guidelines – generally agreed to be at least one hour's moderate-intensity activity each day.
- The time traditionally spent on active play is being spent on sedentary activities such as watching television or playing computer games. More than a quarter of 11–16 year olds watch TV for more than four hours each day.
- Active transport to and from school has decreased. Car journeys to school have doubled in the last 20 years. Just 1 per cent of children cycle to school.

Sport England launched its Sportsmark Award and Activemark to encourage schools to help children adopt more positive attitudes towards physical activity.

### Youth and delinquency

A large body of literature has developed worldwide on this issue, suggesting increasing concern at governmental levels. The general consensus appears to be that sport:

- increases self-esteem, mood and perception of competence and mastery, especially through outdoor recreation;
- reduces self-destructive behaviour (smoking, drug use, substance abuse, suicidal tendencies);
- improves socialisation both with peer group and with adults;
- improves scholastic attendance and performance.

Schemes Several schemes run to help this particular group, but usually they are not long enough and participation is voluntary, suggesting that more hardened offenders will not benefit. An experience of a few days to a few weeks may be of benefit in the short term, but if the individual returns to the same physical and social deprivation, the old values and behaviour patterns will re-emerge. Sport, therefore, may form part of the solution, rather than offering a complete answer.

**IN CONTEXT**

**Young people were a crucial element in London winning the 2012 Games bid. The Games, and volunteering in particular, offer great opportunities to develop citizenship and leadership among young people.**

## Policies to improve school–club links

### Activemark

Activemark is an award scheme for primary schools that recognises good practice within physical education provision. The Activemark and Activemark Gold awards schemes recognise and reward primary, middle and special schools that provide young children with the opportunity of receiving the benefits of physical activity. It has been developed in partnership with the British Heart Foundation (BHF) and has the theme: 'Get Active, Stay Active'. To achieve an award the school needs to:

- offer a broad and balanced physical education programme;
- provide an environment that encourages physical activities;
- teach children the importance of staying active for life;
- provide enhanced curricular provision through some additional opportunities for physical activity;
- have an effective inclusion policy for pupils with disabilities.

Activemark Gold recognises all the above plus:

- realistic, in-depth physical education and physical activity development plans;
- a commitment to providing a range of additional, high-quality opportunities for physical activity.

A team of assessors appointed by Sport England reviews the schools against these rigorous criteria.

Kitemarks will reward delivery of the national PE, School Sports and Club Links strategy in future. They will therefore only be open to schools that are in a School Sport Partnership.

## Sportsmark

The Sportsmark scheme was introduced in the government report *Sport: Raising the Game* in 1995. It recognises and rewards the schools that provide the best physical education and sports provision to their pupils and the local community. The additional Gold Award is presented to those offering exceptional provision. To obtain the award, various criteria have to be achieved.

## Active Sports Programme

This scheme, coordinated by Sport England, is based on four policy headings:

1 Active schools – forms the foundation.
2 Active communities – looks at breaking down the barriers to participation and considers equity issues.
3 Active sports – links participation to excellence, such as participation in the Millennium Youth Games.
4 World Class England – operates four programmes: World Class Start, World Class Potential, World Class Performance and World Class Events.

They are meant to act as building blocks and are not necessarily linear. They also complement the sports councils' participation pyramid of foundation, participation, performance and excellence. The majority of the funding comes from the National Lottery and the regional set-up is strengthened via local authorities. There is a framework around all experiences available to potential participants, such as the National Junior Sports Programme, Sportsmark and Coaching for Teachers.

## Sports Leaders UK Leadership Awards

There are four different awards, catering for different age groups and needs:

- JSLA – The Junior Sports Leader Award is for 14–16 year olds and is taught mainly in schools within the national curriculum for physical education. The award develops a young person's skills in organising activities, planning, communicating and motivating.
- CSLA – For those over 16 years old, the popular Community Sports Leader award is taught in schools, colleges, youth clubs, prisons, and sports and leisure nationwide.
- HSLA – The Higher Sports Leader Award builds on the skills gained through the CSLA to equip people to lead specific community groups, such as older people, people with disabilities and primary school children. The award includes units in event management, first aid, sports development and obtaining a coaching award.
- BELA – The Basic Expedition Leader Award is for those interested in the outdoors, and builds the ability to organise safe expeditions and overnight camps.

## Sport Action Zones

Sport Action Zones (SAZs) are a response by Sport England to address the issue of sporting deprivation in the most socially and economically deprived areas of the country. Participation levels in these areas are considerably below the national average.

Sport is believed to be valuable in contributing to the lives of people in these areas, as well as helping in the regeneration of the communities. Sport is acting in association with many other agencies, across health, education, lifelong learning initiatives, and so on. At the time of writing, 12 such zones have been created, evenly spread around the country, including inner cities and rural areas. Sport England, in association with other partners, helps to fund the zones for an initial five-year period.

Examples of the kind of work the zones are carrying out include:

- working with young people involved in antisocial behaviour;
- working with community health services to support people in poor health;
- providing education, training and support for community sport workers in other sectors who might use sport to meet their objectives;
- setting up local clubs where none exists;
- making local sport centres more accessible;
- engaging with local community groups, especially ethnic minority groups.

## Sporting Ambassadors programme

This programme gives sports heroes and heroines (approximately 200 at present in a wide range of sports) the chance to motivate and inspire young people to participate in sport. They communicate through primary, secondary and special schools, and youth and sport clubs, emphasising the benefits of physical activity and a healthy lifestyle.

The ambassadors:

- visit the different venues;
- present cups, certificates and badges, and show their own achievements;
- speak at school assemblies and to small groups about their experiences as elite performers;
- coach groups of young people.

## Sports colleges

Sports colleges are part of the specialist schools programme run by the DfES. They will have an important role in helping to deliver the government's Plan for Sport:

> They will become important hub sites for school and community sport, providing high-quality opportunities for all young people in their neighbourhood. (Richard Caborn, Minister for Sport)

## School sport coordinators

By 2006, there were 3,200 school sport coordinators, working across families of schools with 18,000 primary link teachers.

The partnership around a sports college starts with an average of four schools, ultimately growing to eight schools. Each partnership receives a grant of up to £270,000 a year. This pays for the full-time partnership development manager.

A primary link teacher (PLT) is located within each of the primary/specialist schools in the partnership, with a remit to improve PE and school sport at the primary school. They have 12 days a year to spend on their work as link teachers.

The school sport coordinator (SSCo) is based around families of schools, with a team comprising a partnership development manager and a PLT. Their role is to enhance opportunities for young people to experience different sports, access high-quality coaching and engage in competition. They are released for two days a week.

The partnership development manager (PDM) is usually located within a sports college, and manages the development of the partnership and the links with other PE and sport organisations.

The overall aim of the partnership is to ensure that children spend a minimum of two hours a week on high-quality PE and school sport. Six strategic objectives have been set:

1. Strategic planning – develop and implement a PE/sport strategy.
2. Primary liaison – develop links, particularly between Key Stages 2 and 3.
3. Out of school hours – provide enhanced opportunities for all pupils.
4. School to community – increase participation in community sport.
5. Coaching and leadership – provide opportunities in leadership, coaching and officiating for senior pupils, teachers and other adults.
6. Raising standards – raise standards of pupil achievement.

## Academies

Academies are a new type of school. The school leadership needs to draw on the skills of sponsors and other supporters in order to develop educational strategies to raise standards and contribute to diversity in areas of disadvantage.

They are all-ability schools, established by sponsors from business, faith or voluntary groups, working in innovative partnerships with government and education. Running costs are met in full by the DfES. Local education authorities are expected to consider the scope for such establishments in areas of disadvantage. They offer a broad and balanced education, specialising in one or more subject areas.

## Sports schools

There is a small selection of specialist sports schools in the UK, but again there is no centralised approach. Some examples are Millfield, Kelly College, Reeds School and Lilleshall. The advantages of such institutions are the combination of top-quality coaching, education, accommodation, medical science, a pool of similar talent, an organised competition structure and links with professional clubs. However, there are some disadvantages. They form a private network of schools which results in an exclusive system, inevitably drawing from a limited pool of talent. Young people may have to experience residential, institutionalised life away from home, and the physical and psychological demands are high.

## PE School Sport and Club Links Strategy (PESSCL)

A high-quality physical education for all children is at the heart of the government's new strategy and brings together a number of existing programmes. PESSCL is to be delivered by the DfES and the DCMS through various programmes (see below). Linked delivery on coaching will also support the strategy, and local authorities need to come together to ensure the effective delivery of these programmes. Over the last few years the government has invested £459 million to transform PE and school sport.

### Gifted and talented

It is part of the government's wider strategy to improve gifted and talented education. It aims to improve the range and quality of teaching, coaching and learning for talented sportspeople, in order to raise their aspirations and improve their performance, motivation and self-esteem. It also aims to encourage young talent to join sports clubs, and to strengthen the relationship between schools and national governing bodies (NGBs). Up to 10 per cent of pupils in primary and secondary schools will be supported. It will include the introduction of talent development camps for pupils in years 6 and 7. Nationally, the programme will include:

- a web-based resource for teachers, coaches and parents;
- a national support network for talented young athletes with disabilities;
- NGB-organised national performance camps for elite young athletes;
- a national faculty of gifted and talented trainers to provide continuing professional development;
- extracurriculum provision for academically able 11–16 year olds in PE and sports studies;
- a school-based profiling and tracking system.

### Step into Sport

Sport relies on 1.5 million volunteer officials, coaches, administrators and managers. Step into Sport is aiming to build on this trend and extend grass-roots interest in this area into a more coordinated strategic approach by NGBs, county sports partnerships and clubs. It should ensure that clubs are ready to receive, develop and deploy a steady supply of volunteers.

Between 2002 and 2004, Step into Sport was delivered in almost 200 school sport coordinator partnerships across all 45 county sport partnership areas, by a consortium of the Youth Sports Trust (via the Top Link programme – see National Junior Sports Programme, below), the British Sports Trust (via Sports Leader Awards) and Sport England, each with their own responsibilities.

This is a new initiative funded by the DCMS and the Home Office Active Communities Unit, which brings together the British Sports Trust and Sport England to encourage young people to become more involved with sport in their local communities. The aim is to provide a structured pathway to attract over 48,000 young people, aged 14–19 years, into voluntary sports coaching. The network of partnerships will be focused mainly around the government's Sport and Education Action Zones.

### National Junior Sports Programme

The National Junior Sports Programme was launched in February 1996 by the Sports Council, working alongside the Youth Sports Trust. Its aim is to encourage young children from the age of four to become involved in sport. It will provide kit, coaching and places to play, and the more talented performers can be identified from a wider base. It is a rolling programme and many teachers are trained. The advantage is that it can fit neatly into the current physical education system. There are five main elements:

**Table 11.2** The FA School Club Links Programme

| Opportunities | Description |
|---|---|
| FA Charter Standard Schools Programme | Involves primary, middle, secondary and special schools, independent and state. Requires as part of the criteria for all schools to form a partnership, with a local charter standard club for boys and girls |
| FA Charter Standard Development Club | Requires clubs which have met the development criteria (minimum of five teams) to create a partnership with a local school or schools as part of their football development plan |
| FA Charter Standard Community Clubs | Requires clubs (minimum ten teams, male and female) to form school club links and appoint a voluntary schools liaison officer |
| FA TOP Sport Football Community Programme | Targets young people aged 7–11 who are less likely to be participating in football for their school due to more limited opportunities and helps them move on to Charter Standard Club |
| Active Sports Girls Football Programme | The Active Sports programme is a fundamental part of the FA's strategy for the development of girls' football. The framework includes a school club link scheme for 10–16 year olds called Kick Start |
| FA Soccability Community Programme | This is an educational programme designed as part of the FA TOP Sport Football Programme to assist young people with disabilities to participate in football |

- Top Play (4–9 year olds);
- Top Sport (7–11 year olds);
- Champion Coach;
- Top Club (11 years+);
- Top Link.

There have been growing calls for more 'inclusive' physical education programmes. These programmes need to cater for the diversity of students, their needs and the schools they attend. It is possible that the government focus on competitive team sports, since the publication of *Sport: Raising the Game*, may not have been successful, as studies suggest these are not the sporting activities which attract this age group (Coalter 1999). Sustaining a broader choice at school is likely to support lifelong participation.

In the New Opportunities Fund, lottery fund money will be available for schemes that encourage the value of sport as character building and diversion, such as summer play schemes and after-school clubs.

The National Junior Sports Programme is intended to support the national curriculum as an additional resource for teachers.

Coaching for Teachers is a joint initiative, funded by Sport England and coordinated by SportsCoachUK, with support from the British Association of Advisers and Lecturers in Physical Education (BAALPE) and the Physical Education Association (PEA), to involve teachers in extracurricular activities.

## School Club Links

The overall aim is to increase the proportion of children guided into clubs from SSCo partnerships. The primary focus is on seven major sports (tennis, cricket, rugby union, football, athletics, gymnastics and swimming). The reasons for their selection included:

- the capacity of the NGB;
- they are central to the national curriculum;
- their ability to help lead other sports;
- popular with both sexes;
- multi skills;
- mix of individual and team sports;
- focus of government initiatives and investment.

# National governing bodies

A national governing body is responsible for its own sport, overseeing competitions and ensuring internationally agreed rules are adhered to. The NGB then affiliates to the International Sport Federation (ISF). An example would be the FA and FIFA. In the past, NGBs in the UK have been very independent, but nowadays they have to demonstrate that they are meeting some of the core objectives of the government if they are to receive lottery funding.

There are approximately 300 governing bodies in the UK. Many are run by unpaid volunteers, although depending on the size of the organisation this has in many cases become the responsibility of paid administrators. They are largely autonomous from the government and are represented by the Central Council of Physical Recreation (CCPR).

Despite the considerable differences between the various governing bodies there are some common aims, including to:

- establish rules and regulations in accordance with the ISF;
- increase participation at the grass-roots level;
- identify and develop talent;
- organise competitions;
- develop coaching awards and leadership schemes;
- select teams for country or UK at international events;
- liaise with relevant organisations such as the CCPR, Sport England, local clubs, British Olympic Association and ISF.

## Changes experienced by national governing bodies

The decline in school sport has led to governing bodies having to consider how best to develop talent. There has been a blurring between amateur and professional sport. The need to compete internationally with countries which have systematic forms of training has made the governing bodies develop the coaching and structuring of competitions.

Funding has become a key issue. NGBs receive money from their member clubs, but elite sport requires huge sums of money. For this governing bodies have had to market themselves in the modern world, especially in trying to attract television coverage which in turn brings in sponsorship deals.

Lottery funding often brings with it certain requirements, such as meeting government targets for participation and developing talent.

NGBs must produce a whole sport plan (WSP), for the whole of a sport from grass roots right through to the elite level, to identify how it will achieve its vision and how it will contribute to Sport England's 'start, stay and succeed' objectives.

WSPs are Sport England's new way of directing funding and resources to NGBs. They will identify the help and resources NGBs need to deliver their WSPs, for example via partners such as county sport partnerships and programmes (e.g. PESSCLS). They provide the opportunity to measure how the NGBs are delivering their sports.

## Key performance indicators

Seven key performance indicators (KPIs) have been agreed which reflect proposals and feedback from Sport England, UK Sport, NGBs and other partners. Sport England will use these high-level KPIs to measure the achievements delivered by the whole sport plans.

The seven KPIs that should be addressed in each plan are:

**Start and stay**

1 Participation – an increase in participation through NGB-driven activity.
2 Clubs – the number of accredited clubs within the sport.
3 Membership – the number of active members of clubs within the sport.
4 Coaches – the number of qualified coaches and instructors delivering instruction in the sport.
5 Volunteers – the number of active volunteers supporting the sport.

**Succeed**

6 International success – performance by teams and/or individuals in significant international championships and world rankings.

7 English athletes representing GB – the percentage of English athletes in GB teams in sports competing as GB.

WSPs will achieve the following:

- In short, 'start, stay and succeed' (Sport Englands objectives).
- They will allow Sport England to give focused investments to NGBs against the resources they need to achieve their objectives.
- Measurable results will give us an indication of how well NGBs are performing and whether Sport England is getting value for money from our investment.
- They will help create more links with regions and partners in all aspects of sport, benefiting us all through shared best practice.

**Key terms**

**Whole Sport Plan [WSP]**
A WSP is a plan for the whole of a sport from grass roots right through to the elite level, which identifies how it will achieve its vision and how it will contribute to Sport England's 'start, stay and succeed' objectives.

## A plan for the development of gymnastics in England 2005–2009

Strategic objectives for English gymnastics are as follows:

- Increase NGB-led participation in gymnastics by 12 per cent by 2009.
- Increase coaches and teachers qualified to deliver quality gymnastics from 31,000 to 45,000.
- Increase the number of trained and active officials and volunteers to support the sport of gymnastics.
- Increase the number of affiliated and accredited clubs.
- Increase support to clubs to enable them to strengthen and develop.
- Ensure equality and child protection standards are implemented in line with British gymnastics policies.
- Raise the level of performance and range of opportunities in each discipline of gymnastics.
- Improve the profile and marketing of gymnastics at home country, regional and local level.

### What you need to know

* Games developed technically in the public schools by refining skills and strategies, creating structure in terms of boundaries and numbers of players, facility and equipment developments and kit to distinguish teams.
* Athleticism was defined as physical endeavour with moral integrity. This became a cult in the nineteenth-century public schools as a fanatical devotion to sport.
* Muscular Christianity was a movement in society which recognised the positive values of rational recreation, not for the sake of sport but by preparing people to serve God with both their minds and bodies.
* The watershed for the state school system of education began in 1870. There was a transition in terminology from drill (military) to physical training (syllabuses) to physical education (*Moving and Growing* and the present-day National Curriculum).

* The level of government control over education changed:
  – from the late nineteenth century to 1933 it was a centralised system;
  – from 1933 to 1988 a decentralised system operated;
  – with the introduction of the National Curriculum in 1988 there was a return to a centralised system but with guidelines for schools rather than being purely prescriptive.
* There are 4 key stages in the National Curriculum, Key Stage 1 and 2 (primary); Key Stage 3 and 4 (secondary).
* There are six sport classifications on the National Curriculum: games; gymnastics; dance; swimming; outdoor and adventurous activities; athletics.
* There are numerous current initiatives to increase participation of young people in competitive school sport such as PESSCLS (Physical Education and School Sport Club Links Strategy) and sports colleges and school sport coordinators.

## Review questions

1 What were the characteristics of the nineteenth-century public schools and the state schools?

2 Describe the process in the technical development of games in the public schools.

3 Define the terms 'athleticism' and 'Muscular Christianity' and discuss their influence on sport and society.

4 Why was athleticism acceptable to the middle classes?

5 Trace the development of gymnastics in state schools from the nineteenth century to the present day.

6 What was the legacy of the public schools in the development of games in state schools?

7 How has the control of government in education changed since the nineteenth century?

8 What are the advantages and disadvantages of having a National Curriculum for Physical Education?

9 Explain the terms 'drill', 'physical training' and 'physical education' and explain how they reflect the changing nature of British society.

10 Briefly outline the major points of PESSCLS policy.

11 How can national governing bodies help to increase participation in their sport?

CHAPTER 12

# Potential barriers to participation and possible solutions

## Learning outcomes

**By the end of this chapter you should understand the following:**

- the terms equal opportunity; discrimination; stereotyping; inclusiveness and prejudice
- the barriers to participation and possible solutions to overcome them for the following target groups:
  - people with disabilities
  - low socio economic social class
  - ethnic minority groups
  - gender;
- the effectiveness of national governing body policies in achieving equal opportunities in active recreation and sport for a variety of social groups.

## Equal opportunities?

In the last section we looked at the different organisations involved in sport and physical activities. We now need to ask the following questions:

- Who are these organisations working for?
- Which groups are they targeting in their aims to increase participation?
- How and why are they trying to develop sporting excellence?
- What's the role of opportunity, provision and esteem for the various social groups in their quest for sporting participation and/or sporting excellence.

We will concentrate on various social groups and the policies developed to increase their levels of physical activity, and try to establish some of the reasons for low participation. We will also study the meaning of excellence in sport and the opportunities available to different social groups.

Many of the qualities assigned to sport are well recognised – opportunity for self-knowledge, personal achievement, good health, enjoyment, skill acquisition, social interaction, responsibility, development of confidence, and so on. We should therefore be concerned that certain sections of the population are missing out on the chance to benefit from such an enriching experience.

It is important to understand the sociological basis for inequality in sport. This is not intended to be a thorough sociological review, but a tool to help us achieve a greater understanding of the issue.

### All men are equal

In the descriptive sense, this is patently untrue: human beings do not possess the same amount of physical, mental or moral qualities. In the prescriptive sense, however, people ought to treat one another with equal respect, dignity and consideration.

## Stratification of society

Society can be divided into layers, just like rocks (i.e. rock strata). The divisions are based on biological, economic and social criteria, such as age, gender, race and social class. The dominant group in society, which controls the major social institutions like the media, law, education and politics, can exercise control over the more subordinate groups. This dominant group need not be the majority – think of previous minority white rule in South Africa. Using this classification, the dominant group in the UK could be described as white, male and middle class; the subordinate groups would be women, ethnic minorities, people with disabilities and those belonging to the working class.

Discrimination can occur when opportunities available to the dominant group are not available to all social groups.

**Key terms**

**Discrimination:** To make a distinction, to give unfair treatment especially because of prejudice. It occurs when a prejudicial attitude is acted on. Discrimination can be overt (e.g. laws which form part of the structure of a society, like the former political system of apartheid, or a membership clause for a private sports club). This can be officially wiped out by changing the law, but covert (hidden or less obvious) discrimination (e.g. people's attitudes and beliefs) can be very hard to dislodge.
**Prejudice:** An unfavourable opinion or attitude often displaying intolerance or dislike of people of a certain race, religion or culture. When acted upon it becomes discrimination.
**Stereotype:** A standardised image or concept shared by all members of a social group. Common stereotypes are based around gender, race and social class.
**Inclusiveness:** All people should have their needs, abilities,and aspiratioons recognised and understood and met within a supportive environment. Inclusive policies are designed to combat the problems associated with social exclusion.

When subordinate groups in society are discriminated against, their opportunities are limited, including opportunities of social mobility (the pattern of movement from one social class to a higher or lower one). This can also be affected by whether the social system is closed (an extreme example is the Hindu caste system in India) or open (a true egalitarian democracy).

## Sport and stratification

Sport is often described by sociologists as a microcosm of society: it reflects in miniature all facets of society. This includes the institutionalised divisions and inequalities which characterise our society. Sporting institutions are equally controlled by the dominant group in society, and stratification in sport is inevitable when winning is highly valued. It is highlighted even more when monetary rewards are available.

Sport is often cited as an avenue for social mobility:

- physical skills and abilities – professional sports requires little formal education;
- sport may create progression through the education system (e.g. athletic scholarships);
- occupational sponsorship may lead to future jobs;
- sport can encourage values such as leadership and teamwork skills, which may help in the wider world of employment.

Although 'sport for all' campaigns are no longer a direct function of Sport England, the groups who are targeted by such initiatives are still under-represented in sport participation. More recently, their participation has been addressed at government level, under the DCMS, using the term 'social exclusion groups'.

### Social exclusion

Aspects of exclusion are:

- ethnicity;
- gender;
- disability;
- youth;
- age;
- sexuality;
- poverty;
- in rural areas/cities.

### Defining exclusion

The Social Exclusion Unit's definition of social exclusion is:

a shorthand label for what can happen when individuals or areas suffer a combination of linked problems such as unemployment, poor skills, low incomes, poor housing, high crime environments, bad health and family breakdown.

So what role can sport play in this situation? Many studies have been carried out and moves are under way for improving the perception of recreation. When considering this area you will need to address the following:

- Descriptive – explain and give examples of how discrimination occurs for the identified groups in society.
- Reformative – suggest solutions to the identified problems.

Table 12.1 shows a summary of the nature and strengths of the benefits of sport, and also the experiences of the excluded groups without direct action by the state or voluntary organisations.

## Constraints and exclusion in sport

These can be broken down into three main categories:

- environmental/structural constraints (economic, physical and social factors);
- personal constraints (internal and psychological);
- attitudes of society and provider systems (policies and managers' practices can act as barriers or enablers).

Sports equity

| Overcoming discrimination: | Can be achieved through: |
|---|---|
| • Recognising your own prejudice<br>• Understanding the difficulty<br>• Talking to people<br>• Receiving support from others<br>• Thinking of alternatives<br>• Going on a training course<br>• Using a policy/ guidelines | • Sharing common values<br>• Promoting equality through sport<br>• Working in partnership<br>• Endorsing the law<br>• Challenging discrimination |

Combinations of aspects of exclusion can be said to lead to double deprivation, for example, being elderly and from an ethnic minority. If exclusion is prolonged in youth it can have lasting effects in terms of playing recreationally, socialising and competing to achieve.

## Race

'Race' refers to the physical characteristics of an individual, while 'ethnicity' is belonging to a particular group (e.g. religious, lifestyle). Racism is a set of beliefs or ideas based on the assumption that races have distinctive cultural characteristics determined by hereditary factors, and that this endows some races with an intrinsic superiority.

The media promote the popular idea of sport enabling many individuals to 'climb the social ladder', as well as highlighting racism in sport and the lack of equal opportunities.

Sport England and governing bodies have sought to encourage non-discriminatory attitudes to combat racism and to open up organisations to equal opportunities.

### Examples of racism in sport

1. Stacking – Refers to the disproportionate concentration of ethnic minorities in certain positions in a sports team, which tends to be based on the stereotype that they are more valuable for their physical skills than for their decision making and communication qualities. In American football there has been a tendency to place ethnic players in running back and wide receiver positions. In baseball, until fairly recently, they have tended to be in outfield positions.
2. Centrality theory (Grusky 1963) – This restricts ethnic players from more central positions which are based on coordinative tasks and require more interaction and decision making. Significantly, coaches who make these decisions are generally white. Sociological studies have revealed the self-perpetuating coaching subculture which exists in American sport (Coakley 1994). When existing coaches need to sponsor a new coach, they are likely to select one with similar ideas to their own.
3. Channelling – Ethnic minorities may be pushed into certain sports, and even certain positions within a team, based on assumptions.

Table 12.1 Constraints and exclusion in sport and leisure

| **Constraint/** | **Youth** | | | **Poor/ unemployed** | **Women** | **Older people** | **Ethnic minority** | **People with disabilities/ learning difficulties** |
|---|---|---|---|---|---|---|---|---|
| | **Children** | **Young people** | **Young delinquents** | | | | | |
| Poor physical/ social environment | + | + | ++ | + + | + | + | + + | + |
| Poor facilities/ community capacity | + | + | + + | + + | + | + | + | + + |
| Poor support network | + | + | + + | + + | + | + | + | + + |
| Poor transport | + + | + + | + + | + + | + + | + + | + | + + |
| Managers' policies and attitudes | + | + | + + | + + | + | + | + + | + + |
| Labelling by society | + | + | + + + | + | + | + | + + | + + |
| Lack of time structure | + | + | + + | + + | | + | | + |
| Lack of income | + | + | + + + | + + + | + | + + | + | + + |
| Lack of skills/ personal and social capital | + | + | + + + | + + + | + | + | + + | + + |
| Fears of safety | + + | + + | + + | + + | + + + | + + + + | + + | + + |
| Powerlessness | + + | + + | + + + | + + | + + | + + | + + + + | + + |
| Poor self-/ body image | + | + | + + | + + | + | + | + + | + + |

*Source*: Department for Culture, Media and Sport

**Note**: The number of + signs shows the severity of particular constraints for particular groups.

## Attempts to overcome racism in sport

'Let's stamp racism out of football' This was a large-scale, national campaign, which began in 1993/94. It was intended to cut racial harassment out of football in the UK. It was supported by the Commission for Racial Equality (CRE) and the Professional Footballers Association (PFA), along with supporters' groups, the FA, the Football Trust, and the Premier and Endsleigh Leagues. In 1994/95, over 10 per cent of clubs took specific action.

The antiracism campaigns were initiated by fans themselves originally, culminating in the national campaign (now called Kick it Out), which has received support from various Ministers for Sport. The focus has now shifted to studying to what extent racism exists at the institutional level.

A recent study by Malcolm and Last at the Centre for Research into Sport and Society at the University of Leicester suggested that at first it would appear that at the elite level there are few barriers for players to overcome. Compared to the number who claim to be of Afro-Caribbean origin on the General Household survey (1 per cent), they seem to be well represented, particularly at the Premiership level (17.5 per cent in 1995/96).

Positional play Over a ten-year period, Malcolm and Last's research found that 50 per cent of black players played in forward positions. These can be glamorous positions, involving high goal scoring and impressive transfer fees. Average black players in the Premier League commanded transfer fees of £1 million more than white players.

However, the main difference occurs in the career paths taken by black footballers. Few break their way into management positions, for example as directors or FA committee members. It is also notable that few Asian players have broken through into the professional ranks.

## Race and education

There has been a tendency for teachers to act on a stereotype, labelling children from ethnic minority groups and developing certain expectations of them. This can be self-perpetuating, as children may internalise these misconceptions and regard the sport side of educational life as the only successful route for them.

Sports Participation and Ethnicity in England 1999/2000 The survey was part of Sport England's commitment to better understand the extent and causes of inequity in sporting opportunities for certain groups in the population, and identify ways to overcome them. The findings have particular relevance to the Active Communities programme, which aims to extend sporting opportunities for all.

The findings were:

- For ethnic minority groups, the overall participation rate in sport was 40 per cent, compared to a 46 per cent national average.
- Only the Black Other group (60 per cent) had participation rates higher than the population as a whole. Black Caribbean, Chinese, Pakistani and Bangladeshi were lower than the national average. These figures were similar for women from the same groups. However, the gap between men's and women's participation was found to be greater among ethnic minority groups than in the population as a whole.

The reasons given for constraining factors in participation were similar to those in the population as a whole, for example, 'work/study demands, home and family responsibilities, lack of money, laziness', but some also quoted negative experiences in sport due to ethnicity. These instances were higher for the Black Other men and less relevant for the Chinese section of the population.

Defining ethnicity is fraught with problems, as it is almost impossible to identify a whole group and presume they will have similar experiences. This is particularly so where religion, culture, values, language, generation, age, gender, length of residency in a country and nationality all play a part in creating considerable diversity of experiences, expectations, way of life and behaviours. However, for the purposes of a national quantitative survey it is required that people be classified into 'broad ethnic groups'. The groups people could choose from were:

- White;
- Black Caribbean;
- Black African;
- Black Other;
- Indian;
- Pakistani;

- Bangladeshi;
- Chinese;
- None of these (17 per cent) became 'Other'.

Participation was defined as 'having taken part in sport or physical activities on at least one occasion in the previous four weeks, excluding walking'. It does not include refereeing or coaching.

An important result of the survey is the complexity of the whole issue. There is considerable variation in the levels of participation between different ethnic groups, between men and women and between different sports. The results also challenge the stereotypical view which suggests that low levels of participation in sport by certain groups are more a reflection of culture and choice than other constraints such as provision, affordability and access.

## Gender

Gender means the biological aspect of a person, either male or female. Gender roles refer to what different societies and cultures attribute as appropriate behaviour for that sex.

We learn our expected role through a process called socialisation, which simply means the learning of cultural values (which is equally applicable to table manners!). We learn first through primary socialisation (mainly from our close family group at an early age), and then through secondary socialisation from the wider world of institutions. What emerges are the terms 'masculinity' and 'femininity', in relation to gender roles.

Gender role models are first asserted in children's play, and early in primary schools there are clear differences in the preferences of girls for less structured activities. Later come matters of self-image and body image, with sportswomen often being portrayed by the media as either muscle-bound superwomen or sleek and fit in a way that seems far beyond the reach of normal women.

Historical factors regarding the role of women cannot be discounted either:

- Sport was always seen as a male preserve. Males developed and controlled most of the modern-day sports.
- Men, as the dominant group in society, denied or limited opportunities for women in relation to the types of sports they could participate in.
- The role of women was stereotypically seen as being the housewife or mother.
- The types of activities women were encouraged to participate in were those considered appropriate to their role and therefore socially acceptable.
- Middle- and upper-class ladies in the nineteenth century began to play sports such as golf, tennis, horse riding, archery, and so on. These activities were not particularly physically demanding and did not involve physical contact or aggression.
- Activities that females could play socially with males were also highly valued, such as croquet followed by lawn tennis.
- Working-class women had the least leisure opportunities of all.

In the present day, opportunities for women have increased in terms of:

- greater independence;
- more disposable income;
- personal transport;
- availability of more sports, clubs and competitions;
- more media coverage;
- more women in positions of responsibility in sports organisations.

The overriding image of female participation in sport is still the emphasis placed on health, fitness and the stereotypical feminine figure.

### Sexism in sport

Sexism is the belief that one sex is inferior to the other, and is most often directed towards women. It is sometimes based on the idea that women are not best suited to roles which carry prestige and influence. Traditionally, women have been denied the same legal, political, economic and social rights enjoyed by men.

It is important not to underestimate the long-lasting effect of attitudes which are handed down through the generations. Sexism against women operates in sport in numerous ways:

## The Sex Discrimination Act 1975

This act made sex discrimination unlawful in employment, training, education and the provision of goods, facilities and services; that is, it set down in law that a female should be treated in the same way as a male in similar circumstances.

Competitive sport is excluded by Section 44 of the Act. Separate competitions for men and women are allowed where 'the physical strength, stamina or physique puts her at a disadvantage to the average man'. Problems have occurred where female referees and PE teachers have been denied promotion on the grounds of being a woman, and some successful appeals have been made.

Private sports clubs can legally operate discriminatory policies, under Sections 29 and 34. After an appeal in 1987, the EC recommended that all clubs which are not genuinely private must remove any barriers which discriminate against men or women.

## Women and professional sport

Professional sport still tends to favour men, even in activities such as pool, where physical strength differences could be questioned.

Only women who are very dedicated and committed move through from participation to a level of excellence. Myths and negative stereotypes still abound, and the media give much less coverage to women's sport:

- Surveys have shown that national newspapers give less than 6 per cent of total sport space to women's sport.
- There are more sport competitions for men.
- Financial constraints affect women more than men, as they attract less sponsorship to help with training, equipment, travelling and general fees.

Female power in sports organisations and higher levels of administration has not matched the rise in female sport participation.

- Few women reach the top levels of coaching: in 1992 there were only 8 female coaches at the Olympics, compared with 92 male coaches.
- Mixed governing bodies, such as swimming, badminton, tennis, riding and cycling, all show a poor ratio of female decision makers in proportion to the number of female participants.

The problem has increased with a more professional and bureaucratic environment, and perhaps reflects the inappropriateness of the male model of sport, women's lack of access to political systems and the poor recruitment mechanisms operating in these institutions.

However, improvements are occurring slowly. The first woman Vice President of the IOC was appointed in 1997.

Female football in the UK is now a professional sport. The Football Association set up a full-time professional league of women's teams in 2000. Millions of pounds were spent and women players can train full-time. Women's football has been confirmed as the UK's fastest-growing sport. In 1993 there were 500 clubs; this figure had risen to 6,200 clubs by 2005. England ladies have a full-time coach and 1,000 players attend 30 regional centres of excellence.

An interesting competition took place in 2003, when Annika Sorenstam became the first female golfer to take on the men in professional competition in 58 years:

> I'm not putting the guys to the test here, or men against women. I would like to emphasise that. I don't want to get into any political things. I don't have anything to do with that. It's not any goal. I don't want to put the guys on the defensive.

Although it caused a storm of protest from certain quarters, the event went ahead. Annika did not make the cut, but she was certainly not outplayed and gave everyone something to think about.

### The Women's Sports Foundation (WSF)

This is a voluntary organisation which promotes the interests of women and girls in sport and recreation. There is a network of regional groups and a wide range of activities and events are organised. Their regular publication is *Women in Sport* Magazine.

### Female participation in recent years

In 1996, the General Household Survey (GHS) reported that men were more likely to participate in a sport or physical activity than women: 87 per cent of men, compared with 77 per cent of women, had taken part in at least one activity during the previous 12 months.

Football is the number one sport for girls and women. There are now 61,000 women competing in clubs affiliated to the Football Association, and there has also been an increase in the number of girls' football teams which are developing within schools. There are 40,000 more under-14 girls playing at school than there were in the mid 1990s.

One problem holding back the amount of girls taking up the sport, however, is the lack of career prospects. There are still only around 19 England-based professional players. The FA has put in place a series of initiatives to increase opportunities for women in football:

- In 1997 it launched its Talent Development Plan for Women's Football.
- Establishment of 42 Centres of Excellence – to develop 10–16 year olds.
- 19 Women's Football Academies – 16 years plus.
- In 2001 the National Women's Player Development Centre was launched at Loughborough University – for the most promising.

Kay (1994) confirmed that women are constrained in their leisure time by the needs of housekeeping and caring for dependants, and by lower car ownership than men. These effects are stronger for women in the lower socio-economic groups. Women's participation in indoor sport has grown, mainly due to the fitness boom and aerobic classes, but participation is still in decline in terms of outdoor sports. In addition to time and transport constraints, fear of attack in urban parks and the countryside have been cited as problems faced by women.

Table 12.2 sets out some of the reasons why women have less time for sport than men.

## Girls and physical education policies

Physical education policies, through the government initiatives in the national curriculum, can still appear to show preferences for competitive team games, sex-differentiated programmes and traditional teaching methods that may alienate many girls.

NIKE and the Youth Sports Trust are cooperating in a scheme that aims to support the delivery of physical education and sport to girls aged 11–14 years, in secondary schools.

## Windhoek Call for Action 1998

*From Brighton to Windhoek: Facing the Challenge* is a document produced by the UK Sports Council and the International Working Group on Women and Sport. The publication charts the progress made from 1994 to 1998 in developing a sporting culture that enables and values the full involvement of women in every aspect of sport. It provides an international overview of strategies and action plans adopted by women and sports in various countries. It considers the challenge that lies ahead and the implementation of the Windhoek Call for Action.

### What women can do

- Develop a positive attitude to a healthy lifestyle; find out what is available locally and encourage a friend to go with them; be determined!
- Having developed an interest, join a club to gain access to coaching and facilities; lobby a governing body, local authority and the media to increase availability and opportunity of coaching, facilities, competition and coverage.
- Attend courses to improve career prospects; apply for senior positions; become a coach or administrator; gain relevant qualifications.
- Be aware that family responsibilities can coexist with other aspirations.

### What organisations can do

- Ensure equality of opportunity to acquire sports skills.
- Adopt policies on child care, transport, access, pricing and programming of facilities.
- Recognise that women do not form an homogeneous group. Women who have disabilities, are members of an ethnic minority, have heavy domestic responsibilities, have busy working lives or are school leavers will all require some specific action directed at them.
- Positive images of women should be widely seen in a variety of sport promotional material, not only the traditionally female sports. This will help provide much-needed role models for young girls.
- Redress inequalities in competition, coaching and financial assistance, and improve the talent identification process.
- Review recruitment practices, establish appropriate training and allow flexible working hours.
- Publicise the achievements of women's contributions to sport.

Table 12.2 How the hours of the week are spent for the average male and female

| | Full-time working male | Full-time working female |
|---|---|---|
| Work and travel to work | 47.2 | 42.3 |
| Household chores, essential cooking and shopping | 12.0 | 24.5 |
| Other non-discretionary activities (other shopping, caring for children personal hygiene) | 13.9 | 18.6 |
| Free time | 45.9 | 33.6 |

*Source*: The Henley Centre 1991

**Note**: This table assumes seven hours of sleep per night.

**IN CONTEXT**

**The Wimbledon Championships introduced equal earnings for men and women in 2007. The Championships declared a percentage increase in the women's prize pot that outstrips the men's, but the tournament chairman defended the earnings contrast, saying, 'We work off the market situation... This is nothing to do with women's rights, it is to do with the marketplace.' He went on to say:**

> **Women tend to win easily in the early rounds, so they are able to play in the doubles. Some of the early round matches last up to three sets, whereas even Sampras could have a first-round five-setter. Seven different people have won the last seven Grand Slam singles titles and that shows how the competitiveness at the top level of the women's game has grown. We also recognise that the top women take away more money from Wimbledon than the men. Last year Venus Williams took away eight per cent more than Pete Sampras, because she won the doubles, in which Sampras did not take part.**

## Activity 1

Discuss the reasons for and against female tennis players receiving equivalent prize money to their male counterparts.

## Sport and people with disabilities

According to the Labour Force Survey 2004, there are 6.5 million adults with disabilities in Britain – 11.1 per cent of the population. Approximately 5 million have a disability severe enough to limit everyday activities, and 1 million have a learning disability. Of these 6.5 million, 69 per cent are over the age of 60, with 5 per cent under 30 years of age.

### Disability sport

This is a term used to suggest a more positive approach towards the participation in sport of people with disabilities. It covers people with a physical, sensory or mental impairment. The term 'disability' is used when impairment adversely affects performance. Other terms used are handicapped sports, sports for the disabled, adapted sport, wheelchair sport and deaf sport.

Many people experience discrimination which effectively excludes them from active social participation. Yet sport can help to integrate people with disabilities into the rest of society and improve their quality of life. DePauw and Gavron (1995) described the barriers as similar to those for women, including a lack of organised programmes, informal early experiences, role models and access, along with other economic, physiological and social factors. Reasons for lower participation are:

- Safety concerns/traditionally considered dangerous.
- Stereotypes – generally society has lower expectations.
- Psychologically, people with disabilities may have less confidence and self-esteem.
- Lack of specialist coaches or leaders who are knowledgeable (e.g. teachers, coaches, leisure managers).
- Lack of access to specialist facilities such as ramps and hoists.
- Discrimination – verbal or institutionalised.
- Fewer opportunities to join clubs or enter competitions.

- Lack of mobility or transport.
- Possibly lower income.
- Lack of media coverage and role models, and therefore a lack of information.

The main barrier to the participation of people with disabilities in the activities of their choice is as much a matter of social attitudes and environmental barriers as their medical condition.

In the UK, the special needs of athletes with disabilities are catered for by six national disability sports organisations:

1. The British Amputee Sports Association;
2. The UK Sports Association for People with Mental Handicap;
3. Cerebral Palsy Sport;
4. The British Les Autres Sports Association;
5. Disability Sport England (formerly the British Sports Association for the Disabled) – probably the most important sports organisation in the UK for people with disabilities;
6. The British Paralympic Association.

The English Federation of Disability Sport (EFDS) acts as the main supporting and coordinating body for the development of sport for all people with disabilities. This is part of a recently restructured disability sport network. In turn, the EFDS has the support and direct involvement of all the major disability sport organisations, and will promote a corporate approach at national and regional level to determine priorities and the implementation of programmes.

Competitive sports have either been designed specifically for people with disabilities, such as goalball, boccia and polybat for the visually impaired, or they have been modified, such as volleyball and wheelchair basketball/tennis.

Current trends tend to focus on the sport rather than on the disability, to allow closer involvement with mainstream sport which previously has not catered for the needs of athletes with disabilities. Increasing participation should provide role models for people with disabilities. It is very important that all these organisations, both mainstream and special needs, cooperate and pool their resources in joint programmes of work; the creation of one umbrella federation might help the situation.

Integration into mainstream sport does not have to mean participating at the same time as everyone else. It is more significant that facilities, competitions, training and coaching should be equally available to people with disabilities as to able-bodied people. However, there is a choice of either participating separately (segregation) to able-bodied people, or participating with the able-bodied (integration). As with many issues, there are advantages and disadvantages to each of these.

## Inclusiveness

Developing an inclusive approach to all aspects of school life, including physical activity, can act as a route into inclusion in the wider community. Goalball is a game developed for people with disabilities, but which can be played by everyone.

Goalball:

- A three-a-side game.
- Aim is to score a goal by rolling the ball along the floor into your opponent's goal.
- Developed for visually impaired people.
- Features which enable visually impaired people to play:
    - The ball has a bell inside.
    - The playing court has tactile markings.
    - All players wear eyeshades to ensure that everyone is equal when it comes to visual perception.
- Goalball is currently played in 87 countries.
- It is a Paralympic sport, and has European and World Championships.
- British Blind Sport (BBS) is the organisation responsible for the sport in the UK.
- Approximately 15 clubs and school teams in the UK.
- The BBS organises 10 one-day tournaments a year, termly national schools competitions, national championships and the British Goalball Cup.
- There are at present no award schemes or coaching courses for goalball.

*Source*: Tutor File Higher Sports Leaders Award British Sports Trust

Advantages and disadvantages of segregated sport

| Advantages | Disadvantages |
|---|---|
| • Security and feeling of safety being among people with similar needs.<br>• Competition may appear fairer when competing against people with similar abilities.<br>• Appropriate modifications can be used.<br>• Specialist staff can focus on the needs of disabled individuals.<br>• Reaching levels of excellence may be more viable. | • Can reinforce the sense of being different to main society – sport may be the one chance they have to socialise within wider society.<br>• Use of facilities at different times.<br>• Does not raise public awareness of the capabilities of people with disabilities.<br>• Can be overprotective. |

## Activity 2

1 Research the sport of polybat or boccia.
2 What modifications have been made to tennis and basketball for wheelchair athletes?

## Improving opportunities

### Disability Sport England

www.euroyellowpages.com/dse/dispengl.html

This organisation was formally known as the British Sports Association for the Disabled, which was founded in 1961 by Sir Ludwig Guttman, a neurosurgeon who worked at Stoke Mandeville hospital.

Disability Sport England is about:

- promoting the benefits of sport and making it accessible to everyone, regardless of ability;
- helping talented athletes reach the highest levels, such as the Paralympic Games.

Liaison with the sports councils will mean a more coordinated approach towards laying the foundations for developing young people, talent development, coaching, national governing bodies, local authorities, membership services and management administration.

The aims of Disability Sport England are:

- To provide opportunities for people with disabilities to participate in sport.
- To promote the benefits of sport and physical recreation for people with disabilities.
- To support organisations in providing sporting opportunities for people with disabilities.
- To educate and make people aware of the sporting abilities of people with disabilities.
- To enhance the image, awareness and understanding of disability sport.
- To encourage people with disabilities to play an active role in the development of their sport.

## Activity 3

Visit your local leisure facility and note down the positive and negative aspects in relation to people with disabilities using that facility.

Sport England Sport England has supported the development of national bodies for disability sport and the appointment of specialised regional and local development officers. The organisation has implemented various projects aimed at improving sporting opportunities for people with disabilities:

1 The campaign 'Every Body Active' was set up following research which highlighted several major problems encountered by people with disabilities; in particular a lack of awareness among mainstream leisure providers and PE teachers as to the special needs of this group.
2 The 'Pro-motion' campaign established in 1990 is now a national programme, intending to increase awareness, training, liaison and resources.

The Sports Council's policy document *Sport and People with Disabilities* was published in 1993, and is a national statement of intent for which it will be accountable.

Local authorities Local authorities play a crucial role at local level because of their leisure departments. The planning and architects departments are also important when trying to build functional and imaginative facilities. When facility tenders are reviewed and renewed, the needs of people with disabilities must be considered.

## Excellence and disability sport

Excellence in sport performance has grown substantially, in both the number of competitions and the variety of activities. The Paralympics (so called because it runs parallel to the Olympics) and the World Championships are notable examples.

As knowledge about training, coaching and the input of sport science increases, the performance levels of athletes with disabilities will undoubtedly improve.

**IN CONTEXT**

**As part of the Essex legacy of the 2012 London Games, a statement of equity and inclusion affirms that: 'The high profile that will be given to disabled people at the Paralympic Games offers an unparalleled opportunity to raise awareness of disability issues and to ensure that disabled sports people are offered the same opportunities as their able-bodied colleagues'.**

## Classification

This is an attempt to group sports competitors to enable fair competition. It was initially used for sport by gender, where separate competitions developed for men and women, and by weight in sports such as boxing. It is now used to include individuals with disabilities.

Two types of classification are employed:

- Medical classification: this developed in the 1940s and was dominant into the 1990s. It was based on the level of spinal cord lesion. It was designed to enable individuals with similar severity of impairment to compete against one another. It was used for wheelchair athletes and amputees. Many other disability sport federations adopted this system, resulting in a multiple classification system.
- Functional classification: an integrated classification system that places emphasis on sport performance by disability groupings rather than by specific disability. This has enabled disability sport to move on from its original rehabilitation base to elite competitive sport. Wheelchair basketball was the first Paralympic sport to experiment with this system. This system demands that athletes be evaluated on what they can and cannot do in a particular sport.

## Facilities

Facilities are gradually improving for users with disabilities, partly under the Safety at Sports Grounds Act 1975, and also through a growing desire to provide access. The programming of activities and the attitudes of staff are also important considerations.

Outdoor facilities are increasing provision, for example, those run by the Calvert Trust and Scope. Several important sports centres exist, such as the Ludwig Guttman Sports Centre at Stoke Mandeville and the Midland Sports Centre for the Disabled in Coventry.

### EXAMINER'S TIP

When mentioning facilities and coaching in relation to disability sport, make sure you are specific and mention accessible facilities or specialist coaching.

## Future trends

Competitive sport opportunities have increased due to a number of factors:

1. More focus in society on equal opportunities through legislation such as the Disability Discrimination Act.
2. Increasing number of modified or adapted activities, as well as the development of sports specifically designed for people with disabilities, such as goalball.
3. The increase in expectations within society and among disabled people themselves.

| Sport for all | Elite level |
|---|---|
| • Increasing numbers of individuals with disabilities will participate at all levels in the sport pyramid.<br>• Equity issues will continue to be addressed for groups who suffer the lowest levels of participation, particularly females and low income groups.<br>• Public awareness and acceptance of disability sport will increase. | • Structured competitive programmes will operate at local, regional, national and international levels.<br>• Coordination between sport organisations concerned with disability sport and those that are more sport-specific.<br>• Athletes with disabilities will continue to specialise in sport events, with classification and competitions becoming sport-specific. This will result in improved standards of performance.<br>• People with disabilities will participate more as coaches and officials, especially as current athletes retire from competition. |

Source: Adapted from K. DePauw and S. Gavron (1995) *Disability and Sport*, Human Kinetics

4 More specialist staff.
5 Increase in organisations that focus specifically on disability sport, such as Disability Sport England and specialist governing bodies.
6 A growth in clubs and consequent competitions, culminating in the Paralympic Games.
7 Increasing media coverage and the emergence of certain role models.
8 Increase in technology, such as prosthetics and wheelchairs.

In summary, we can conclude that:

- Societal attitudes are changing towards wider participation and competition by athletes.
- The original purpose of rehabilitation through sport has given way to sport for sport's sake.
- The Olympic sport movement will continue to shape the future direction of disability sport.
- Classification, drug testing, advances in technology, and improved training and coaching, techniques and sports medicine will further influence disability sport.

## What you need to know

* The broader the base of sport participation, the greater the talent pool from which to draw in order to increase the chances of sporting excellence.
* Unequal access to the 'sport for all' ideal will negatively affect the sports pyramid.
* Sport initiatives must take careful note of the complex nature of the various groups they seek to help.
* Discrimination can be overt, e.g. membership clause of a sports club and covert, e.g attitudes and prejudices.
* Constraints which affect participation can be the environment, lack of facilities or access to facilities; societies attitudes; lack of time or income; lack of relevant skills and power and poor self image.
* Attemps to raise participation need to address the structural problems as well as people's attitudes.

## Review questions

1 What is meant by the 'dominant group' in society and how can this group affect sporting opportunities?

2 How can sport be an avenue of social mobility?

3 What does the term 'stacking' refer to in sporting situations?

4 Suggest four strategies which organisations can implement in order to improve the participation of women in sporting and recreational activities.

5 What does the term 'social exclusion' mean and what measures can be taken to address the issues?

6 What is the significance of the emergence of the term 'disability sport'?

7 What is the significance of the term 'inclusiveness' when referring to disability and sporting participation?

8 How can elite athletes be used to inspire and motivate young people to participate and continue in sport?

9 Suggest reasons why ethnic minorities participate less in sport and physical recreation than the white population?

10 What barriers have women faced in trying to increase their levels of sport participation?

# The analysis and evaluation of physical activity as a performer and/or an adapted role/s

SECTION

D

CHAPTER 13

# An introduction to practical coursework

## Learning outcomes

**By the end of this chapter you should understand the following:**

- understand the requirements of the practical assessment;
- select your optimum activity considering all relevant factors;
- understand how you will be assessed;
- analyse your own performance, identifying strengths and weaknesses;
- formulate a plan to optimise your performance.

## CHAPTER INTRODUCTION

The practical coursework is your opportunity to demonstrate your skills in two of the three optional roles of performer, coach/leader or official in your chosen activity or activities. You have the opportunity to dictate how well you do because you know exactly the areas in which you will be assessed.

The purpose of this chapter is to outline how you will be assessed and help you to understand the requirement of the published specification. It is not intended to inform you how to become a better technical performer, coach/leader or official. There are many more resources available to help you with the specific knowledge of each activity and it would not be feasible to attempt to outline all the details required for each one in this chapter. You should read relevant coaching manuals and rule books as well as watch appropriate videos to enhance your knowledge and understanding of your own activity.

The chapter will outline advice on assessment and preparation for the moderation, the roles you are expected to master and details of how to analyse your performance. Many of you will relish the opportunity to master the skills previously developed through physical education lessons, the GCSE course and extra-curricular activities. However, the requirements of the course at AS level demand a technical competence via demonstration and execution through conditioned practices rather than playing in a competitive situation. Both of these require practice and concentration to achieve high marks.

The aim of the practical coursework component is not only to assess the physical skills and application of strategies and tactics but to bring together all the various theoretical components, allowing the optimisation of performance. The task facing you is to use your knowledge and understanding of the theoretical aspects of the course to identify weaknesses in performance and possible causes, and to use the acquired knowledge to address the faults.

Table 13.1 outlines the AQA Examination Board requirement for AS and A2 levels of study. It is useful to have some understanding of the A2 course because if you develop a clear understanding of the correct technique during the first year of study, it will make your studies easier the following year.

Table 13.1 Requirements for AS and A2 levels of study

| AS level | A2 level |
|---|---|
| Demonstration of skills in two out of three roles:<br>• Practical performer<br>• Coach/leader<br>• Official/referee.<br>Demonstration of core skills in isolation and conditioned practice.<br>Roles may be assessed in:<br>• one activity<br>• two activities.<br>The only restriction is that you may not be assessed in the same role in two different activities. | Demonstration of skills in one role:<br>• Practical performer<br>• Coach/leader<br>• Official/referee.<br>Assessment is based on performance in a competitive situation or equivalent.<br>See the individual specification criteria for exact assessment requirements.<br>Plus an analysis of the weaknesses of performance when compared with an elite performer, possible causes of the weaknesses and solutions.<br>Practical performer – assesses their own performance.<br>Coach/leader – assesses another performer.<br>Official/referee – assessed their own performance. |

## Structure of the course and preparation advice

This element of the course aims to develop many skills and prepare students to fulfil a number of roles. Figure 13.1 outlines such roles.

In order to complete each of these roles successfully, time must be devoted to practice and development of knowledge about the rules, scoring systems, tactics, strategies, technical skills, specific terminology, physical preparation, psychological requirements and any other areas that may hinder or promote performance.

It may be easier to view this section of the course as progressive, with the foundation skills and knowledge being laid during the AS year and the refining and optimising of performance occurring during the A2 year. Many of the skills developed via practices at AS level will be examined in more detail during full competitive situations at A2 level.

Many students neglect the practical element of the course and tend to focus on the theoretical aspects. However, a large percentage of the final marks – up to 40 per cent – is allocated to this section. Therefore time should be devoted to developing the skills required from the onset of the course; this should not be left until close to the final assessment or moderation.

To fully understand the nature of performance and how to facilitate improvement, links should be made with the theoretical components as frequently as possible. Individual strengths and weaknesses should be identified and, as the

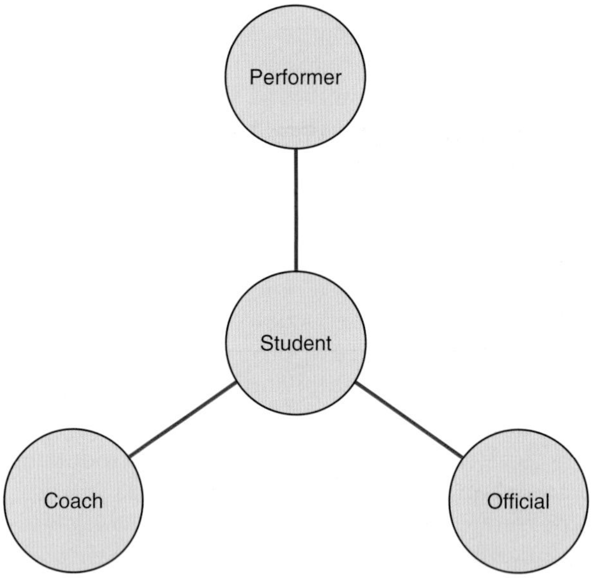


Figure 13.1 A student will fulfil a number of roles

course progresses, possible causes and corrective measures can be implemented.

The selection of activities must be carefully considered, as there may be restrictions. In addition to your own experience, other factors may include the time available to complete extra training, the opportunity for extra-curricular activities, the accessibility of facilities and resources, plus the expertise of teachers and coaches.

The nature of assessment requires a demonstration or applied knowledge (depending on your chosen roles) of named core skills related to a specific activity, the difficulty of which gradually increases due to the requirement of executing effectively in more pressurised or demanding situations.

The activities available for assessment are outlined in Table 13.2. The categories are sub-divided to allow for easier application of the criteria. You do not have to choose a particular combination of activities. The purpose of dividing the activities into groups will become clear as you continue to read through the chapter and begin to understand how you will be assessed.

The marking of the practical activities is conducted through continual assessment. This allows for ongoing development of performance and caters for students who may have an 'off day' during a moderator's visit. There are several key terms that need to be outlined in order to fully understand the assessment procedure:

Table 13.2 Activities available for assessment

| **Category 1** |
| --- |
| Association Football Badminton Basketball Boxing Canoeing/Kayaking (moving/inland water)<br>Climbing Cricket Fencing Gaelic Football<br>Goalball Golf Handball Hockey (Field/Roller/Ice)<br>Horse Riding Judo Karate Lacrosse<br>Mountain Activities Netball Orienteering<br>Rowing and Sculling<br>Rugby Union/League<br>Sailing/Windsurfing/Kitesurfing<br>Skiing/Snowboarding<br>Softball/Baseball/Rounders<br>Squash<br>Table Tennis<br>Tae Kwon Do<br>Tennis<br>Track/Road Cycling/Mountain Biking<br>Volleyball<br>Water Polo |
| **Category 2** |
| Athletics<br>Olympic Weightlifting<br>Swimming |
| **Category 3** |
| Dance Contemporary/Creative/Ballet<br>Diving<br>Gymnastics<br>Trampolining |

- *skills in isolation* – the demonstration of specific core skills, which will be compared with a correct technical model (see later for full explanation);
- *conditioned practice* – the demonstration of core skills and some tactical awareness in a more pressured practice situation, but not a full game or equivalent competitive situation;
- *competitive situation* – demonstration of core skills, strategies and tactics, the application of the psychological and physiological qualities needed within a fully competitive environment or appropriate alternative. This is not actually assessed until the A2 year of the course.

To facilitate development, the various skills need to be analysed to identify personal strengths and weaknesses. More detailed advice to complete this process is outlined in the next section.

Each activity is different in terms of core skills. Examples from different categories are shown below in Figure 13.2, which illustrates the diverse nature of each activity.

Once this process has been completed for all the core skills, time should be devoted to rectify faults or develop an awareness of the correct techniques or rules related to each one. The assessment is based on competence of performance in comparison with a correct technical model (see next section for further details) and marks are awarded to sub-routines of the skill as well as the end result. For example, the sub-routines for a badminton stroke may be the grip, footwork and preparation, shot positioning and timing, follow-through and recovery, and finally effectiveness.

To develop the necessary skills and tactical awareness, time must be given to practice or observation of practice. It is of no use simply reading books or watching videos informing you how to complete the skills correctly. They may be useful as a reference resource but there is no substitute for actually performing or analysing the skills.

Training sessions are always easier with others, not just because it is more sociable but because they can actually help to improve your performance by observing and coaching. If the practice takes place with another student who has limited knowledge of the activity, outline the identified weaknesses of the skills and prepare a sheet of the correct techniques and coaching points required.

However, if time can be spent with a teacher or another student who is experienced and is able to identify your weaknesses, this may be of greater benefit. Allocated time for development may be available during either lessons or extra-curricular activities.

Further development may take place at a local club and the expertise of the coaches and officials may be utilised. If this is the case, it may be advisable to inform them of the specification criteria so that they are aware of your aims and the specific skills that need to be developed.

When possible, video record any practice sessions and analyse your development. Evaluate any progress and restructure your training schedule as required.

To develop the effective application of your skills in a competitive situation, set targets for each game or event and ask someone to evaluate your performance. Do not set too many each time, possibly two or three, but try to concentrate on these, and do not become over-concerned with other areas of weakness – they can be targets next time.

When developing your personal skills, do not try to change everything at once or expect a huge improvement in performance overnight. The process may take months or years to complete. Many elite performers/coaches/officials strive to make minor modifications to their technique/knowledge/performance in order to achieve the optimum performance. The aim of the AS/A2 course is not to make you compete at this level but to be competent performers. Try to remember that when developing your practical performance.

## Requirements of a practical performer

You are being assessed on your ability as a performer in the selected activity and will be required to demonstrate a mastery of sport-related skills in both isolation and conditioned practices. During the conditioned practices you will also be assessed on your tactical awareness and ability to participate in set plays, as well as show your analysis and evaluation skills to critically appraise your performance, suggesting how it could be improved.

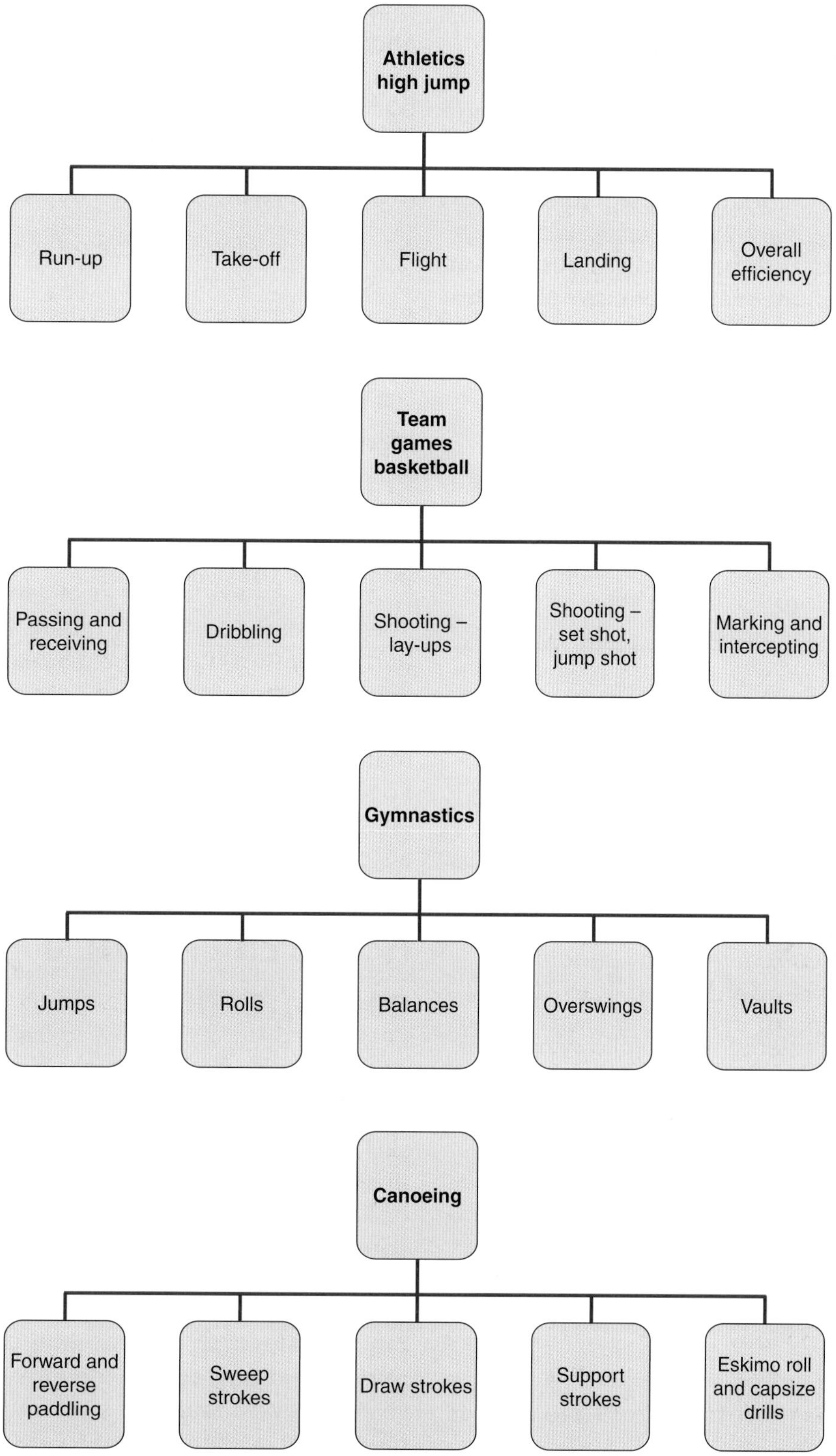


**Figure 13.2** The core skills differ depending on which activity is undertaken

## What do the specification criteria actually mean?

**Category 1 Activities** (refer to Table 13.2 to remind yourself of these activities).

For the demonstration of the five named core skills in isolation there are 25 marks available. You need to fully understand the criteria to ensure you are able to access all the marks. For example, if the core skill is 'passing' you will be required to show a range of passing techniques, not just one or two methods, to be awarded full marks.

There are 15 marks awarded for application of those core skills in the conditioned practice. These are mainly sub-divided as follows:

- attacking situations
- defensive situations
- set plays or specific situations.

Each of these areas is worth 5 marks.

For some activities these sub-divisions may be different – you need to refer to the published specification for full details. These activities include canoeing/kayaking, climbing, horse riding, mountain activities, orienteering, rowing and sculling, sailing/wind surfing, skiing/snowboarding and track/road cycling.

The final 10 marks are awarded for:

- your ability to implement and follow the rules, your effort and efficiency;
- your ability to analyse your performance and suggest appropriate measures to improve performance.

Each of these areas is worth 5 marks.

## What do the specification criteria actually mean?

**Category 2 Activities** (refer to Table 13.2 to remind yourself of these activities).

The difference between these and the Category 1 activities is that due to the nature of those listed in Category 2 you have to demonstrate only two events, strokes or lifts. Each one is sub-divided into three specific sub-routines and awarded up to 5 marks each, making a total of 15 marks per event and 30 marks in total for your demonstrations.

In terms of the conditioned practice requirement you have to demonstrate your ability in only one event, and this is assessed out of 12 marks. The final marks, worth up to 4 each, are awarded for:

- your knowledge of the rules, strategies and effort;
- your ability to analyse your performance and suggest appropriate measures to improve performance.

## What do the specification criteria actually mean?

**Category 3 Activities** (refer to Table 13.2 to remind yourself of these activities).

The final category is very different to the previous two categories due to the diverse nature of the activities listed. In order to fully understand the requirements of a particular activity you should read the specification criteria carefully. Most of the advice offered in the previous pages of this chapter can then be adapted to ensure you can access all the marks.

# Requirements of a coach/leader

If you are being assessed in this role you will be required to observe, analyse and suggest improvements a performer can make to their core skills/techniques. This will be a test of your understanding of the relevant techniques and basic tactics depending on the situation, as well as your ability to ensure all the participants involved are safe and that you can implement key elements of the theoretical aspects of this section in a practical situation. For example, you must understand how to provide effective feedback, select the best teaching style and modify the method of guidance used to ensure learning takes place. The final aspect of the assessment will involve you evaluating your own performance and suggesting aspects that you too could improve upon to become a better coach/leader.

Remember, this role is worth a total of 50 marks.

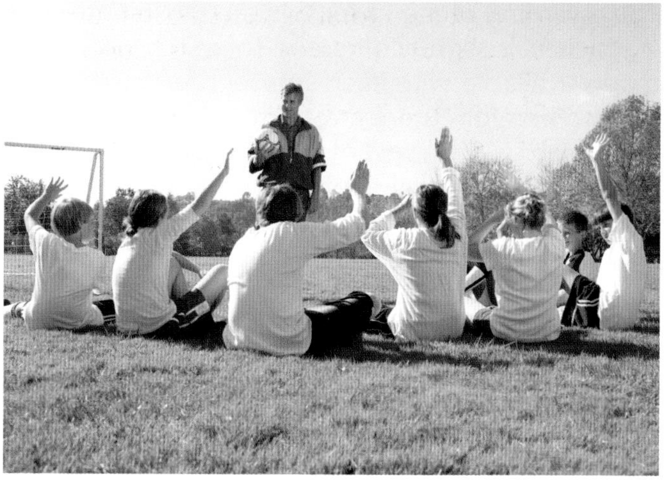

Figure 13.3 Coach working with players

## What do the specification criteria actually mean?

**Category 1 Activities** (refer to Table 13.2 to remind yourself of these activities).

You will be assessed on your ability to analyse and evaluate the strengths and weaknesses of a performer in a variety of named core skills in isolation and suggest corrective practices. This is worth 25 marks – 5 marks per named core skill. For example, in Association Football the named core skills for an outfield player are passing and receiving, dribbling and moving with the ball, shooting, heading (attack and defence) and finally tackling and jockeying a player. You will be expected to analyse a variety of specific techniques within each of these groups and provide specific feedback to the player about their performance, using specialist technical vocabulary.

The second section of marks assesses your ability to analyse the core skills/techniques, not in isolation but during conditioned practices or a modified game situation. Another 15 marks are available for the following criteria, each of which is worth 5 marks:

- ability to analyse the relevant skills/techniques during attacking phases of play;
- ability to analyse the relevant skills/techniques during defensive phases of play;
- ability to analyse the relevant skills/techniques during set play phases of play.

For each of these areas you should be able to comment on basic strategies and tactics, outlining what the performer did well and what they did poorly. Comments should also cover the impact of the performance on other players or the outcome of the activity.

Some of the activities will have alternative criteria if those highlighted above are not relevant. For example, mountain activities and horse riding do not have attacking and defensive phases of play, therefore an alternative aspect of the sport will be assessed. You should check the assessment criteria carefully to ensure you understand which aspects of the activity you need to develop knowledge of.

The final 10 marks (each of which is worth 5 marks) are awarded for your:

- ability to commuicate effectively with the performer to implement change as required;
- ability to analyse your personal performance as a coach/leader.

The first bullet point refers to your ability to implement the various theoretical aspects of coaching you have studied to produce an effective performance from the person you are working with. For example, are your instructions and feedback clear and accurate? Do you use the appropriate methods of guidance? Do you use the correct teaching style?

The second bullet point assesses your ability to evaluate your own performance and suggest ways in which you could become a better coach/leader. It is very hard to become a perfect coach! Ask yourself, does the 'perfect coach' actually exist? There are numerous examples of good quality, experienced coaches and leaders saying they didn't get everything right, whether they are referring to tactics, preparing their athletes in terms of fitness or generally not making a decision quick enough to cause a change which may have affected the final result. Bear this in mind and don't think you have to be perfect. There is always room for improvement. You may like to ask yourself, 'does the performer understand me?' If not, why not?

## What do the specification criteria actually mean?

**Category 2 Activities** (refer to Table 13.2 to remind yourself of these activities).

The requirements within this category are similar to Category 1 but rather than analyse five core skills/techniques you are now required to develop your knowledge of two events. For example, from the sport of athletics you may choose the high jump and hurdles, or swimming the front crawl and the butterfly stroke.

Your ability to analyse and evaluate a performer's strengths and weaknesses is worth 15 marks per event (30 marks in total). The remainder of the marks are awarded for your effectiveness within a conditioned practice/modified competition. However, you have to analyse only one event and comment on three named core skills/techniques which are clearly outlined in the criteria. For example, if you specialised in the high jump, the three core skills would be:

- run-up
- take-off
- flight and landing.

If you chose swimming and the front crawl, the three core skills would be:

- starts, turns and finish
- head action, breathing action and body position
- arm action and leg action.

The awarding of marks for this section in Category 2 activities is slightly different. There is a total of 20 marks available, with each sub-section worth 4 marks. Therefore there are 12 marks available for your analysis of the event based on the three core skills as outlined above, plus an additional 8 marks for your:

- ability to communicate effectively with the performer to implement change as required;
- ability to analyse your personal performance as a coach/leader.

The advice outlined in the previous section relating to these two bullet points also applies.

## What do the specification criteria actually mean?

**Category 3 Activities** (refer to Table 13.2 to remind yourself of these activities).

The third category requires exactly the same skills of analysis and evaluation. Due to the different nature of Dance there are specific requirements which are outlined in the criteria which refer to the performance and choreography of a solo sequence, worth 30 marks and 20 marks respectively. You are able to offer a variety of genres depending on your strengths and personal interests.

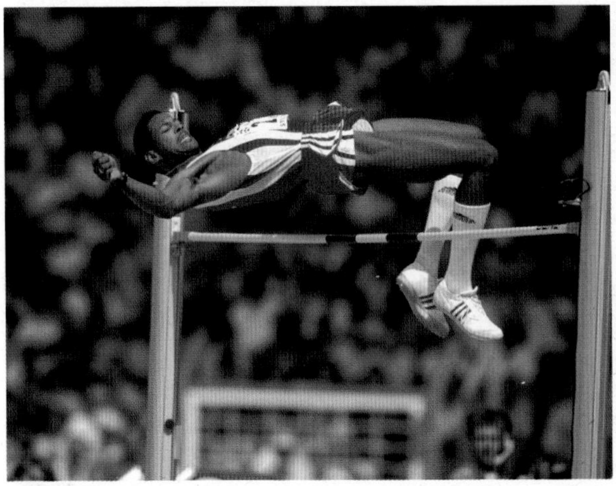

**Figure 13.4** A picture of a high jumper

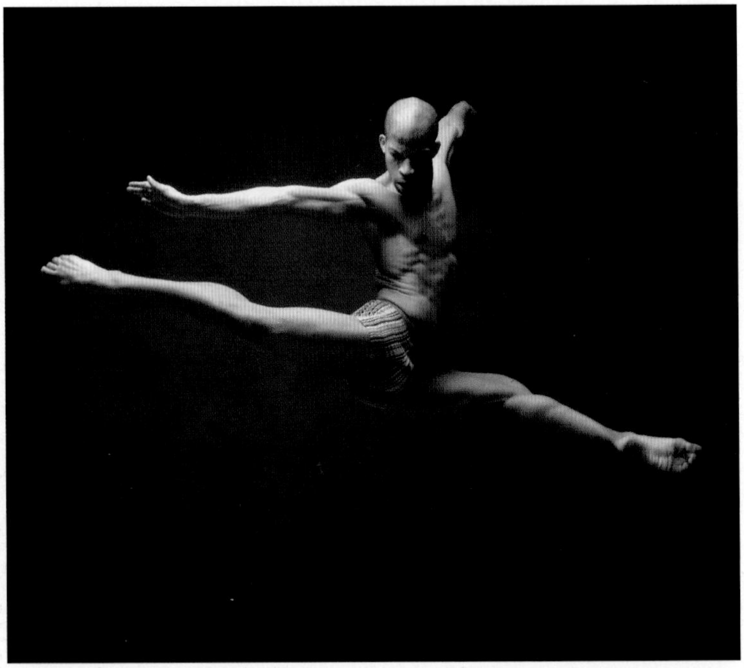

**Figure 13.5** A picture of a dancer

The other activities have 25 marks available for analyis and evaluation of the demonstration of core skills. A further 15 marks are available for your ability to assess a performer during a conditioned practice or modified competitive practice.

The final 10 marks (each of which is worth 5 marks) are awarded for your:

- ability to communicate effectively with the performer to implement change as required;
- ability to analyse your personal performance as a coach/leader.

## Requirements of an official

If you choose to be assessed in this role you will be required to fulfil three main objectives. The first involves you demonstrating your ability to apply the rules relating to the various core skills both in isolation and within conditioned practices. The second aspect of being an official requires you to show you have a good understanding of the requirements and expectations associated with the role. For example, an awareness of safety issues and the ability to apply the rules fairly and consistently. The final aspect assesses your ability to apply the correct scoring systems and justify the decisions made to players and other officials as required.

Remember, the skill of being an official is to be fair and consistent. The nature of sport relies on officials, referees and umpires making decisions immediately to ensure fair play and the safety of all participants. Officials do not get every decision correct and at the elite level they are increasingly added by new technology . For example, just look at how the introduction of technology is now such an important aspect of many sports and often final decisions are referred to the fourth official for clarification or confirmation. Therefore, bear this in mind when developing the skills required to be an official – you cannot get every decision correct, but try to get as many right as possible.

Although each of the activity categories may have slightly different requirements, the structure is broadly the same. More detail will be outlined in terms of the mark allocation in the specific sections below, but the following bullet points show the main skills you will need to develop.

The first section of marks focuses on the core skills, general awareness of requirements for an official and personal preparation. This includes:

- the ability to explain any relevant rules relating to the named cores skills;
- the ability to demonstrate an awareness of safety issues relating to equipment, players' clothing and the playing area;
- the ability to understand and explain the scoring and/or judging system;
- the ability to undertake the various roles associated with the activity;
- the ability to be physically and mentally preparated to officiate and be suitably equipped.

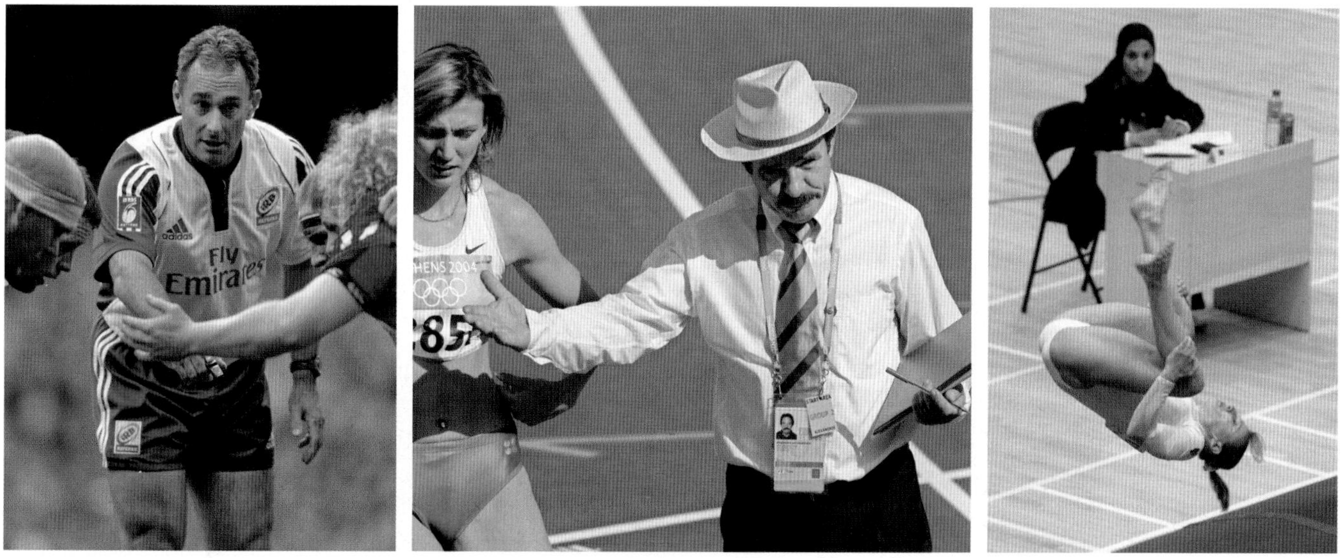

**Figure 13.6** A picture of a rugby referee, athletic judge and gymnastic judge

The second section of marks relates to your ability to execute the knowledge shown above in a conditioned practice or modified competitive situation when officiating the named core skills. This includes:

- the ability to apply the rules or judging criteria correctly;
- the ability to be consistent;
- the ability to communicate decisions correctly;
- the ability to demonstrate a rapport with the performers to maintain fair play;
- the ability to analyse and evaluate your own performance and suggest appropriate methods to improve.

As you can see from the lists above you will be assessed in a similar manner to how you would evaluate an official if you were watching a sporting contest.

The following information outlines in more detail how the marks are awarded depending on the nature of the activity.

### What do the specification criteria actually mean?

**Category 1 Activities** (refer to Table 13.2 to remind yourself of these activities).

25 marks are available (5 per sub-section) for the first group of bullet points outlined above.

25 marks are available (5 per sub-section) for the second group of bullet points outlined above.

### What do the specification criteria actually mean?

**Category 2 Activities** (refer to Table 13.2 to remind yourself of these activities).

30 marks are available (5 marks per sub-section). The additional 5 marks are available because you have to outline the rules relating to two events rather than five core skills.

20 marks are available (4 marks per sub-section) for the second group of bullet points outlined above.

### What do the specification criteria actually mean?

**Category 3 Activities** (refer to Table 13.2 to remind yourself of these activities).

25 marks are available (5 per sub-section) for the first group of bullet points outlined above.

25 marks are available (5 per sub-section) for the second group of bullet points outlined above.

## Assessment procedures

The school/college will be assigned an external moderator to ensure the marking criteria are applied correctly by the teachers when compared with recommended national standards. The moderation may involve either:

- one school/college
- a group of schools/college
- video evidence.

The moderator may not see all the activities being offered by the school/college due to time restrictions, availability of facilities or numbers involved. However, the assumption must be made that they will observe any possible combination of activities and as a consequence you should be fully prepared. This may involve not only the actual practical performance but also any analysis of performance requirements. The best way to prepare for the moderation is to start practising the core skills as early in the course as possible and give yourself the opportunity to experience as many conditioned situations as possible to develop your skills.

The moderation usually involves both AS and A2 students. Consequently, it may be easy to lose focus and concentration. Many students assume the moderator is not watching them because they are at the other end of the sports hall or far side of the playing field. They may be assessing you at any time.

A common error during the moderation visit involves a lack of concentration during the demonstrations of the core skills. Many students appear to not apply themselves fully and produce weaker demonstrations compared with their actual ability. This may be due to the misconception that they are easy, do not require much attention and are less intense compared with the conditioned practice or competitive situation.

It also helps to make the effort to dress appropriately and 'look the part'. This will at least give the moderator the impression that some preparation and thought have been given to the assessment rather than simply turning up on the day.

The nature of physical activity inevitably involves mistakes being made during performance; it is almost unavoidable. Even performers at the highest level make errors of judgement or are influenced by the environment, occasion and opponents. If mistakes are made, do not worry about them, redirect your attention and concentrate on the task ahead. The moderator will look at the overall performance, not just one small part.

If the selected activity is a team game or one that involves other performers, do not try to be the centre of attention all the time. The assessment is based on your ability to fulfil a role within a specific position. Marks may be lost because of the inability to implement certain tactics, strategies and systems of play.

The moderator may require the analysis of your performance and a comparison with another student. If this does happen, further advice is outlined in the next section covering all aspects of preparation for this assessment.

## Analysis of skills and performance

As the course progresses, there will be a requirement to analyse your performance and that of others in greater detail. In order to achieve this, a coaching cycle should be used ensuring a consistent approach – an example is shown in Figure 13.7.

Understanding each element is crucial if the coaching process is to be effective and actually develop skills and their application.

- *Performance* – these are the actions of the performer either in isolation, practice or competitive situation.
- *Observation* – the actions of the performer are either watched by another person or video recorded.
- *Analysis* – the actions of the performer are assessed. Notes should be taken when possible to highlight key strengths and weaknesses.
- *Evaluation* – the actions of the performer are compared with a correct technical model, competent performer or past performances.
- *Planning* – possible causes of weaknesses are identified and corrective measures devised to eradicate the problems. These may be in the form of physical practices, physiological adaptations or psychological preparation. It is also important at this stage not to neglect the strengths of the performer but to maintain a level of training to ensure the strengths do not decline at the expense of improving the weaknesses.
- *Feedback* – the identified training adaptations are discussed with the performer and implemented during the forthcoming performances.

When the coaching and analysis process occurs, there are many factors that may need to be considered and knowledge of each must be established if the outcome is to be successful. Many students can identify basic faults in technique and performance but not expand their responses with the use of detailed technical information or appropriate terminology. Figure 13.8 highlights some of the knowledge that may be required to successfully complete the coaching cycle.

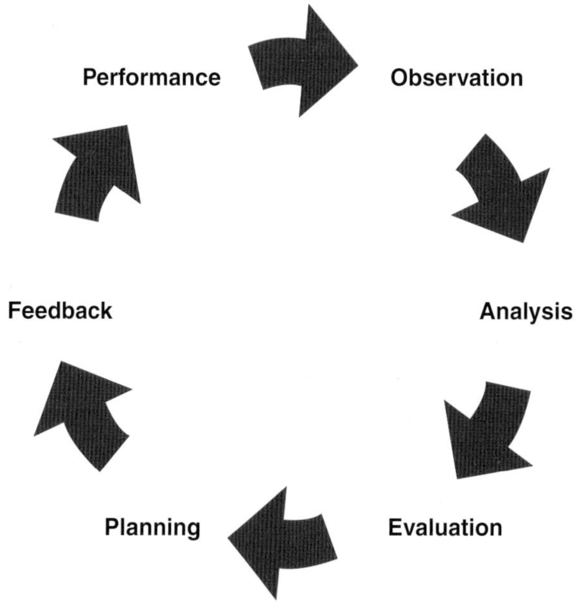


**Figure 13.7** An example of a coaching cycle

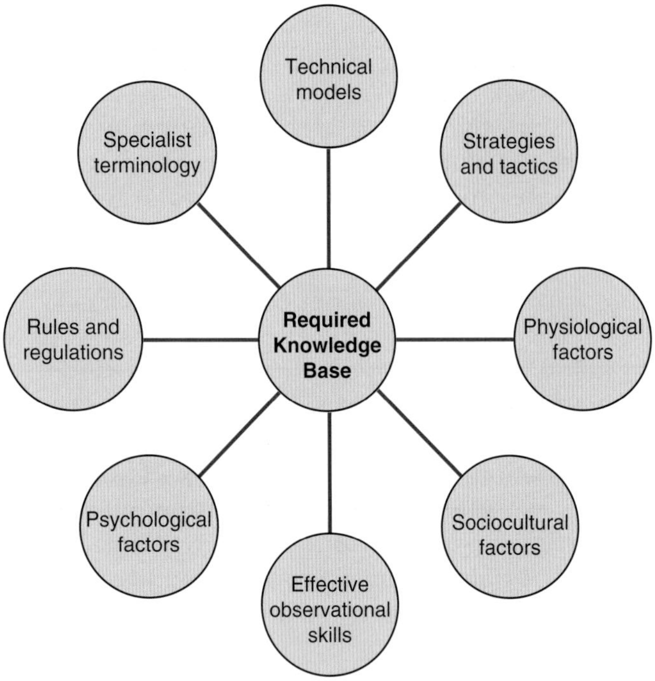


**Figure 13.8** Required knowledge for successful completion of the coaching cycle

As you can see, the knowledge base required to be an effective coach who is able to observe and analyse performance is wide ranging and varied. During the course of your studies, you should aim to improve each of them.

## Technical models

Often reference will be made to your performance compared with or knowledge of a 'correct technical model'. This term refers to the performance of a skill that is considered to be of a very high standard. There may actually be several variations of a skill and different performers may have their individual peculiarities but still be highly successful. Similarly, as many activities become exposed to scientific and technological support, alterations in techniques are becoming more common as actions and techniques are refined.

As a consequence, it is advisable to base your comparisons on the most recent information or a performer who is generally accepted as being close to the norm. The technique of many international competitors may be considered unique and inadvisable to coach to developing athletes.

There are many resources for appropriate technical models, often published by the national governing bodies. Suitable sources include:

- coaching manuals
- photographs
- instructional videos
- CD-ROMs
- the Internet
- television recorded performances with expert commentary
- live events.

When studying and developing an awareness of each skill, refer to the specific sub-routines identified previously. A thorough knowledge and understanding of each phase of the skill is vital if the observation and analysis process is to be effective. For each skill, make diagrams and notes of the key points for each sub-routine. Initially, concentrate on the major technical points, including the correct terminology, but later, once these are well learned and easily recognised, develop an awareness of the more advanced technical points.

### Activity 1

Research and find relevant resources to identify the key technical points or rules for each of the core skills.

A useful aid to developing this understanding is a chart containing all the basic information for each sub-routine of the specific skill. Often an A3 piece of paper divided as shown in Table 13.3 can be easily constructed and will contain all the information required.

### Activity 2

Complete a chart for each core skill using the resources identified above.

Table 13.3 Basic information for each sub-routine

| Sub-routine 1 | Sub-routine 2 | Sub-routine 3 | Sub-routine 4 | Sub-routine 5 |
|---|---|---|---|---|
| Diagram or photographs of this phase<br>Correct technique<br>*Include two or three points* | | | | |
| Common faults<br>*Include two or three points* | | | | |
| Corrective practices<br>*Include one per fault* | | | | |

## Observation advice

When observing any performance, the various viewing angles may provide different information about the effectiveness of performance. Imagine when watching a sporting event on television the numerous camera angles employed by the editor and the different impressions and information produced by each. It is now common practice in many high-level sporting events to use such technology to aid referees in their final decision. This approach should be employed to aid your observation and analysis.

Different views give very different perspectives and the aim of the observation should be identified clearly. The actual execution of skills may require a position as close to the action as possible from the side, front and rear, while the observation of tactical awareness and effective implementation may require a location further away. However, a view from behind the field of play may provide different information than one from the side or elevated in a stand. It may be advisable to vary your position to maximise the information upon which to base your judgements.

When observing, either live or from video evidence, make notes to remind you of specific instances or actions. Divide the observation sheet into sections covering the areas required. For example, when observing a game, the sheet may consist of sections for attacking skills, defensive skills, tactics and set plays.

## Analysis of personal performance

Before any personal development of skill and technique can occur, your own performance must be analysed and evaluated. This can be achieved in a number of ways:

- teacher/coach observing performance and providing feedback;
- another student observing performance and providing feedback;
- video recording of performance and personal analysis.

If possible, the third is in many ways the most useful as you can see the faults (via visual guidance) and develop a better understanding of the exact modifications needed. Video footage is also useful as a means of stopping the action and making specific comparisons with the technical model, which may be more difficult during live or full-speed actions.

Once the performance has been analysed, the next stage in the process involves the evaluation of the effectiveness of its application during either conditioned practices or competitive situations. For game activities, these are often split into the following sections:

- effectiveness of attacking skills;
- effectiveness of defensive skills;
- effective implementation of strategies and tactics;
- effective implementation of physiological and psychological factors that affect performance.

Other activities have alternative categories which are more appropriate, for example swimming and athletics may require the comments to be based on two events and gymnastic events on agilities and twists. Detailed requirements need to be obtained from the specification criteria.

### Activity 3

Observe and analyse your personal performance in the selected two roles for the various core skills and conditioned practices.

Once this process has been completed, a structured programme should be followed to develop the identified weaknesses in the skills or enhance your effectiveness when analysing the skills in context. Frequently assess your development either via a teacher/coach or by video recording again. Do not just assume because practice is taking place an improvement will occur – you may be practising the wrong technique, giving the wrong advice or interpreting the rules incorrectly.

## Key points to remember

The following points should be applied from the start of the course.

- Start preparation for the final assessment at the beginning of the course – do not leave it until the last few weeks.
- Learn the correct techniques and rules for the chosen activities.
- Take time to analyse your strengths and weaknesses.
- Set realistic targets for performance development.
- Evaluate progress regularly and revise targets.
- Look for the links between the theoretical aspects of the course and personal practical performance.
- Keep notes updated regularly and use them as a revision resource.
- Enjoy it – the practical aspect of the course is supposed to be fun!

# CHAPTER 14

# Applied exercise physiology and skill acquisition in practical situations

## Learning outcomes

**By the end of this chapter you should be able to:**

- name and explain the principles of training and apply them to a given performer;
- calculate optimal training intensities through use of heart rate, the Borg scale and 1 rep max percentages;
- explain the physiological value of a warm-up and cool-down;
- design and justify a warm-up and cool-down for a given performer which includes a range of different stretching activities;
- critically evaluate a number of different training methods and apply them to a given performer;
- identify and outline the testing procedure for at least one fitness test for each component of fitness;
- discuss the reasons for fitness testing and the limitations of fitness tests;
- comment on the validity and reliability of each fitness test;
- outline the factors to consider when organising a training session;
- describe Mosston and Ashworth's teaching styles and outline when to use each effectively;
- understand the various ways of presenting practices;
- explain the different types of practices and when to use each one;
- outline various forms of guidance and how to optimise their use;
- explain the importance of feedback and outline the different types of feedback that can be used.

## Preparing for Section B – Application of theoretical knowledge for effective performance

Much of the content of this chapter you will acquire through your practical lessons in your school or college. However, this theoretical content will be assessed via an extended question in Section B of your Unit 1 written examination paper. You will be expected to apply your acquired knowledge to a practical scenario and the question will focus on the application and justification of that knowledge in the context of a performer, coach or official.

## Section 1 Applied exercise physiology

This section seeks specifically to investigate how training can improve and enhance fitness and performance levels. The chapter consists of two main sections. The first discusses the principles and types of training that can be employed in a training regime, while the second focuses on the assessment of fitness strengths and weaknesses of a performer by means of a battery of fitness tests available to the coach and athlete.

In order to maximise your performance in this aspect of your examination, it will be necessary for you to have an awareness and understanding of the factors that underpin a range of performers and use the knowledge gained from this chapter to identify and justify strengths and weaknesses in their performance and suggest appropriate strategies to enable an improvement in their performance.

# The principles of training

The principles of training are essentially the rules or laws that underpin a training programme. If these rules are not followed then any training undertaken will become obsolete and worthless. There are many principles of training that the coach and athlete must bear in mind in the design of an effective training regime.

## Specificity

The law of specificity suggests that any training undertaken should be relevant and appropriate to the sport for which the individual is training. For example, it would be highly inappropriate for a swimmer to carry out the majority of his/her training on the land. Although there are certainly benefits gained from land-based training, the majority of the training programme should involve pool-based work.

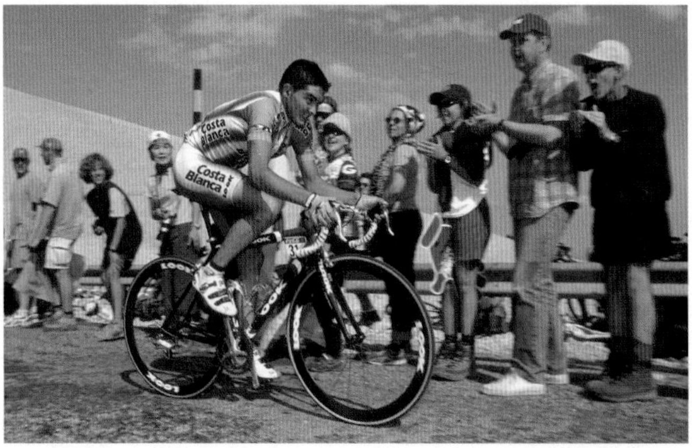

Figure 14.1 A cyclist will follow the principle of specificity as most training undertaken will focus on the legs

The specificity rule does not govern just the muscles, fibre type and actions used but also the energy systems which are predominantly stressed. The energy system used in training should replicate that predominantly used in the event. The energy systems should also be stressed in isolation of each other so that high-intensity work (stressing the anaerobic systems) should be done in one session, whereas more aerobic and endurance-based work should be completed in a separate session.

**IN CONTEXT**

**When designing a weight training programme for a shot-putter, for example, the coach will ensure specificity by using weights or exercises (such as an inclined bench press) that replicate the action of shot-putting. He will ensure that the exercises use the same muscle group and muscle fibres that the athlete recruits during the event and that the repetitions are undertaken explosively, using the alactic (ATP-Pc system) energy pathway, which of course is the predominant energy system used during the shot-putt.**

## Progressive overload

This rule considers the intensity of the training session. For improvement and adaptation to occur, the training should be at an intensity where the individual feels some kind of stress and discomfort. This signifies overload and suggests that the old adage 'no pain, no gain' has some truth in it, especially for the elite athlete. Overload for the shot-putter may therefore involve lifting very heavy weights, or indeed using a shot that is heavier than that used in competition. If exercise takes place on a regular basis the body's systems will adapt and start to cope with these stresses that have been imposed. In order for further improvement to occur, the intensity of training will need to be gradually increased – this is progression and can be done by running faster, lifting heavier weights, or training for longer.

## Reversibility

Also known as 'regression' or detraining, this explains why performance deteriorates when training ceases or the intensity of training decreases for extended periods of time. Quite simply, if you don't use it you lose it!

Seven weeks of inactivity has been shown to give significant decreases in maximum oxygen uptake up to 27 per cent, which reflects a fall in the efficiency of the cardiovascular system. In particular, stroke volume and cardiac output can decrease by up to 30 per cent. During exercise, increases in both blood lactate and heart rate have been shown to increase for the same intensity of exercise. Muscle mass and therefore strength also deteriorate but at a less rapid rate. Now you may be able to understand why pre-season training feels so tough even after just 6–8 weeks of inactivity.

## Individual difference

This suggests that the benefits of training are optimised when programmes are set to meet the needs and abilities of an individual. What may help one athlete to improve may not be successful on another. The coach must therefore be very sympathetic to the needs of the individual athlete and adjust training programmes accordingly.

## Overtraining/moderation

Overtraining is a common problem to elite athletes as they strive for greater improvement. It is caused by an imbalance between training and recovery, which usually occurs when insufficient time has been left for the body to regenerate and cause adaptation before embarking upon the next training session. In their search for the best possible performance in competition, elite athletes are often tempted to increase training loads and frequency of training above optimal levels, which can lead to symptoms of overtraining. These symptoms include enduring fatigue, loss of appetite, muscle tenderness, sleep disturbances and head colds. The coach can identify overtraining syndrome by physiological testing, which may show the athlete having an increased oxygen consumption, heart rate and blood lactate levels at fixed workloads. In order to combat overtraining the coach should advise prolonged rest, and a reduction in training workloads for a period of weeks or even months. This should restore both performance and competitive desire.

Furthermore, by ensuring adequate rest days and following the 3:1 hard:easy ratio the coach and athlete should avoid falling into the overtraining trap. To prevent overtraining it is essential that the training programme is planned sufficiently well to include a variation in training intensities and to include regular rest days. By simply following a ratio of three hard sessions to one easy session, overtraining should be avoided.

## Variance

Variety is the spice of life. So to prevent boredom, staleness and injury through training it is necessary to ensure that the training programme employs a range of training methods and loads so as not to impose too much psychological or physiological stress on the performer.

## The F.I.T.T. regime

The coach may also wish to consider the F.I.T.T. regime when designing the training programme. These letters stand for:

- F = frequency of training;
- I = intensity of exercise;
- T = time or duration of exercise;
- T = type of training.

### 'F'

The frequency of training. The elite athlete will need to do some sort of training most days, depending upon the activity being undertaken. Endurance or aerobic type activities can be performed five or six times per week, but more intense or anaerobic activities such as strength or speed work should be performed three or four times per week, as sufficient rest days are required for the body tissues to repair themselves following this high-intensity work-out.

### 'I'

The intensity of the exercise. This also depends upon the type of training occurring and can be quite difficult to measure objectively. Some ways of gauging the intensity of exercise are outlined below:

- calculating the training zone;
- calculating the performer's $VO_2$max and working at a percentage of it;
- calculating the respiratory exchange ratio;
- using lactate tests;
- also more basic tests such as the 'talk test';
- perceived exertion scales such as the Borg scale.

For aerobic work, exercise intensity can be measured by calculating an individual's 'training zone'; this is represented by the training heart rate and so involves observing heart rate values. This has become much easier with the advent of the heart rate monitor.

The most established method of calculating the training zone is known as the Karvonen Principle. Karvonen developed a formula to identify correct training intensities as a percentage of the sum of the maximum heart rate reserve and resting heart rate. Maximum heart rate reserve can be calculated by subtracting resting heart rate (HRrest) from an individual's maximum heart rate (HRmax):

Maximal heart rate reserve = HRmax – HRrest

Where an individual's maximal heart rate can be calculated by subtracting their age from 220:

Maximal heart rate = 220 – age

Karvonen suggests a training intensity of between 60–75% of maximal heart rate reserve for the average athlete, although this can obviously be adapted to account for individual differences.

We might expect an elite performer to work at values nearing 85% of max HR reserve for example.

Training heart rate 85% = 0.85 (maxHR reserve) + HRrest

Consider the following example to illustrate the value of this measure of intensity.

A 20-year-old rower, with a resting heart rate of 65 bpm, is aiming to build up his endurance capacities for a forthcoming event. He is advised to train between 60–75% of his training heart rate reserve in the weeks prior to the event. To calculate his training zone, the rower used the Karvonen formula as follows:

Training heart rate 60 per cent = 0.60 (HRmax – HRrest) + HRrest
= 0.60 (200 – 65) + 65
= 81 + 65
= **146 beats per minute**

Training heart rate 75 per cent = 0.75 (HRmax – HRrest) + HRrest
= 0.75 (200 – 65) + 65
= 101 + 65
= **166 beats per minute**

Thus the rower now has some precise figures to use to ensure that he is training at the correct intensity.

In order for some kind of aerobic adaptation to occur, the rower must be exercising within his target zone, between 146 and 166 beats per minute.

Another method of monitoring the intensity of training is through working the athlete at a % of $VO_2$max. For the elite endurance athlete, this should be no less than 70% of $VO_2$max, while those exercising for health-related reasons will see benefits from training at just 50% of their $VO_2$max. Figure 14.2 shows the linear relationship between heart rate and oxygen consumption ($VO_2$). If the athlete's HRmax is known, then it is possible for the coach to extrapolate the $VO_2$max from the graph in Figure 14.2.

A coach could also use lactate tests to ensure the athlete is working sufficiently hard and analyse oxygen consumption and carbon dioxide production to determine the respiratory exchange ratio. The Respiratory Exchange Ratio (RER) or Respiratory Quotient is a method of determining which energy providing nutrient is predominantly in use during exercise. It is represented as follows:

$$\frac{\text{Volume of } CO_2 \text{ expired per minute}}{\text{Volume of } O_2 \text{ per minute}}$$

The closer the value is to 1.0 the more likely it is the body is using glycogen as a fuel, whereas the expected value for fats is 0.7. Intermediate figures suggest that a mixture of fuels is being utilised which is obviously the expected norm. Obviously the harder the athlete is working the more he or she relies on using glycogen as a fuel.

**The Borg Scale** is a subjective evaluation of how hard you are working during exercise. Essentially the performer rates their level of exertion on a scale of 6-20. At the bottom of the scale is 6, meaning that there is no exertion. Between 7 and 8 is extremely light exertion. Eleven is a light level of exertion. As you go up the scale to 15, you reach a heavy workload. By the time you reach 20, you are working so hard you cannot sustain it for very long.

This is a simple measure of intensity. It does not require any equipment, just an honest assessment of how hard you're exerting yourself. Despite it's simiplicity the Borg scale has a suprisingly high correleation to the measures of intensity such as % $VO_2$max and the training heart rate.

Table 14.1 The Borg perceived exertion scale

| Exertion | RPE |
|---|---|
| no exertion at all | 6 |
| extremely light | 7 |
| | 8 |
| very light | 9 |
| | 10 |
| light | 11 |
| | 12 |
| somewhat hard | 13 |
| | 14 |
| hard (heavy) | 15 |
| | 16 |
| very hard | 17 |
| | 18 |
| extremely hard | 19 |
| maximal exertion | 20 |

Note: RPE = ratio of perceived exertion

'T'

The time or duration that the exercise is in progress. For aerobic type activities, the athlete should be training within his/her training zone for a minimum of 20–30 minutes. However, duration should not be considered in isolation since intensity of training often determines the duration of the training session.

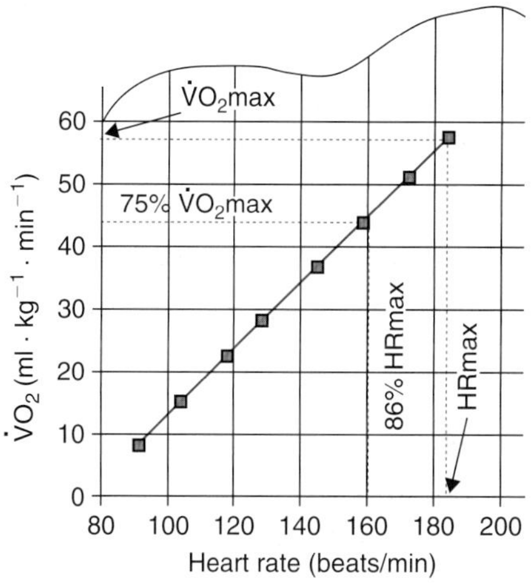


Figure 14.2 The linear relationship between HR and $VO_2$

## Activity 1

- Use the table here in this activity and Figure 14.3, calculate your training zone (between 60 and 75% of your maximum heart rate reserve).
- Now complete a 15-minute run, ensuring your heart rate lies at 70% of your MHR.
- Sketch the heart rate curve expected.

| Age | | 20 | 25 | 30 | 35 | 40 | 45 | 50 | 55 | 60 | 65 | 70 | 75 | 80 |
|---|---|---|---|---|---|---|---|---|---|---|---|---|---|---|
| 55% | 19 | 18 | 18 | 17 | 17 | 17 | 16 | 16 | 15 | 15 | 14 | 14 | 13 | 13 |
| 60% | 21 | 20 | 19 | 19 | 19 | 18 | 18 | 17 | 17 | 16 | 16 | 15 | 15 | 14 |
| 70% | 24 | 23 | 23 | 22 | 22 | 21 | 20 | 20 | 19 | 19 | 18 | 18 | 17 | 16 |
| 80% | 27 | 27 | 26 | 25 | 25 | 24 | 23 | 23 | 22 | 21 | 21 | 20 | 19 | 19 |
| 90% | 29 | 28 | 28 | 27 | 26 | 26 | 25 | 24 | 23 | 23 | 22 | 21 | 21 | 20 |

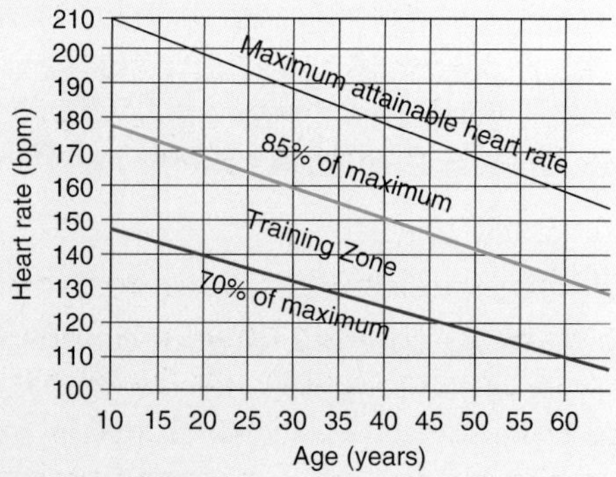


Figure 14.3

Use the table here in this activity as a calculator to work out your target training zone at various intensities. All scores reflect your heart rate for a 10 second count. Don't forget to start counting from zero! If you fall between age ranges take the next group up. For example, if you are 18 and wish to train at 70% of your maximum heart rate, find the age group 20 along the top of the table and move down until you come to 70% of MHR. Your target 10s pulse rate should be 23 beats. You may wish to convert this to beats per minute, in which case multiply the figure in the box by six.

'T'

The type or mode of training that is undertaken. This really relates to the principle of specificity as discussed earlier in this chapter.

# Warm-ups and cool-downs

## Warm-up

One might not immediately think of warm-ups and cool-downs as a principle of training, but as they should be undertaken prior to and following every training session and will improve the effectiveness of training, it seems highly appropriate to discuss them here.

Before embarking upon any type of exercise, it is imperative to perform a warm-up, as it is fundamental to safe practice.

A warm-up should prepare the body for exercise. It can prevent injury and muscle soreness, and has the following physiological benefits:

- The release of adrenaline will increase heart rate and dilate capillaries, which in turn enable greater amounts and increased speed of oxygen and blood delivery to the muscles.
- The speed of oxygen delivery is further improved as a result of the decreased viscosity of the blood which occurs as a consequence of the increase in muscle temperature.
- Increased muscle temperatures associated with exercise will facilitate enzyme activity as well as encourage the dissociation of oxygen from haemoglobin. This increases muscle metabolism and therefore ensures a readily available supply of energy through the breakdown of glycogen.

### Activity 2

An investigation into training intensities – the training zone!

- Using the Karvonen Principle, calculate your training zone.
- Record your resting pulse rate
- In groups of three work on a given method of aerobic exercise (eg, running, step-ups, rowing, cycling). One person should be exercising at a steady pace, the second keeps an eye on heart rate and the third records the results.
- Record heart rate at the following times:
  a) Immediately prior to exercise
  b) 2mins after exercise commences
  c) 5mins after exercise commences (ensure you are in the zone!)
  d) 7mins after exercise commences (still in the zone?)
  e) 10mins after exercise commences (stop exercise now!)
  f) 1min after exercise stops
  g) 3mins after exercise stops
  h) 5mins after exercise stops
- Copy out and record your results in the table below

| HRrest | Prior to Ex | 2 mins during | 5 mins during | 7 mins during | 10 mins during | 1 min after | 3 mins after | 5 mins after |
|---|---|---|---|---|---|---|---|---|
| | | | | | | | | |

- Draw a graph to illustrate your heart rate before, during and after exercise. Identify on your graph your training zone.

- Increased temperatures also lead to decreased viscosity within the muscle. This enables greater extensibility and elasticity of muscle fibres which ultimately leads to increased speed and force of contraction.
- Warm-ups also make us more alert, due to an increase in the speed of nerve impulse conduction.
- Increased production of synovial fluid ensures efficient movement at the joints.
- A warm-up may also result in limiting the effects of DOMS (Delayed Onset of Muscle Soreness), which is characterised by tender and painful muscles often experienced in the days following heavy and unaccustomed exercise. The explanation of this soreness is quite simple and results from the damage to muscle fibres and connective tissue surrounding the fibres. The soreness is usually temporary and goes within a couple of days as the muscle fibres repair themselves. DOMS is most likely to occur following eccentric contraction and can result from weight training, plyometrics or even walking down steep hills.
- Certain psychological benefits can also occur through a warm-up, particularly if the individual has certain superstitions or rituals they follow. Think of the New Zealand All Blacks Rugby Team performing the Haka, prior to kick-off.

Furthermore, it should not be forgotten that warm-ups should be *specific* to the activity that follows and should include exercises which prepare the muscles to be used and activate the energy systems required for that particular activity.

To ensure the athlete gains as much from the warm-up as possible, the following stages should be followed:

**Stage 1** The first phase of a warm-up has the purpose of raising the heart rate, increasing the speed of oxygen delivery to the muscles, and of course raising the body temperature. This can be achieved by performing some kind of cardiovascular exercise such as jogging.

**Stage 2** Now that muscle temperature has increased, the athlete can perform some mobility or stretching exercises. It is essential that both static and dynamic stretches are performed where the muscle is working over its full range. Press-ups, squat thrusts and lunges are good for this.

**Stage 3** The final stage of a warm-up should involve a sport-specific or skill-related component where the neuromuscular mechanisms related to the activity to follow are worked. For example, practising serving in tennis, tumble turns in swimming or shooting baskets in basketball.

### Activity 3

Design a warm-up programme for a sport of your choice. What activities would you include in your programme, and why?

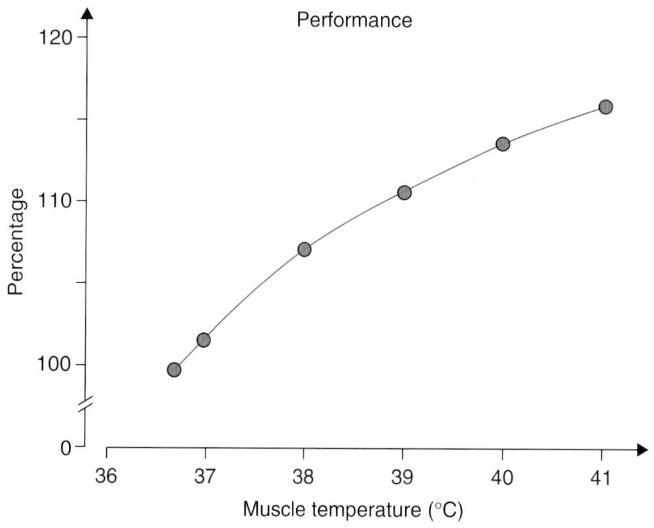


**Figure 14.4** The relationship between performance and muscle temperature

## Cool-down

Following exercise, a similar process must be followed in order to prevent unnecessary discomfort; this is a cool-down. It involves performing some kind of light continuous exercise where heart rate remains elevated. The purpose is to keep metabolic activity high, and capillaries dilated, so that oxygen can be flushed through the muscle tissue, removing and oxidising any lactic acid that remains. This will therefore prevent blood pooling in the veins which can cause dizziness if exercise is stopped abruptly. The final part of the cool-down period should involve a period of stretching activity, which should hopefully facilitate and improve flexibility as the muscles are very warm at this stage. As with a warm up, cool-downs may also limit the effects of Delayed onset of muscle soreness (DOMS).

Now that we understand the basic laws which govern training, the next stage in our search for a beneficial training programme is to determine the method or type of training that is best employed.

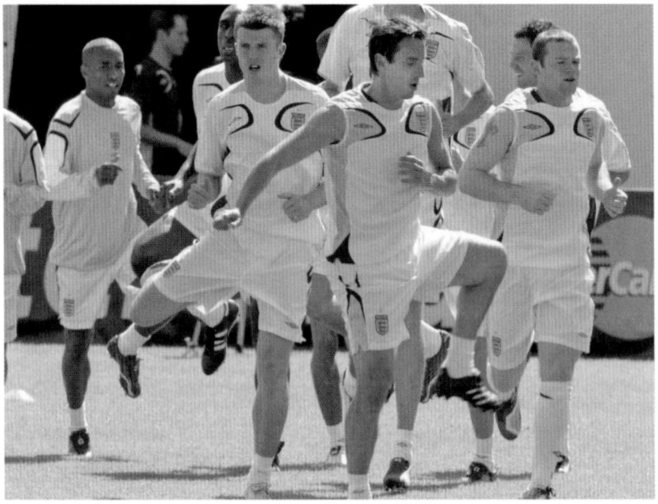

Figure 14.5 A cool-down helps to promote recovery following exercise

# Training methods

## Continuous methods

Continuous methods of training work on developing endurance and therefore stress the aerobic energy system. Central to this method of training is the performance of rhythmic exercise at a steady rate or low intensity which use the large muscle groups of the body over a long period of time (between 30 minutes and two hours). Good examples of such activities include jogging, swimming, cycling or aerobic dance. The intensity of such exercise should be at approximately 60–80% of HRmax, as outlined in the Karvonen Principle, so the body is not experiencing too much discomfort while exercising.

The great advantage of this type of training, however, is that great distances can be covered without the lactate build-up associated with anaerobic training methods. Distance runners, for example, may total up to 140 miles per week, a distance equivalent of London to Lincoln.

With such high mileage comes the danger of injury, particularly to the muscles and joints, so any programme should be thoroughly scrutinised. Other disadvantages of this type of training are that it can be quite monotonous, and although good in developing an aerobic base for all activities, it is not necessarily sport specific when it comes to team games. The health-related benefits of continuous training have been well documented; jogging and aerobics are very popular, and as long as individuals are made aware of the injury risk factors, there is no reason why the majority cannot participate safely.

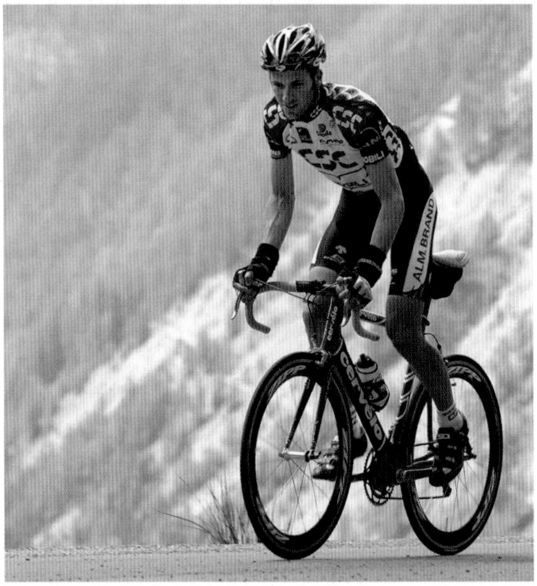

Figure 14.6 Continuous training will form the main part of a cyclist's training programme

## Fartlek, or speedplay

This is a slightly different method of continuous training. It is a form of endurance conditioning, where the aerobic energy system is stressed due to the continuous nature of the exercise. The only difference, however, is that throughout the duration of the exercise, the speed or intensity of the activity is varied, so that both the aerobic and anaerobic systems can be stressed. Fartlek sessions are usually performed for a minimum of 45 minutes, with the intensity of the session varying from low-intensity walking to high-intensity sprinting. Traditionally Fartlek training has taken place in the countryside where there is varied terrain, but this alternating pace method could occur anywhere and you could use your local environment to help you; for example:

- easy jog for three lamp posts;
- sprint for one lamp post;
- easy jog for three lamp posts;
- sprint for one lamp post;
- repeat three further times;
- walk for one minute;
- jog at 75 per cent of MHR for five minutes;
- repeat four times.

This method of training, devised by a Swede, Gosta Holmer, has been adapted by many physiologists.

A few examples now follow.

The Gerschler method involves jogging for 10 minutes followed by 30 seconds of long, fast strides followed by 90 seconds jogging recovery. The jogging recovery decreases by 15 seconds after each 30 second stride-out. For example, the next bout of exercise would involve 30 seconds fast followed by 75 seconds jog recovery, the next 30 seconds of work is followed by 60 seconds of jog recovery and so on until the athlete has only 15 seconds of recovery. Having completed this one set of 30 second strides the athlete will repeat once more 30 seconds fast followed by 90 seconds jogging, etc.

The Saltin method involves a 10-minute warm-up jog followed by three minutes of sustained fast running with 60 seconds of jog recovery, repeated six times. This is useful for middle distance and cross country runners, and perhaps for boxers, who must sustain all-out effort over three-minute rounds.

This type of training can be very individual and the athlete can determine the speed or intensity at which he/she wishes to work. It can also be fun and offers variety to what some regard as the monotony of continuous jogging. Since both aerobic and anaerobic systems are stressed through this method of training, a wealth of sportspeople can benefit. It is particularly suited to those activities that involve a mixture of aerobic and anaerobic work, e.g. field games such as rugby, hockey or soccer. However, to make the session more sport specific for games players, the direction of running should be altered to mimic the running pattern within a game – for example, side to side and backward running should be included as well as running forwards in a straight line.

## Intermittent training

Intermittent methods of training involve periods of work or exercise interspersed with periods of recovery. Athletes appear to be able to perform considerably more work when the session is broken down into short intense periods of effort and recovery breaks, and the physiological benefits are great.

## Interval training

This is probably the most popular type of training used in sport for training the elite athlete. It is very versatile and can be used in almost any activity, although it is most widely used in swimming, athletics and cycling. Interval training can improve both aerobic and anaerobic capacities.

In order for the correct capacity to be stressed, several variables have been identified which can be manipulated. These variables include:

1. Distance of the work interval (duration)
2. Intensity of the work interval (speed)
3. The number of repetitions within a session
4. The number of sets within a session
5. Duration of the rest interval
6. Activity during the rest interval.

In order to train the relevant energy system, the coach must ensure that the variables have been adjusted appropriately.

1. For anaerobic speed fitness, the duration of the work period should last for 3–10 seconds, or an equivalent distance that can be covered in that time at the highest intensity (depending upon the activity being performed).
2. Intensity should be assessed by the athlete working at a percentage of their maximum effort or personal best time for the distance. For improvements in anaerobic speed this should be 90–100 per cent.
3. Generally, the number of repetitions depends upon the length of the work period. For anaerobic speed, the work interval is relatively short and we can expect to perform up to 50 short, intense bouts within a session.
4. These 50 repetitions may be divided into a number of sets (a group of work and rest intervals), to ensure that the athlete does not get unduly fatigued, e.g. 5 sets × 10 reps.

5 Between each repetition is a period of rest which can be determined by the time it takes for the heart rate to return to about 150 beats per minute. It can be compared to the work interval time, expressed as the work:relief (rest) ratio. For anaerobic speed where the work interval is relatively short, the rest period may take three times that before the heart lowers to 150 bpm. This would be expressed as a work:relief ratio of 1:3.
6 The type of activity that takes place during these rest intervals differs, depending upon the energy system being trained. When developing anaerobic speed no activity apart from perhaps some light stretching during the recovery phase, while the lactic acid system will require active recovery involving light jogging or walking.

## Anaerobic speed development

eg, 3 × 10 × 30 m (wbr) 5 mins rest between sets

Where:

3 = No sets
10 = No of repetitions
30 m = Distance of work interval
wbr = Walk back recovery

## Anaerobic speed endurance development or lactate training

eg, 8 × 300 m runs 3 mins work relief

Where:

8 = No of repetitions
300 m = Distance of work interval
3 mins = Recovery period

## Aerobic development

eg, 4–6 × 2–5 min runs work:relief ratio = 1:1 (2–5 min)

Where:

4–6 = No of repetitions
2–5 mins = Duration of work period
W:R = 1:1 (2–5 mins) = Recovery period

For anaerobic speed endurance, an exercise period of between 15 seconds and 90 seconds should be performed at a moderate intensity. Up to 12 repetitions may be completed over two or three sets with a work to relief ratio of 1:2. This should give time for some although not all lactic acid to be removed. Thus in successive work intervals, the body must work with some lactic acid already present within the system, which should improve the buffering capacity of the body. To speed up the removal of lactate during the relief period, some light exercise should be performed, such as rapid walking or jogging – this is known as work relief.

To train the aerobic system, the work interval should be much longer, perhaps up to 7 or 8 minutes in duration. The intensity should again be moderate (and certainly faster than any pace undertaken during continuous training) and measured as a percentage of personal best times for the distance. The longer exercise periods mean that fewer repetitions are needed, maybe only three or four in one session, which can be performed in one set. In order to put extra stress on the aerobic system the recovery time is usually much shorter in comparison to the work period. A work:relief ratio of 1:1/2 may be used where the athlete rests for half the time it took to complete the work period.

The requirements of an interval training session can be expressed as the interval training prescription. For example, a swimmer may have the following session prescribed:

2 × 4 × 200 m W:R 1:1/2

where: 2 = number of sets
4 = number of repetitions
200 m = training distance
1:1/2 = work to relief ratio.

Some examples of interval training regimes are outlined in Table 14.2.

Sprint interval training sessions are specifically designed to stress the ATP-PC system, improving its capacity and increasing the muscle stores of ATP and PC. This obviously has a direct effect upon sprinters or any activity where bursts of speed are required.

Fast interval training sessions develop anaerobic endurance and therefore stress the lactic acid system. The buffering capacity of the body improves, which delays the onset of fatigue and decreases the effect of lactic acid. This training is of particular importance to 400m runners and sprint swimmers.

The aerobic system is stressed by performing slower intervals which improves the oxidative capacity of the body. Any endurance-based event such as distance running or swimming will benefit from this type of training, in addition to field games such as rugby and hockey.

Again, as with other training methods, it is important to ensure that where possible the session is adapted to suit the requirements of the game. For example, a squash player may adapt the work period to include running to one corner of the court and returning to the 'T' then running to the second corner and back to the 'T', running to the third, etc., until all four corners have been touched – this might represent on repetition of a work period which can then be followed by a period of rest.

Table 14.2 Interval training prescriptions

| **Major energy system** | **Training time (min:sec)** | **Repetitions per workout** | **Sets per workout** | **Repetitions per set** | **Work: relief ratio** | **Type of relief interval** |
|---|---|---|---|---|---|---|
| ATP-PC | 0:10 | 50 | 5 | 10 | | rest-relief (eg, walking, flexing) |
| | 0:15 | 45 | 5 | 9 | | |
| | 0:20 | 40 | 4 | 10 | 1:3 | |
| | 0:25 | 32 | 4 | 8 | | |
| ATP-PC/LA | 0:30 | 25 | 5 | 5 | | work-relief (eg, light to mild exercise, jogging) |
| | 0:40–0:50 | 20 | 4 | 5 | 1:3 | |
| | 1:00–1:10 | 15 | 3 | 5 | | |
| | 1:20 | 10 | 2 | 5 | 1:2 | |
| LA/$O_2$ | 1:30–2:00 | 8 | 2 | 4 | 1:2 | work-relief |
| | 2:10–2:40 | 6 | 1 | 6 | | |
| | 2:50–3:00 | 4 | 1 | 4 | 1:1 | rest-relief |
| $O_2$ | 3:00–4:00 | 4 | 1 | 4 | 1:1 | rest-relief |
| | 4:00–5:00 | 3 | 1 | 3 | 1:1/2 | |
| **Major energy system** | **Training distance (M)**<br>**Run Swim** | | | | | |
| ATP-PC | 50 10 | 50 | 5 | 10 | 1:3 | rest-relief (eg, walking, flexing) |
| | 100 25 | 24 | 3 | 8 | | |
| ATP-PC/LA | 200 50 | 16 | 4 | 4 | 1:3 | work-relief (eg, light to mild exercise, jogging) |
| | 400 100 | 8 | 2 | 4 | 1:2 | |
| LA/$O_2$ | 600 150 | 5 | 1 | 5 | 1:2 | work-relief |
| | 800 200 | 4 | 2 | 2 | 1:1 | rest-relief |
| $O_2$ | 1,000 250 | 3 | 1 | 3 | 1:1/2 | rest-relief |
| | 1,200 300 | 3 | 1 | 3 | 1:1/2 | |

## Circuit training

Circuit training involves performing a number of calisthenic exercises in succession, such as press-ups, abdominal curls, step-ups, etc. Each exercise is usually performed for a set amount of time or a set number of repetitions, and the circuit can be adapted to meet the specific fitness requirements of a given sport or activity (see Figure 14.8).

When planning a circuit there are several factors that need consideration. The first of these is the most fundamental – what exactly do you require the circuit for? Once you have answered this you can choose the exercises to include. You will also need to consider:

- the number of participants;
- their level of fitness;
- the amount of time, space and equipment available.

Having considered all these points you can now go ahead and plan the layout of your circuit.

One golden rule when devising the layout of the circuit is that *the same body part should not be exercised consecutively*. Therefore the sequence of the exercises should be as follows: arms, trunk, cardiovascular, legs, arms, trunk, cardiovascular, etc. The exception is for experienced athletes performing an 'overload' circuit where the endurance of one muscle group is being trained.

The great benefit of circuit training is that it is extremely adaptable, since exercises can be included or omitted to suit almost all activities. It also enables large numbers of participants to train together at their own level. With regular testing, improvements in fitness are easily visible through circuit training as current work can be compared to previous test scores. Figure 14.8 illustrates a 3 in 1 circuit, whereby each participant completes

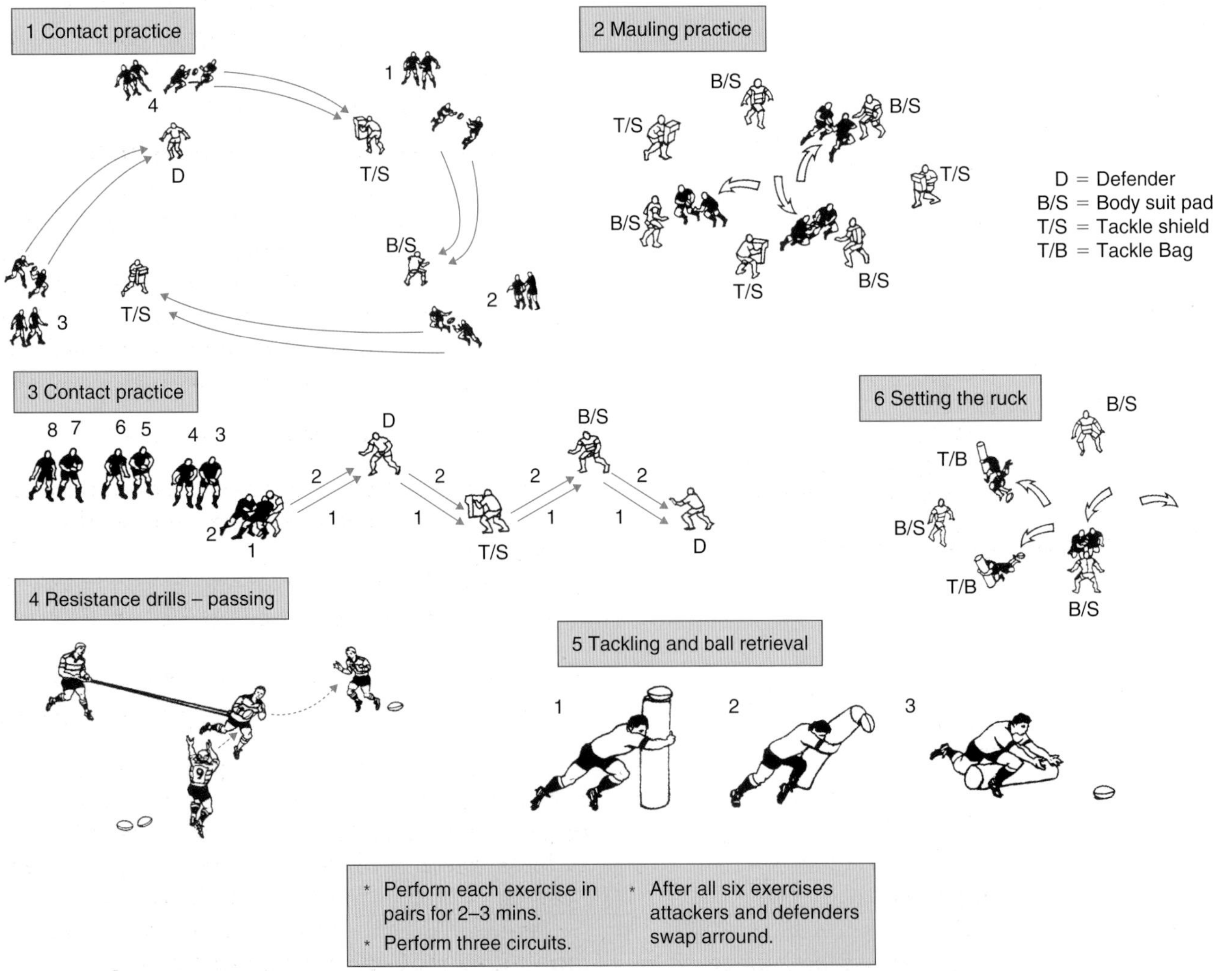


**Figure 14.7** Rugby contact circuit

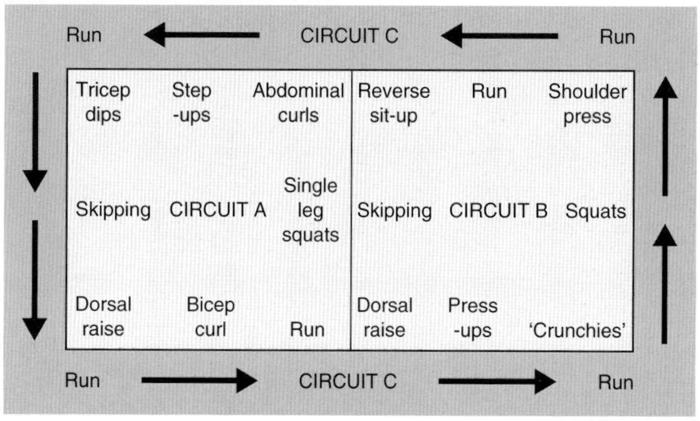


Each participant is to complete each circuit.

Circuit A = 8 exercises × 30 secs = 4 mins
Circuit B = 8 exercises × 30 secs = 4 mins
Circuit C = Run around outside = 4 mins
Repeat 2 or 3 times

Each participant is to complete circuit A, B and C with 60 secs walking recovery between circuit.

**Figure 14.8** A general fitness circuit

circuits A, B and C. This circuit is particularly good for general conditioning and enables large numbers to participate.

## Activity 4

Design a circuit training session for an activity of your choice. Give reasons for the exercises you have chosen and explain how the principle of progressive overload could be applied. Table 14.3 might help in the selection of some exercises.

**Table 14.3** Exercises to include in a circuit

| | |
|---|---|
| Cardiovascular exercises | running around the gym<br>skipping<br>step-ups<br>cycling on an ergometer<br>bounding exercises on a mat |
| Trunk exercises | abdominal curls<br>crunchies<br>dorsal raises<br>trunk twists |
| Arm exercises | press-ups/box press<br>bicep curls<br>tricep dips<br>shoulder press<br>squat thrusts<br>chin-ups to beam |
| Leg exercises | single leg squats<br>any of the cardiovascular exercises outlined above |

## Strength training

Strength gains are sought by many athletes and usually occur either through weight or resistance training methods, or through a further type of training known as plyometrics.

With advances in technology and the improvement in the quality of weight machines, weight training has increased in popularity in both athletic and recreational training regimes. It can be used to develop several components of fitness, including strength, strength endurance and explosive power. Which of these are stressed at a particular time is determined by manipulating the weight or resistance, the number of repetitions and the number of sets. Central to the devising of an effective weight training programme is the principle of one repetition maximum (1RM). The 1RM is the maximum amount of weight the performer can lift with one repetition. Once this has been found for each exercise the coach can design a programme adjusting the resistance as a percentage of the athlete's maximum lift. Take a moment to study Table 14.4 which is a simple guide to strength development.

For activities where maximum strength is required, such as power lifting or throwing the hammer, training methods which increase muscle strength and size will be required. Essentially this will involve some form of very high resistance, low repetition exercise. For example, performing 3 sets of 2–6 repetitions at 80–100 per cent of maximum strength, with full recovery between sets.

Key points for power development are:

1 The movement and contraction period must be explosive to ensure the muscle works rapidly.
2 The use of very high loads or resistance which will encourage the muscle to recruit all its motor units.
3 Ensuring the muscle recovers fully between sets, enabling the relevant energy system to recover.

To train for activities which require strength endurance, such as swimming or rowing, a different approach to training will be required. In order to perform more repetitions, a lighter load or resistance is needed and the following programme might be prescribed: 3 sets of 20 repetitions at 50–60 per cent of maximum strength with full recovery between sets.

One aspect of strength that is difficult to improve through regular resistance training is core strength. Core strength is the combined strength of all the muscles from your hips to your armpits – and is responsible for many things including posture. An increase in core strength can lead to increases in virtually all other types of strength and dramatically reduces the chance of injury during strength training. The best method of improving core strength and stability is with the use of a Swiss ball. Simply performing abdominal crunches or leg raises on the Swiss ball will strengthen the abdominal and lower back muscles, the 'core' of the body's strength.

## Plyometrics

Power is the ability to produce maximal muscular forces very rapidly. It is determined by the force exerted by the muscle (strength) and the speed at which the muscle shortens: Power = Force × Velocity. It thus follows that by improving either strength or speed of shortening, power may be improved. One method of training which may improve the speed at which a muscle shortens is plyometrics.

It has long been established that muscles generate more force in contraction when they have been previously stretched. Plyometrics enables this to occur by taking the muscle through an eccentric (lengthened) phase whereby elastic energy is stored before a powerful concentric (shortening) phase. This stimulates adaptation within the neuromuscular system whereby the muscle spindles within the muscle cause a stretch reflex, which prevents muscle damage and produces a more powerful concentric contraction of the muscle group. This has important consequences for sprinting, jumping and throwing events in athletics, as well as in games such as rugby, volleyball and basketball where leg strength is central to performance.

Exercises that might form part of the plyometrics session include:

- bounding
- hopping
- leaping
- skipping
- depth jumps (jumping off and onto boxes)
- press-ups with claps
- throwing and catching a medicine ball.

Taking the example of depth jumping (Figure 14.9), here the athlete drops down from a box or platform 50–80cm high. On landing the quadricep muscle group lengthens, pre-loading the muscle. A stretch reflex causes the muscle to give a very forceful concentric contraction driving the athlete up onto a second platform. Furthermore the exercise becomes more effective if the athlete spends as little time as possible in contact with the ground when landing. This particular plyometric activity can also be made sport specific. For example, a basketball player could perform a rebound after dropping down from the box or a volleyball player could perform a block, etc. Due to the high impact nature of the plyometrics individuals would need to be screened for injury and participants would need to undergo a thorough warm-up.

Key points to consider when undertaking plyometric training:

- warm up thoroughly;
- use a flat, non-slip landing surface that has good shock absorbing properties, such as a grass field;
- make sure any boxes or benches used are sturdy and safe;
- ensure you follow guidelines on technique of the exercises, i.e. landing on the ball of your foot, then rocking back onto your heel and then taking off from the ball of the foot again. The sequence should therefore be 'ball-heel-ball';
- progression in exercise should be gradual to avoid soreness;
- if you experience joint or muscular pain stop immediately.

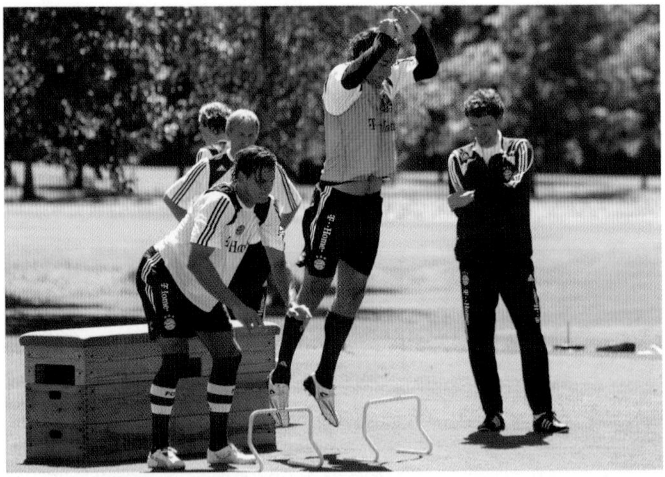

**Figure 14.9** Depth-jumping, a plyometric activity

Table 14.4 The development of different types of strength

| Objective | Intensity of training load | Repetitions in each set | Number of sets | Recovery between sets | Evaluation procedures | Training of value for |
|---|---|---|---|---|---|---|
| development of maximum strength | 85–95% | 1–5 | normal 2–4 advanced 5–8 | 4–5mins | maximum lift dynamometer | weight lifting, shot, discus, hammer, javelin, jumping events, rugby and contact sports, men's gymnastics |
| development of elastic strength | 75–85% | 6–10 | (4–6) | 3–5mins | standing, long and vertical jump capability | all sports requiring 'explosive' strength qualities – sprinting, jumping, throwing, striking |
| development of advanced level of strength endurance | 50–75% of maximum | 15–20 | (3–5) | 30–45 secs | maximum reps possible | rowing, wrestling, skiing, swimming, 400m, steeplechase etc. |
| development of a basic level of strength endurance | 25–50% of maximum | 15–20 | (4–6) | 60 secs | maximum reps possible | generally required for all sports suitable for young and novice competitors and fitness participants |

The strength gains and muscle hypertrophy associated with strength training may only start to become evident after about eight weeks of training, and are largely due to the increase in size and volume of the myofibrils.

## SAQ training

SAQ stands for speed, agility and quickness. It is a relatively new type of training that is used in many team games such as rugby and football and is designed to improve the speed, agility and reactions of a performer. Central to this activity are resistance drills, perhaps using bungy ropes, ladder drills to improve leg speed and jumping activities to improve leg speed and strength.

**Activity 5**

A triple jumper requires some advice on improving leg strength. Design a strength programme, stating which type of strength is being developed.

## Mobility training

Mobility training is the method employed to improve flexibility. It is often a neglected form of training, but should be incorporated into every athlete's training programme. Effective flexibility training can improve performance and help prevent the occurrence of injury.

The method of stretching used in mobility training should centre on the connective tissue and the muscle tissue acting upon the joint, as these tissues have been shown to elongate following a period of regular and repeated stretching. Several types of stretching have been identified and outlined below.

### Active stretching

The athlete performs voluntary muscular contractions, and holds the stretch for a period of 30–60 seconds. By consciously relaxing the target muscle at the limit of the range of motion, muscle elongation may occur following regular contraction.

### Passive stretching

This refers to the range of movement which can occur with the aid of external force. This is generally performed with the help of a partner who can offer some resistance, although gravity and body weight can also be used.

One method of flexibility training that has emerged from passive stretching is proprioceptive neuromuscular facilitation (PNF). This seeks to decrease the reflex shortening of the muscle being stretched, which occurs when a muscle is stretched to its limit. A simple PNF technique is now outlined.

1 Move slowly to the limit of your range of motion with a partner aiding (passive stretch). Hold for a few seconds.
2 Just before the point of discomfort, isometrically contract the muscle being stretched for between 6 and 10 seconds.
3 After the hold, the muscle will release, having stimulated a Golgi tendon organ (GTO) response which causes further relaxation of the muscle and enabling further stretching of the muscle with the aid of a partner.

PNF stretching relies on the fact that when a muscle contracts isometrically, when stretched, the stretch reflex mechanism of the muscle spindles is switched off. The GTO causes relaxation of the muscle and therefore enables the muscle to stretch further than previously. A second PNF method is known as the CRAC method (Contract–Relax, Antagonist–Contract).

With continued practice of PNF, a new limit of the muscle stretch may occur, but don't forget that pain is the body's signal that damage is occurring, and athletes should not stretch beyond the slight discomfort.

### Static v Dynamic stretching

Static stretching involves the lengthening of the target muscle and holding for a period of 15-20 seconds whilst dynamic stretching involves taking the muscle through its full range of motion such as when performing lunges for example.

Furthermore, stretching and mobility training should only be performed after a thorough warm-up where an increase in body temperature has occurred. This is easily achieved by performing a period of light cardiovascular exercise, centring upon those muscle groups that are to be stretched. In addition, wear warm clothing while

Table 14.5 A critical evaluation of a range of types of training

| Type | Advantages | Disadvantages |
|---|---|---|
| Continuous | • time efficient<br>• trains cardiovascular and muscular endurance<br>• easy to follow routine programme<br>• can be sports-specific, eg, distance running<br>• less chance of injury because lower intensity | • only trains the aerobic system<br>• athletes may need higher intensity<br>• training can be monotonous<br>• may not be specific to some activities, eg, team sports<br>• can lead to overuse injuries |
| Fartlek | • develops aerobic and anaerobic systems<br>• adds variety of pace<br>• train at higher intensity than in continuous training | • may not be sports-specific<br>• higher intensity training may increase risk of injury |
| Interval | • many variables can be manipulated to stress *all* energy systems<br>• adds variety of pace and duration<br>• can be very sports-specific, eg, sprinting, swimming, cycling | • more time is needed<br>• increases risk of injury due to higher intensity |
| Circuit | • trains cardiovascular and muscular endurance as well as strength<br>• time efficient/many performers<br>• can be very sports-specific | • not maximal improvements in endurance and strength<br>• need access to equipment<br>• individuality may be lost |
| Aerobic circuit | • time efficient/many performers<br>• can train at high intensity<br>• can be very sports-specific | • need access to equipment<br>• higher risk of injury<br>• individuality may be lost |

Adapted from Abernethy *The Biophysical Foundations of Human movement*, Human Kinetics, 1997

performing the stretches to maintain body temperature; if possible, perform in a warm environment.

**EXAMINER'S TIP**

For each component of fitness make sure you can give the name of a recognised test, briefly outline the testing protocol and state the method to evaluate the test results.

# Fitness testing

## Measuring strength

Strength can be measured with the use of dynamometers which give an objective measure of the force generated within various muscles or muscle groups. The easiest strength test to administer is using the Handgrip Dynamometer which measures grip strength generated by the muscles in the forearm. Record the maximum reading from three attempts for both left and right hands.

### Advantages

- a simple and objective measure.

### Disadvantages

- the validity of the handgrip test has been questioned, since it only indicates strength of muscles of the forearm.

Another common test of strength is the one repetition maximum test (1RM test). This assesses the maximal force a subject can lift in one repetition using free weights or other gym equipment.

### Advantages

- weight training equipment is easily accessible.

### Disadvantages

- when performing maximal lifts the threat of injury is more apparent and so safety is essential;
- it can be difficult to isolate individual muscles.

**EXAMINER'S TIP**

Make sure you use the correct units of assessment for each fitness test you perform.

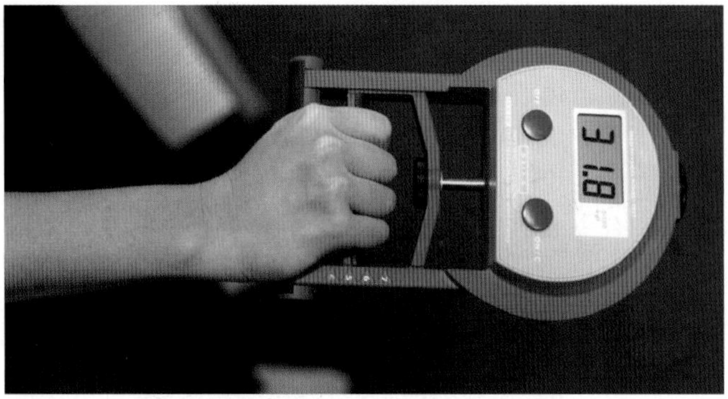

**Figure 14.10** The handgrip dynamometer test

**Table 14.6** Grip strength norms

| Classification | Non-dominant (Kg) | Dominant (Kg) |
|---|---|---|
| **Women** | | |
| Excellent | >37 | >41 |
| Good | 34–36 | 38–40 |
| Average | 22–33 | 25–37 |
| Poor | 18–21 | 22–24 |
| Very poor | <18 | <22 |
| **Men** | | |
| Excellent | >68 | >70 |
| Good | 56–67 | 62–69 |
| Average | 43–55 | 48–61 |
| Poor | 39–42 | 41–47 |
| Very Poor | <39 | <41 |

For persons over 50 yrs of age, reduce scores by 10%.

Source: Data from Corbin, Lindsay and Tolson (1978) Concepts in Physical Education.

## Measuring muscular endurance

A test for muscular endurance will assess the ability of one muscle or a group of muscles to continue working repeatedly. A simple test to measure the endurance of the abdominal muscle group is the NCF Abdominal Conditioning Test.

### Equipment

- NCF abdominal conditioning tape
- tape recorder
- stopwatch
- gym mat.

Follow the instructions given on the tape. Subjects are required to perform as many sit-ups as possible, keeping in time to the bleeps emitted from the tape. Get a partner to count the number of sit-ups completed correctly, and time the duration of the work period. Subjects should withdraw from the test when they can no longer keep in time to the bleeps, or when technique deteriorates noticeably.

### Advantages

- easy to administer with little equipment;
- large groups can participate in the test at once;
- the abdominal muscles can be easily isolated.

### Disadvantages

- correct technique is essential for successful completion of the test.

**Table 14.7** Normative scores for the abdominal curl conditioning test

| Stage | Number of sit-ups | Standard | |
|---|---|---|---|
| | Cumulative | Male | Female |
| 1. | 20 | Poor | Poor |
| 2. | 42 | Poor | Fair |
| 3. | 64 | Fair | Fair |
| 4. | 89 | Fair | Good |
| 5. | 116 | Good | Good |
| 6. | 146 | Good | Very good |
| 7. | 180 | Excellent | Excellent |
| 8. | 217 | Excellent | Excellent |

## Measuring stamina/aerobic capacity

Aerobic capacity can be assessed by measuring a person's $VO_2$max: a simple prediction of $VO_2$max can be made through the **NCF multistage fitness test.** This is a progressive shuttle run test which means that it starts off easily and gets increasingly difficult.

### Equipment

- 20m track (or flat non-slippery surface);
- NCF cassette tape;
- tape player;
- tape measure and marking cones.

Follow the instructions given on the tape. Subjects are required to run the 20m distance as many times as possible, keeping in time to the bleeps emitted from the tape. Each shuttle of 20m should be run so that the individual reaches the end line as the bleep is emitted.

**EXAMINER'S TIP**

Try to critically evaluate each fitness test you perform.

The difficulty increases with each level attained, and speed of running will need to be increased accordingly. Continue to run as long as possible until you can no longer keep up with the bleeps set by the tape. If you fail to complete the 20m shuttle before the bleep is emitted you should withdraw from the test, ensuring that the level and shuttle number attained has been recorded.

### Advantages

- scores can be evaluated by referring to published tables;
- large groups can participate in the test at once;
- limited equipment required.

### Disadvantages

- the test is maximal and to exhaustion and therefore relies, to a certain extent, on subject's levels of motivation;
- the test is only a prediction and not an absolute measure of $VO_2$max;
- the test may favour subjects more used to running. Swimmers for example may not perform as well as they might in a swimming pool.

Another test of aerobic capacity is the PWC170 Test. PWC stands for 'Physical Work Capacity' and this is sub-maximal test. Subjects are required to perform three consecutive workloads on a cycle ergometer, while the heart rate is monitored. Initially a workload is set that increases the subject's heart rate to between 100 and 115 beats per minute. The heart rate is measured each minute until the subject reaches steady state. The test is repeated for a second and third workload which increases the heart rate to between 115 and 130, and 130 and 145 beats per minute respectively. Each steady state heart rate and respective workload is graphed and used to predict a workload that would elicit a heart rate response of 170 beats per minute. The score can then be compared to standard tables and a prediction of $VO_2$max given.

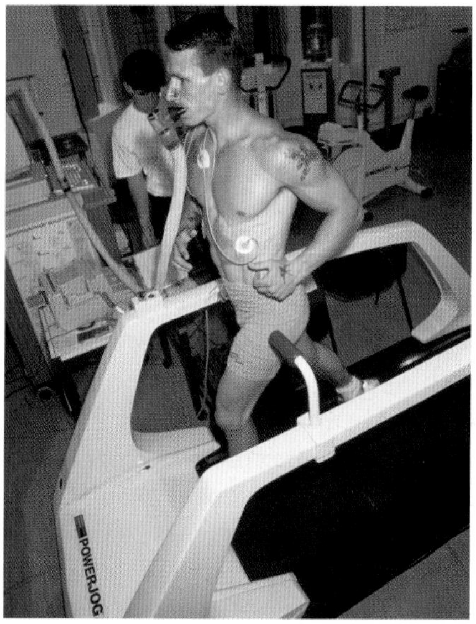


Figure 14.11 Measuring $VO_2$ max through direct gas analysis

### Advantages

- cycle ergometers often contain a pulse monitor, and therefore the heart rate is easily monitored;
- this is a sub-maximal test.

### Disadvantages

- as the test is performed on a bicycle it may favour cyclists;
- this is only a prediction of $VO_2$max based on heart rate scores;
- the test is maximal and therefore relies upon participant's motivation;

Table 14.8 Classification of aerobic fitness ($Vo_2$ max in ml Kg[1] MCN[1])

| Age (yrs) | Low | Fair | Average | Good | High |
|---|---|---|---|---|---|
| **Women** | | | | | |
| 20–29 | <24 | 24–30 | 31–37 | 38–48 | 49+ |
| 30–39 | <20 | 20–27 | 28–33 | 34–44 | 45+ |
| 40–49 | <17 | 17–23 | 24–30 | 31–41 | 42+ |
| 50–59 | <15 | 15–20 | 21–27 | 28–37 | 38+ |
| 60–69 | <13 | 13–17 | 18–23 | 24–34 | 35+ |
| **Men** | | | | | |
| 20–29 | <25 | 25–33 | 34–42 | 43–52 | 53+ |
| 30–39 | <23 | 23–30 | 31–38 | 39–48 | 49+ |
| 40–49 | <20 | 20–26 | 27–35 | 36–44 | 45+ |
| 50–59 | <18 | 18–24 | 25–33 | 34–42 | 43+ |
| 60–69 | <16 | 16–22 | 23–30 | 31–40 | 41+ |

Source: Data from American Heart Association (1972).

- full sit-ups are not recommended to be undertaken on a regular basis, due to excessive strain being placed on the lower back region.

Direct gas analysis is by far the best of $VO_2$max as it gives a truly objective measure of oxygen consumption. Subjects are measured at progressively increasing intensities until exhaustion on a laboratory ergometer (treadmills, cycle or rowing machines tend to be the most popular). A computer analyses the relative concentrations of oxygen inspired and expired and by performing simple calcuation the maximum volume of oxygen consumed by the muscles can be worked out when performing the test to exhaustion.

**EXAMINER'S TIP**

The units of measurement for $VO_2$max is ml/kg/min for weight bearing activities such as running and L/min for non or partial weight bearing activities such as cycling.

## Measuring flexibility

The sit and reach test can be easily administered. It gives an indication of the flexibility of the hamstrings and lower back.

### Equipment

- sit and reach box.

Sit down on the floor with your legs out straight and feet flat against the box. Without bending your knees, bend forwards with arms outstretched and push the cursor as far down as possible and hold for two seconds. Record your score.

### Advantages

- easy to administer;
- there is plenty of data available for comparison.

### Disadvantages

- the test measures flexibility only in the region of the lower back and hamstrings, so it cannot give an overall score of flexibility;
- the extent to which a subject has warmed up may well affect results, when comparing with norms.

Another test of flexibility involves the use of a goniometer, a piece of equipment used to measure the range of motion at a joint. The 'head' of the goniometer is placed at the axis of rotation of a joint while the arms are aligned longitudinally with the bone. A measurement in degrees can be taken which gives a very objective reading that can be used to assess improvement. One small disadvantage of this piece of equipment is that it is not always easy to identify the axis of rotation of a joint.

Table 14.9 Sit and reach test ratings

| Male | Female | Rating |
|---|---|---|
| >35 | >39 | Excellent |
| 31–34 | 33–38 | Good |
| 27–30 | 29–32 | Fair |
| <27 | <29 | Poor |

## Measuring speed

The simplest measure of speed is a 30m sprint. Mark out 30m on a non-slip surface and sprint as hard as you can from a flying start over the course. Record the time taken.

### Advantages

- equipment is readily available.

### Disadvantages

- timing can be affected by error;
- effects of weather and running surface may affect the results;
- this does not test the speed of individual body parts.

Table 14.10 30m sprint test

| Time (secs) | | Rating |
|---|---|---|
| Male | Female | |
| <4.0 | <4.5 | Excellent |
| 4.2–4.0 | 4.6–4.5 | Good |
| 4.4–4.3 | 4.8–4.7 | Average |
| 4.6–4.5 | 5.0–4.9 | Fair |
| >4.6 | >5.0 | Poor |

## Measuring power

Power can be measured with the help of a jump metre.

### Equipment

- jump metre.

Standing with your legs straight on the mat of the jump metre, pull the string taut. In one smooth movement, bend the knees and explode upwards. Record the score. Repeat and take the highest score. If a jump metre is not available, the vertical jump test is similar.

Table 14.11 Vertical jump test scores

| Distance (cm) | | Rating |
|---|---|---|
| Male | Female | |
| >60 | >47 | Excellent |
| 51–59 | 36–46 | Good |
| 41–50 | 29–35 | Average |
| 27–40 | 25–34 | Poor |
| <26 | <24 | Very poor |

## Measuring agility

Agility is most commonly measured via the Illinois agility run.

### Equipment

- tape measure
- cones
- stopwatch.

Set up the course as illustrated in Figure 14.12. Lie flat on the floor at the start position. On the command 'go' get to your feet and complete the course in the quickest time possible. Ask your partner to time you and record your results.

### Advantages

- the testing procedure is simple to administer with little equipment required;

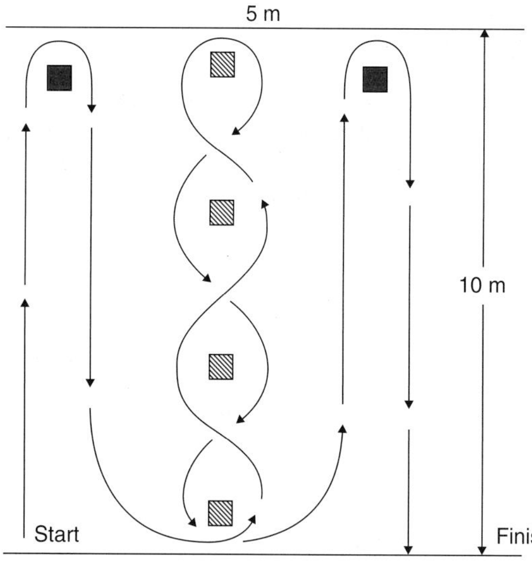


Figure 14.12 The Illinois agility run test

- a widely used test with easily accessible rating.

### Disadvantages

- since agility is influenced by many other factors such as speed, balance and coordination, the validity of test scores could be questioned;
- this test is not sport specific. The agility demanded for different sports is very specific. For example, in some games such as hockey the player must be agile while using a stick to control the ball. Where possible, agility tests should show relevance to the particular activity for which the athlete is being tested.

Table 14.12 Illinois agility run test

| Time (secs) | | Rating |
|---|---|---|
| **Male** | **Female** | |
| <15.2 | <17.0 | Excellent |
| 16.1–15.2 | 17.9–17.0 | Good |
| 18.1–16.2 | 21.7–18.0 | Average |
| 18.3–18.2 | 23.0–21.8 | Fair |
| >18.3 | >23 | Poor |

## Measuring reaction time

Although the most accurate measures of reaction time will involve the use of a computer program, a simple test is the stick drop test.

### Equipment

- a metre ruler.

A partner holds a metre rule in front of you. Place your index finger and thumb either side of the 50cm calibration without making contact with the ruler itself. Without warning the partner should release the ruler, and you must catch it with your finger and thumb as quickly as possible. Record the calibration at the point your index finger lies.

### Advantages

- the testing procedure is simple and easy to administer with little equipment required.

### Disadvantages

- the relevance of a stick drop test to sporting activity is questionable. Where possible the testing environment should reflect the environment of the game or activity for which the athlete is being tested;
- the test only measures visual reaction time, but in many sporting situations, such as the 100m sprint, reaction time to an audio cue is required.

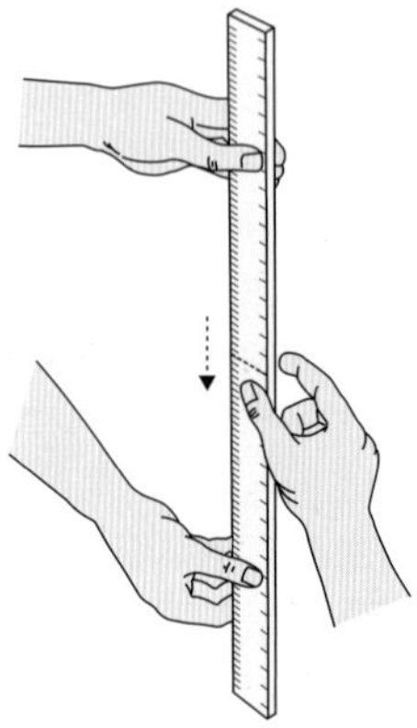

Figure 14.13 The stick-drop test of reaction time

Table 14.13 Stick drop test

| Reaction time | Rating |
|---|---|
| >42.5 | Excellent |
| 37.1–42.5 | Good |
| 29.6–37.0 | Average |
| 22.0–29.5 | Fair |
| <22 | Poor |

# Issues in the testing of fitness

## Why test?

In order to measure fitness levels, a battery of recognised tests has been developed, which are easily administered and evaluated. These tests have been outlined earlier. Through testing it is possible to:

- identify the strengths and weaknesses of the athlete;
- provide baseline data for monitoring performance;
- provide the basis for training prescriptions;
- assess the value of different types of training and help to modify training programmes;
- predict physiological and athletic potential;

- provide comparisons with previous tests and other elite performers in the same group;
- identify overtraining syndrome;
- identify talent;
- enhance motivation;
- form part of the educational process.

## Validity and reliability of testing

Validity of testing is concerned with whether the test measures exactly what it sets out to. We have discussed for example, that the sit and reach test is a valid test for the assessment of flexibility in the lower back and hamstrings but not at the shoulder. The validity of a test is further improved if the test is sport specific, i.e. the testing environment should resemble the activity being tested, so that specific muscle groups and fibres together with specific actions from the sport are actually being assessed.

A further question of validity is, are the tests truly replicating the sporting environment accurately? We would have to question therefore the validity of the multi-stage fitness test to a swimmer. A much more appropriate test of $VO_2$max for a swimmer would be conducted in the confines of a swimming pool. Reliability, meanwhile, questions the accuracy of the test results. If a test is reliable it should be possible to gain the same or similar result during a retest, i.e. the results should be consistent and reproducible. The testers should be experienced and equipment should be standardised. The sequencing of tests is also important since if more than one test is to be conducted during the same session, the order of the tests could affect results.

When any type of testing is undertaken, it must be remembered that many things contribute to performance and fitness tests look solely at one aspect. In order to maximise the reliability of a specific test, it may be necessary to repeat the test several times in order to minimise the possibility of human error. The ability to interpret the results and standardising testing procedures and protocols will also contribute to the validity and reliability of a test.

### EXAMINER'S TIP

For your examination make sure you are able to comment on its validity and reliability.

### Key terms

**Validity:** Does the test measure what it claims to assess.

**Reliability:** The consistency and repeatability of the test results.

## Maximal v sub-maximal tests

One other factor to be considered when testing includes the subjects level of motivation – is the athlete really pushing him/herself in the tests, particularly when some tests require the athlete to work to near exhaustion? Submaximal tests are therefore often favoured over maximal tests since they do not require the athlete to undergo the duress and strain of maximal tests and therefore increase the reliability of the results. Additionally, maximal tests could interfere with an athlete's training programme.

## Other issues in measuring fitness

When planning fitness tests it is important to follow a few simple guidelines:

- ensure (where possible) that the variables tested are relevant to that sport;
- ensure that the tests selected are valid and reliable;
- ensure that the testing administration and protocol are strictly adhered to;
- ensure that all tests are carried out with due regard for health and safety;
- ensure that results are interpreted in the correct manner;
- ethical considerations such as human rights need to be taken into account.

### Activity 6

Complete the measuring tests outlined above and record your results. Make sure you warm up thoroughly and perform the tests under the guidance of your teacher.

### Activity 7

See the table below for each of the components of fitness. Give a recognised test, a brief description of the test and how each test can be evaluated.

| Fitness component | Recognised test | Description of test | Evaluation |
|---|---|---|---|
| aerobic fitness | | | |
| anaerobic fitness | | | |
| strength | | | |
| muscular endurance | | | |
| flexibility | | | |
| body composition | | | |
| speed | | | |

### Activity 8

Discuss the merits of fitness testing. Outline some tests you may use to assess an athlete's level of fitness and how you would evaluate them.

### Activity 9

Compare and contrast the relative merits and limitations of the multi-stage fitness test and direct gas analysis in the assessment of aerobic capacity.

# Section 2 Applied skill acquisition

## Considerations in motor learning

There are many different factors called learning variables which you have to be aware of, understand and consider. These can influence the effectiveness of the learning process.

There are four main categories of learning variables. In considering these categories you may come across unfamiliar terms; these are explained in later sections.

### Category 1: variables associated with the learning process

The basic process that learners go through when faced with a new situation to which they have to respond is usually similar for everyone. The learner will:

- observe the situation;
- interpret the situation;
- make decisions as to what they have to do;
- decide on plans of action;
- generate movement plans;
- take in further information (feedback) which becomes available in some form as the result of actions.

The learner can experience success or difficulty in any part of this process. Understanding it helps a teacher in the task of presenting useful information to the learner.

### Category 2: variables associated with individual differences

A sensitive teacher or coach would try to develop good knowledge of the individual differences listed below, and consider how they might affect the learner, in order to help the learning process:

- ability;
- age (chronological and maturational);
- gender;
- physiological characteristics such as physique (size, shape, weight linked to maturity, fitness);
- psychological characteristics, such as motivation, attitudes, personality;
- previous experience;
- sociological aspects.

### Category 3: variables associated with the task

A teacher would need to consider:

- the complexity of the task (e.g. simple or complex?);
- the organisation of the task (e.g. high or low?);
- the classification of the task (e.g. open/closed? fine/gross?);
- the transfer possibilities.

An understanding of task analysis is essential in order that the appropriate teaching strategies can be developed.

### Category 4: variables associated with the instructional conditions

Teachers and coaches can manipulate the learning environment in a variety of ways:

- through styles of teaching;
- through mode of presentation;
- by using different forms of guidance;
- by choosing appropriate types of practice.

All the above approaches will have a considerable effect on the learning experience of the individual or group.

## Teaching styles

What style of teaching should you use? It is important that you are aware that the style of teaching adopted by a teacher or coach can considerably affect the learning environment. In planning strategies using the various methods already discussed a teacher or coach is trying to create a favourable learning environment. An effective style of teaching aims to present information and thus develop effective learning by promoting achievement, satisfaction and motivation. Teachers invariably adopt different styles in various situations. A teacher's or coach's style of teaching is developed as a result of many factors.

### Mosston and Ashworth's spectrum

In looking at the decisions to be made over what, when and how to teach and learn, Mosston and Ashworth (1986) developed their spectrum of teaching styles.

The more teacher orientated position, 'A', is referred to as the command style. The other end of the spectrum, where the learner makes more of the decisions, is referred to as discovery learning. There are obviously variations between the two extremes. For example:

- practice
- reciprocal
- self-check
- inclusion
- guided discovery
- problem solving
- discovery.

### Command style (A)

This style tends to see the teacher adopting a very authoritarian style! Within this rather behaviouristic approach there is little consideration given to the individual with all learners being treated in generally the same way. This style is thought to inhibit cognitive learning as thinking and questioning are not encouraged by the teacher. The teacher makes all the decisions. The learner is not allowed to develop responsibility for their own learning and is in danger of becoming a clone of the teacher by following movements, decisions and strategies dictated by the teacher. It can also lead to poor self discipline. This type of learning has limitations for developing open skills as these require the performer to be able to adapt and make their own decisions.

In addition, due to the formality of the situation there is little opportunity for any social interaction. This traditional approach helps to establish: pupil control, clear objectives/models for pupils, routine/organisation/rules, and safety procedures. It is useful when working with beginners, large groups and in dangerous and limited time situations. It is often adopted in the early stages of learning as a starting point from which other styles develop.

## Reciprocal style (C/D)

Developing further along the spectrum than command style this approach is based more on cognitive theories. Although what is to be taught or covered is still decided by the teacher, it allows learners to take slightly more responsibility and become more involved in the decision-making process. The sessions are structured in order that the objectives are clearly stated to the learners. The learners work in pairs taking alternative goes at being observer and performer. Although there is regular general and specific input from the teacher, the situation lends itself to more social interaction than the command style. Learners are encouraged to give feedback as a result of their own analysis and evaluation of the performer's progress. In analysing and evaluating their partner's performance the learner is developing a greater understanding of the movement and passing this on to the partner. They should also be able to transfer this to their own performance when their partner has to reciprocate, giving additional individual feedback.

This style of teaching is useful in developing a learner's:

- self image
- confidence
- communication skills (encourage interaction)
- cognitive strategies (encourage decision making).

The teacher does, however, need to monitor the process carefully and interject regularly to ensure that incorrect techniques are not being developed and reinforced. It is also important that the learners are at the appropriate maturational level of development and can cope with both giving and receiving constructive criticism from their peers and not merely focus on the negative or destructive aspects.

## Guided discovery

This much more individualistic style of teaching is rather time consuming as the teacher sets a problem and leads the learner to the correct answer. In guided discovery the teacher generally has to lead the performer by providing the appropriate information, cues and questions in order to get the learner to 'discover' effective and correct movement skills or the understanding associated with certain techniques. The teacher needs to have an in-depth knowledge of each pupil and be constantly evaluating progress. Due to inevitable time limitation, learning will not be uniform for all. Students will progress at different rates, creating extra demands on the teacher.

By using progressive question and answer techniques in association with reinforcement, teachers can guide a learner's greater understanding. In developing greater understanding in one area the performer will also learn to adapt decision making and reasoning processes from previous or correct skills (pro-active positive transfer) to future learning situations. In being more involved with their own learning the learner is thought to gain greater personal satisfaction together with a more positive self image which in turn will help to develop even greater motivation.

## Problem-solving approach

Very often associated with the guided discovery method discussed above, the problem-solving approach encourages students to be creative and develop their individual cognitive and performance processes. According to their different sizes, shapes, abilities and capabilities learners can approach problems set by the teacher individually. For example:

- Find a way to dribble past your opponent in 1v1 situation.
- How could you gain the attack from this situation?

These more 'cognitive perspective' approaches are believed to have long-term benefits as learners are encouraged to think about, understand and adapt performance according to a variety of situations. Variety of practice is therefore important, particularly if the effects of positive transfer are to be developed. The development of schemas relies heavily on variety of practice and are a more cognitive explanation of how learners deal with new or novel situations.

### Activity 10

Consider the styles discussed above and decide which style of teaching would be best suited to the following situations:

- abseiling on an adventure trip
- a group of well-motivated students with sound technical knowledge of the skills
- a teacher coaching four students per session
- a teacher of dance developing creativity.

## Whole or part method of practice

The whole method of learning is when the activity or skill is presented in total and practised as a full/entire skilled movement or activity.

The part method of learning is when the activity or skill is broken down into its various components or sub-routines, and each sub-routine is practised individually.

Additional variations have been developed whereby whole-part, part-whole and progressive part methods have been used. Whether it is more effective to teach a skill as a whole or to break it down into its various sub-routines depends very much on the answers to several questions:

1. Can the skill/task be broken down into its sub-routines without destroying or changing it beyond all recognition?
2. What is the degree of transfer from practising the parts (sub-routines) back to the main skill or activity?
3. What is the performer's level of experience or stage of learning?

### Whole approach

It is argued that if a whole approach is used, a learner is able to develop their kinaesthetic awareness, or total feel for the activity. The learner is usually given a demonstration or explanation of what is required, builds up a cognitive picture and then becomes acquainted through practice with the total skill. They are then able to positively transfer the actions/skills more readily to the competitive or 'real' situation. By being able to link the essential spatial and temporal elements of the skill, the activity/skill quickly becomes meaningful to the performer.

This approach is seen as a more effective use of time when skills have:

- low levels of complexity;
- high levels of organisation;
- rapid movement patterns (discrete or ballistic in nature).

Although it might be possible to break down the parts, they are usually very much interrelated, so breaking the skill down would change it out of all recognition – with possible negative effects on transfer (e.g. hitting a soft ball).

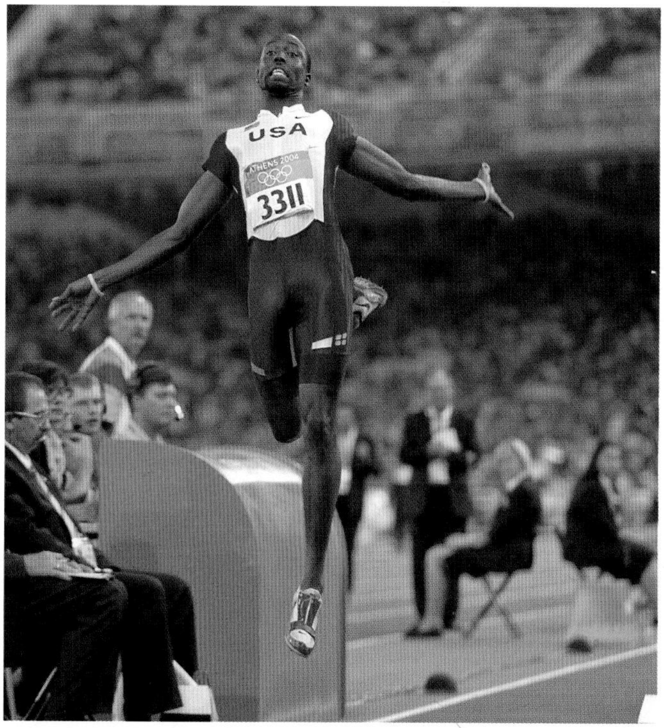


**Figure 14.14** The long jump can be taught using the whole method

When a skill is complex, highly organised and thus difficult to break down, an easier way to present it to beginners often has to be found. Simplifying the activity/task enables the performer to experience the whole activity, but with less information and decision making to deal with. Equipment is very often made lighter or bigger/smaller, and less technical rules are imposed, or fewer physical demands and dangers (e.g. uni-hoc, mini hockey, short tennis).

In general, this method is better with:

- experienced performers;
- motivated performers.

## Part approach

This approach is seen as a more effective use of time when skills have:

- high levels of complexity;
- low levels of organisation;
- elements of danger.

Skills which are very complex, but low in organisation, lend themselves to being practised and learned more effectively by the part method. An additional consideration, again, is how interrelated or independent the various sub-routines are. Just because sub-routines are easily separated does not mean that they have to be practised by themselves. The part method, while allowing teachers and coaches to work on areas of the skill that a beginner finds difficult, also tends to be more time-consuming.

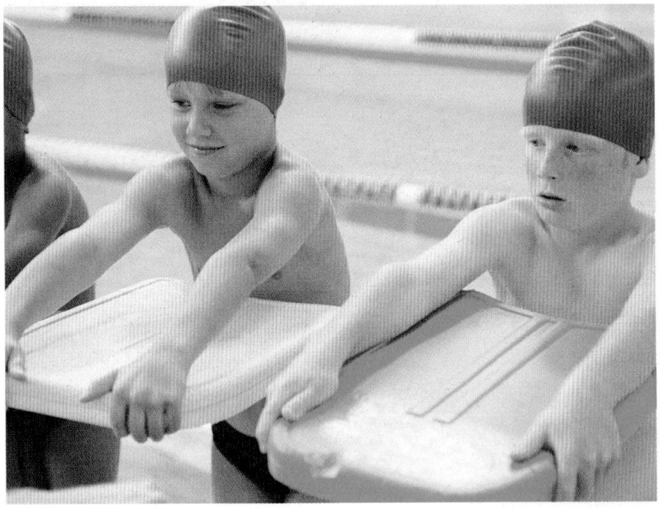

**Figure 14.15** Swimming can be taught using the part method

Activities such as front crawl in swimming, which are not too complex, and low in organisation, lend themselves to being taught by the part method. The arm action, leg action, breathing pattern and body position can all be analysed and taught individually. While each can be (and usually is) practised independently, allowing the performer to experience success and thus gain confidence, it is important that the performer is able to practise synchronising the various sub-routines. If the beginner does not experience the whole stroke, there is a possibility that the kinaesthetic feel for the entire action could be lost (e.g. the timing of breathing in coordination with the arm action). In breaststroke, where the kick, glide and pull have to be synchronised exactly, this is even more important.

When teaching the skills of passing in major team games, such as football, rugby and hockey, it is essential that they are not taught in isolation. The beginner needs time for the interrelated units or sub-routines to be practised together so that they can make the natural link between the parts. Therefore, this becomes a more progressive part method, with combinations of the whole.

In general, this method is better with:

- inexperienced performers;
- performers with a limited attention span or low motivation.

## The progressive part method

The progressive part method involves the learner being taught complex skills by gradually linking one part of the skill to another. This approach is seen as a more effective use of time when skills are:

- complex;
- serial;
- potentially dangerous.

Once one stage has been mastered, the next can be added. For example, a coach trying to develop a gymnast's routine would often follow a progressive part method. All the relatively

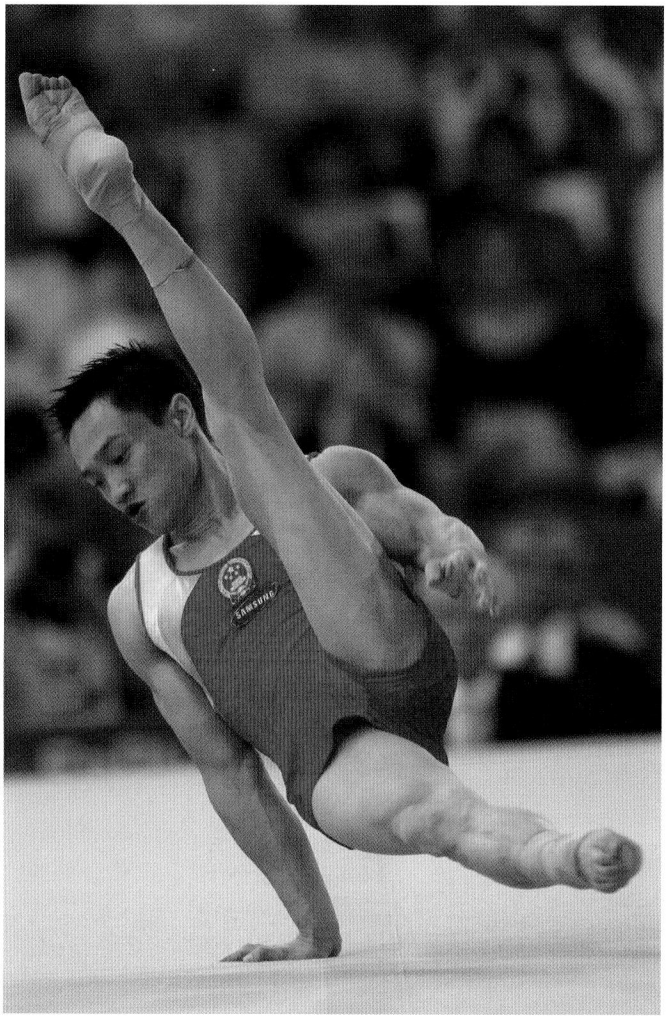

Figure 14.16 A gymnast completing a floor routine would use the progressive part method

complex but independent parts of the routine (e.g. handstand, cartwheel, handspring, somersault) are learned and practised in isolation, then joined together in small units so that the gymnast can experience and learn how to fluently link (sequence) the individual skills. These blocks of skills are then linked again, until the various parts of the action have been built up into the whole routine (the chain is completed).

This method is generally effective when:

- performers are novices (giving them a sense of achievement);
- performers have limited attention span.

However, this method can be time-consuming, and the performer may become overly concerned with mastering one particular sub-routine rather than viewing the skill in its overall context.

## Whole-part-whole method

A variation on the whole and the part methods is the whole-part-whole practice. The teacher/coach introduces the complete skill, highlighting the important elements. The performer then attempts to carry out the skill. As a result of any problems or faults observed, the teacher breaks down the whole skill into various sub-routines to allow the learner to practise appropriate areas of difficulty.

The isolation of the difficult elements may differ for individuals. Once the teacher is satisfied that the problem areas have been mastered, the parts are integrated back into the whole skill. For example, a high jumper may be experiencing a problem with their lay-out position while passing over the bar. The coach would isolate this aspect of the skill and develop a particular practice to rectify the fault; then the athlete would attempt to incorporate the new lay-out position into the full jumping technique.

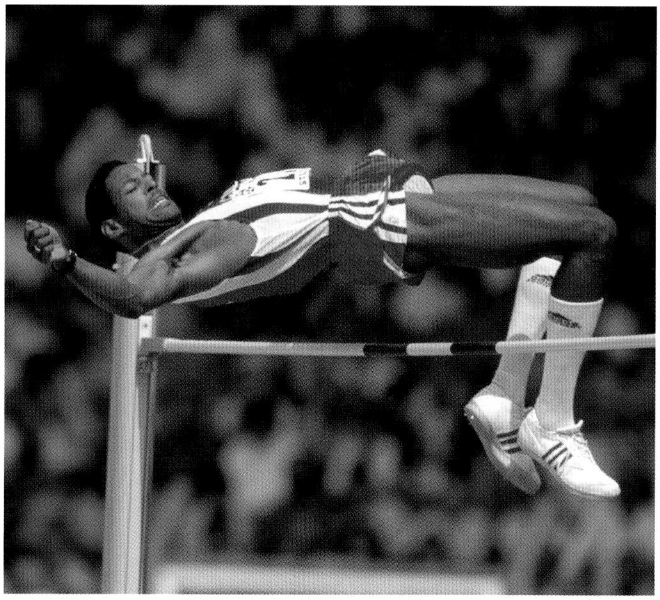

Figure 14.17 A high jumper could use the whole-part-whole method

Teaching by any specific method is not guaranteed to work and the best teachers and coaches are generally flexible, using various combinations of the different methods at different times. Many teachers begin an activity by allowing the beginner to experience the sequencing of the whole movement. They will then analyse strengths and weaknesses, enabling them to develop a part method to deal with any problem areas. Then a progressive part process may develop, where chunks or units of actions are practised together in a simplified task or small-sided game. The performer is then allowed to return to the whole movement. Small problem areas may continue to be practised in isolation in order to refine technique. Complete adherence to one or other method is not advisable or useful.

Table 14.14 Summary of methods of practice

| Whole method | Part method | Progressive part method |
|---|---|---|
| • Low level of complexity/simple task<br>• High levels of organisation<br>• Interrelated sub-routines<br>• Discrete skills<br>• Short duration/rapid ballistic<br>• Lacks meaning in parts<br>• Allows coordination of important spatial/temporal components | • High levels of complexity<br>• Low levels of organisation<br>• Independent sub-routines<br>• Serial tasks<br>• Slow tasks<br>• Lengthy or long duration<br>• Dangerous skills | • Complex task<br>• Helps 'chaining' of complex skills learned independently<br>• Allows for attention demands to be limited<br>• Allows for coordination of spatial/temporal components to be experienced<br>• Helps with transfer to whole |
| | **Performer is:** | |
| • experienced;<br>• someone with high levels of attention;<br>• in the later stages of learning;<br>• older;<br>• highly motivated;<br>• using distributed practice. | • a beginner;<br>• someone with a limited attention span;<br>• in the early stages of learning;<br>• having problems with a specific aspect of skill;<br>• someone with limited motivation;<br>• using massed practice. | |

Table 14.15 Advantages of whole and part method

| Whole method | Part method |
| --- | --- |
| • Wastes no time in assembling parts<br>• Useful for quick, discrete skills where a single complete action is required<br>• Better for time-synchronised tasks if the learner can cope with the level of the skill (e.g. swimming stroke)<br>• The learner can appreciate the end product<br>• The movement retains a feeling of flow/kinaesthetic sense<br>• The movement can be more easily understood (the relationship between sub-routines)<br>• The learner can develop their own schema/motor programme through trial-and-error learning<br>• Transfer from practice to real situations is likely to be positive<br>• Good for low organisational tasks which can be broken down easily | • Allows serial tasks to be broken down and learned in components (e.g. gymnastic movement)<br>• Reduces the demand on the learner when attempting complex skills<br>• Allows confidence and understanding to grow quickly or be built up gradually with more complex skills<br>• Helps to provide motivation to continue if progress can be seen to be being made<br>• Especially important with skills which can be seen as potentially dangerous (e.g. some gymnastic skills)<br>• Can reduce fatigue in physically demanding skills<br>• Allows the teacher to focus on a particular element and remedy any specific problems<br>• Provides stages of success<br>• Good for low organisational tasks which can be broken down easily |

Table 14.16 Disadvantages of whole and part method

| Whole method | Part method |
| --- | --- |
| • Ineffective with complex tasks<br>• Not appropriate in tasks with an element of danger<br>• Not always appropriate if group/performer has very little experience<br>• May overwhelm a performer and produce little success at first<br>• Could lead to learner losing confidence | • Transfer from part to whole may be ineffective<br>• Highly organised skills are difficult to break down into parts<br>• Loss of awareness of end product<br>• Loss of continuity/feel of flow<br>• Loss of kinaesthetic sense<br>• Can have a demotivating effect when not doing full movement<br>• Can be time-consuming |

## Activity 10

Explain how you would introduce the skills listed below to a group of inexperienced performers, justifying your answer in each case:

- sprint start;
- basketball lay-up;
- triple jump;
- netball shot;
- tennis serve;
- cricket bowling action;
- rugby tackle;
- hockey dribble;
- gymnastic vault;
- volleyball spike/smash;
- golf shot;
- paddling a kayak.

## Massed and distributed practice

The two main forms of practice available for a coach to use are massed and distributed practice. Massed practice is seen as being almost continuous practice, with very little or no rest between attempts or blocks of trials. Distributed practice is seen as practice with relatively long breaks or rest periods between each attempt or block of attempts.

Other forms of practice may include fixed and variable practice. Fixed practice involves repetition of the same skill to reinforce learning. Varied practice involves using a mixture of massed and distributed practice within one session.

### Practice and the learner

Although massed practice may appear to save time, as the teacher or coach does not have to spend time after long breaks either reintroducing the performer to the task or reducing psychological barriers (fear, anxiety, etc.), this may be a short-sighted policy, as distributed practice is seen as being a more effective learning process for beginners.

The length of the practice session should be appropriate to both the physical and the psychological maturity of the performer.

Beginners are more likely to be affected by a lack of attention/concentration and a lack of appropriate physical and mental fitness to sustain long periods of practice. Therefore, distributed practice with beginners, allowing for greater variation of practice, is seen as essential, as it not only allows for better schema developments and transfer possibilities, but also helps to maintain motivation. Random practice is seen as being more effective than ordered practice.

There is evidence to support the view that for the more experienced/older/fitter performer, massed practice is more effective.

### Practice and the task

Practice sessions need to be long enough to allow for improvement, but should not be overly long. While the effect of fatigue in relatively dangerous situations (gymnastics, outdoor pursuits) could be potentially serious, the effect of fatigue in massed practice can hinder performance in the short term, although not necessarily skill learning in the long term.

Alternatively, distributed practice for discrete skills may lead to a lack of motivation due to the performer's frustration at having delays between attempts. Group or team activities can be practised for longer than individual tasks as players can have rests in between, thus lessening fatigue and frustration. At the same time, groups should not be so big that rest intervals or waiting times become too long, thus demotivating learners or allowing opportunities for ill discipline.

The use of rest periods or intervals needs to be considered within distributed practice. They can be used for the following:

- to reduce fatigue;
- to reduce short-term inhibition;
- to give feedback (knowledge of results and knowledge of performance);
- to offer an alternative activity/novelty game

**Table 14.17** Practice and the individual

| Massed practice | Distributed practice |
|---|---|
| Better when the individual is:<br>• experienced;<br>• older;<br>• fitter;<br>• more motivated. | Better when the individual is:<br>• a beginner;<br>• less experienced;<br>• limited in their preparation (physical/mental);<br>• less motivated. |

**Table 14.18** Practice and the task

| Massed practice | Distributed practice |
|---|---|
| Better when the task is:<br>• discrete, brief in nature (e.g. hitting a golf ball, shooting baskets);<br>• simple. | Better when the task is:<br>• continuous, requiring repetition of gross skills (e.g. swimming, cycling, running);<br>• complex – precision-orientated;<br>• dangerous. |

(must ensure no negative transfer);
- to develop positive transfer;
- to re-motivate;
- to offer mental practice/rehearsal.

## Variability of practice

Repetition of skills is important in order to reinforce the correct movement patterns, particularly at the early stages of learning and with closed skill, that is, fixed practice. However, the nature of the skill should be considered. If a skill is classified as an 'open' skill, it would be better to vary the practice to allow a performer to become familiar with the demands of executing the skill in a situation similar to that found in the competitive situation.

The characteristics of varied practice are:

- skills practised in new/different situations;
- useful for open skills;
- helps development of schema (see page 173);
- helps performer successfully adapt to meet the demands of the situation;
- practice should be similar to 'real game' situation;
- practice should be meaningful;
- variety of massed and distributed practice;
- will maintain motivation.

## Mental practice

The definition of mental practice is the mental or cognitive rehearsal of a skill without actual physical movement.

When looking at the various types of practice available for a teacher or coach to use, mental practice or mental rehearsal is an area frequently overlooked. We have mentioned already that time intervals or rest periods between practice can be used for mental practice.

Mental practice or rehearsal is seen as being very beneficial. In the early stages of learning (cognitive phase), mental rehearsal is seen as the learner going through a skill/task and building up a mental picture of the expected performance in their mind (a cognitive process). This may involve an individual deciding how to hold a hockey stick, or a gymnast going over the sequence of a simple vault in their mind. More advanced performers can use mental practice to rehearse possible alternative strategies or complex actions/sequences, almost pre-programming their effector systems and possibly helping with response preparation, reactions and anticipation.

Mental practice can be a powerful tool in the preparation of the highly skilled performer. Top-class skiers regularly use it to rehearse turns, and to imagine the approach to gates and certain aspects of the terrain. A traditionally held view is that through mental practice a performer can slightly stimulate (below optimum threshold) the neuromuscular systems involved in activities and thus simulate (practise) the movement. In addition, mental practice is used regularly by more experienced performers in learning to control their emotional states. Optimum levels of arousal can be reached and maintained for effective performance. Wider developments in sports psychology have meant that mental rehearsal is being used increasingly to reduce anxiety and increase confidence, by getting the performer to focus their attention on winning or performing successfully.

Although mental rehearsal is now seen as an important element of practice (better than no practice at all), it is not seen as a type of practice to be used exclusively; rather, it is much more effective when used in conjunction with physical practice. In being aware of the effects of mental rehearsal, it is important that teachers and coaches not only plan their sessions to allow time for it to take place, but also that they teach performers how and when to use it effectively. Practice is essential.

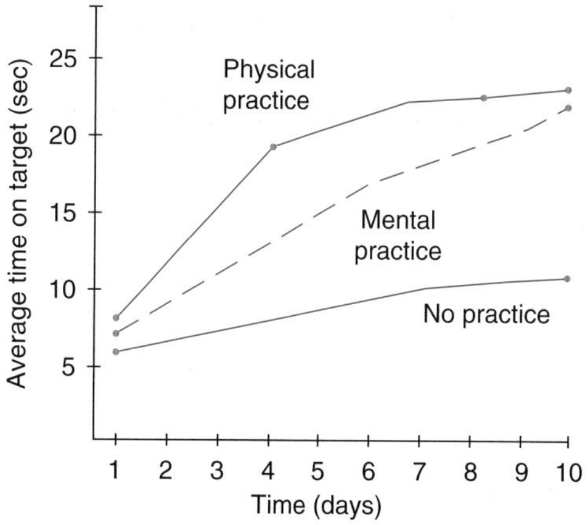


**Figure 14.18** Comparison of effects of mental and physical practice on performance
*Source*: Rawlings, Rawlings, Chen Yilk, The facilitating effects of mental rehearsal in the acquisition of rotary pursuit tracking, (1972) *Psychonomic Science* 26, p.71 (Copyright 1972 Psychonomic Society Inc.)

## The use of mental practice prior to performance

The performer needs to be advised to seek out a relatively quiet situation where they can focus mentally on the task. This will probably involve moving away from the competitive or performance situation. The learner or performer needs to:

- go somewhere quiet;
- focus on the task;
- build a clear picture in their mind;
- sequence the action;
- imagine success;
- avoid images of failure;
- practise regularly.

## The use of mental practice between practices

When used in between physical practices, a performer must try to recreate the kinaesthetic feeling and mental image they have successfully experienced (remembering what was good). Equally, when a performer makes a mistake, stopping for a few seconds to reason why and then rehearsing a good performance may have a positive effect on future performances.

This mental review of good and bad practice both during and after performance will help in building up positive images. A golfer, when playing a practice swing, is very often mentally rehearsing the positive feel for the shot, imaging distance, angles of trajectory and power needed.

As we have seen already, more experienced performers can plan ahead, particularly in situations requiring adaptation or performance strategies. Questions (Where…? What if…?) can be considered, determined and possibly prepared for.

Mental practice within the associative phase (motor stage) can enhance learning, helping the performer to develop the decision-making and conceptual aspects of the skill which link to the specific skills being taught. Tactics and strategies can be combined with the sequencing of skills. It can also be used to help create effective random practice.

## The uses of mental rehearsal in sport and physical education

- Mental rehearsal creates a mental picture of what needs to be done.
- Mental rehearsal evaluates possible movements and can mentally experience their outcomes (success/failure).
- Mental rehearsal can build self-confidence.
- Mental rehearsal can be used as a mechanism to focus attention.
- It has been proved that mental rehearsal produces small muscle contractions, simulating actual practice.
- Performers at the cognitive stage of learning can use mental rehearsal to focus on the basics of a skill/the whole movement.
- Performers in the autonomous stage of learning can use mental rehearsal to control arousal level/to focus attention on immediate goals.
- Mental rehearsal provides mental warm-up.
- Mental rehearsal must be practised regularly in order to be useful.
- Mental rehearsal can be used before competition and in rest periods during competition.
- Mental rehearsal must be as realistic as possible in order to be effective.

### Activity 7

1 Divide your group into three and record the results of ten attempts of a skill. The skill can be anything you wish (e.g. a basketball shot, volleyball serve or badminton serve).

2 After the first round of trials, each group experiences a different form of practice:

- Group A – mentally practise the skill for five minutes.
- Group B – no practice, actually perform a totally different skill.
- Group C –practise the same skill for five minutes.

3 Complete a second set of trials and record the results.

4 Calculate the average scores for each set of trials, sketch a graph and discuss the results.

- The performer can use all the senses during mental rehearsal.
- The performer can use mental rehearsal to envisage images of both success and failure.
- Mental rehearsal may be used in rest periods during distributed practice.
- Mental rehearsal may prevent physical wear and tear (e.g. triple jumpers use mental rehearsal to save joints).

## Types of guidance

Guidance is information given to the learner or performer in order to help them limit possible mistakes (incorrect movement), thus ensuring that the correct movement patterns are carried out more effectively. While guidance or instructions are usually given to beginners when skills/tasks are unfamiliar, they are obviously used continually in various forms at all stages of learning and performance. The form of guidance given, together with its effectiveness, will depend on several aspects:

- the learner – motivation; stage of performer's experience/learning linked to their information-processing capacities and capabilities;
- the type/nature of the skill/task;
- the environment or situation.

In order to facilitate the acquisition of skill, formal guidance can take several forms:

- visual guidance;
- verbal guidance;
- manual/mechanical guidance.

If formal guidance does not serve to improve performance through the long-term retention of learning, it cannot be called guidance.

### Visual guidance

Visual guidance can be given in many different ways in order to facilitate the acquisition of skill:

- demonstration;
- video/film/TV/slow motion;
- posters/charts;
- OHTs/slides;
- modify the display (see page 152 for a discussion of the term 'display').

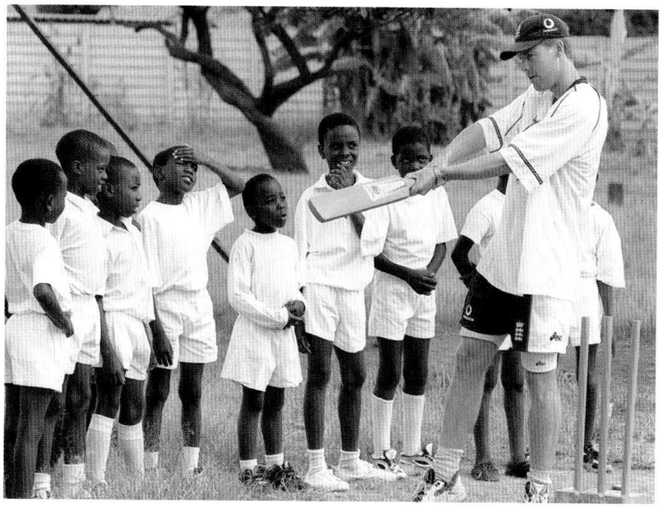

Figure 14.19 A coach uses visual guidance to demonstrate the correct technique

Visual modes of receiving information are valuable at all levels. Visual guidance is particularly useful, however, in the early stages of learning (cognitive phase), by helping the learner establish an overall image or framework of what has to be performed. This modelling of the elements involved in skills is an important aspect of skill acquisition. However, when presenting the learner, particularly a beginner, with effective visual guidance, it is important that:

- accurate/correct models of demonstration are used/given (usually provided by the teacher or an experienced performer);
- attention be directed in order that major aspects of the skill are emphasised/reinforced;
- demonstrations/models should not be too complex/lengthy (usually whole skill first, then parts later);
- demonstrations/models should be realistic/appropriate;
- demonstrations must be repeated or referred back to;
- demonstrations can be combined with verbal guidance to highlight key points.

There are considerable differences of opinion with regard to the long-term effectiveness of visual guidance. However, for the more advanced performer, specific and complex information can generally be provided more readily by modern technology, such as biomechanical analysis and use of slow-motion playback.

Visual guidance can also be used to highlight certain cues or signals from the display, helping the selective attention processes of beginners in particular. Equipment in infant and junior schools is often brighter or bigger in order to help performers to 'see things' more clearly.

The teacher or coach can modify the display more specifically by highlighting areas of the court or pitch that shots should be played into, or by making target areas bigger. Routes of movement can also be indicated by markers, and so on.

It is very difficult in reality to consider visual guidance in isolation, as verbal explanations very often have to accompany the demonstration or visual image being presented.

The disadvantages of visual guidance are:

- It depends on the coach's ability to demonstrate the correct model.
- It can be dependent on expensive equipment (e.g. video).
- It has limited value to a group coaching situation regarding technical skill.
- It is dependent on the coach's ability to demonstrate problems within skills.
- Some skills may be too complex to be absorbed by the performer.
- Some information presented may not be relevant.
- Some images may be rather static and therefore give little information about movement patterns.
- It is difficult to use in isolation.

## Verbal guidance

Verbal guidance is another common form of guidance used by teachers or coaches and can be either very general or specific. A teacher may talk through a particular strategy in team games in order to give players a general picture of what is required before putting the move into practice. It is also useful to draw learners' attention to specific details of certain movements by giving verbal cues alongside visual demonstrations. Verbal labelling of specific aspects of a movement by a performer is also thought to facilitate learning. A teacher may help the beginner to link their visual image of the task to certain verbal cues.

It is important that the learner does not become too heavily reliant on verbal guidance, thus reducing their ability to pay attention to aspects of performance, process information, make decisions and solve their own problems when guidance is removed.

Verbal guidance is thought to be more effective with advanced performers who, because of increased experience and wider movement vocabulary, are able to translate verbal comments into visual images more readily. Teachers or coaches may therefore find it difficult to simply describe certain movements to beginners, particularly those involving more complex or highly organised skills. They will have to use a combination of both visual and verbal guidance in order to help the learner internalise the information being presented.

When considering verbal guidance, it is important that it is:

- clear/precise;
- relatively short;
- appropriate to the level of the learner;
- not overused.

It is important not to overload the learner. Only a few important points will be taken in during the first few attempts. Children have very short attention spans.

It is also useful to note that when giving verbal guidance:

- everybody should be able to hear;
- the pitch and tone of the voice should be varied in order to encourage or emphasise a specific point;
- a sense of humour is a great help.

The disadvantages of verbal guidance are:

- It is heavily dependent on the coach's ability to express the necessary information.
- It is less effective in early stages of learning.
- It is dependent on the performer's ability to relate the verbal instruction/information to the skill under practice.
- Some techniques are very difficult to describe verbally.
- Verbal guidance can become boring if it is too lengthy.

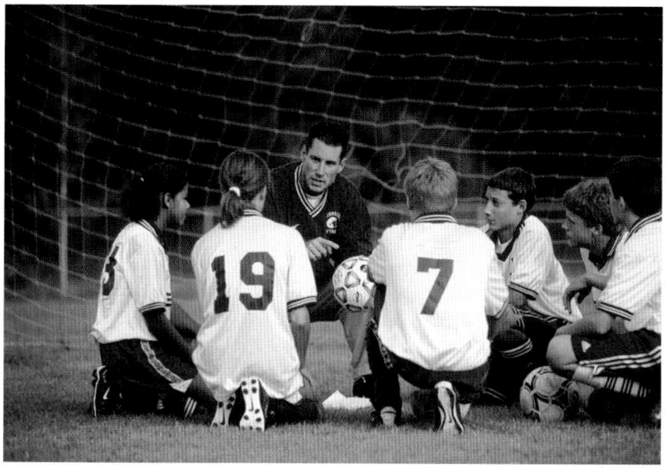

Figure 14.20 A coach uses verbal guidance to highlight key points to the players

## Activity 11

In discussion with a partner, try to think of ways you could verbally guide a performer through learning a gymnast vault.

## Manual/mechanical guidance

This type of guidance involves trying to reduce errors by physically moving (forced response) or restricting/supporting (physical restriction) a performer's movements in some way.

This form of guidance is particularly useful in potentially dangerous situations. A performer may need physical or mechanical support initially in order to develop the confidence necessary to perform the skill themselves. In trampolining, a coach may stand on the bed and physically support the beginner through the stages of a somersault. With more advanced performers they may also use a twisting belt, which would provide mechanical guidance by physically restricting the performer.

A performer may have their response or actions forced by the coach or teacher. In taking a performer through an action in tennis, for example, a coach will very often take hold of the racket arm, forcing the performer to carry out certain movements (e.g. a backswing for early preparation).

While in the initial stages of learning, mechanical aids, such as floats and armbands in swimming, serve a very useful purpose, although it is important that beginners do not become over-reliant on them and lose their own kinaesthetic feel for the movement. There has to come a time, in gymnastics for example, where support for the learner is gradually removed, once the teacher or coach is sure that the performer is safe.

By producing his or her own movements, and not relying on what has been termed a 'crutch', the performer can develop their own kinaesthetic awareness. This will help in reducing possible bad habits (negative transfer), and by increasing confidence should serve to develop the performer's motivation and self-confidence.

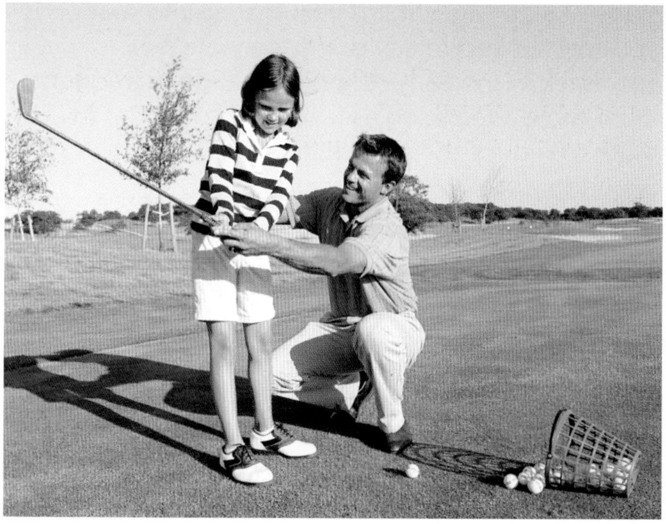
Figure 14.21 A coach uses manual guidance to develop the correct movement patterns

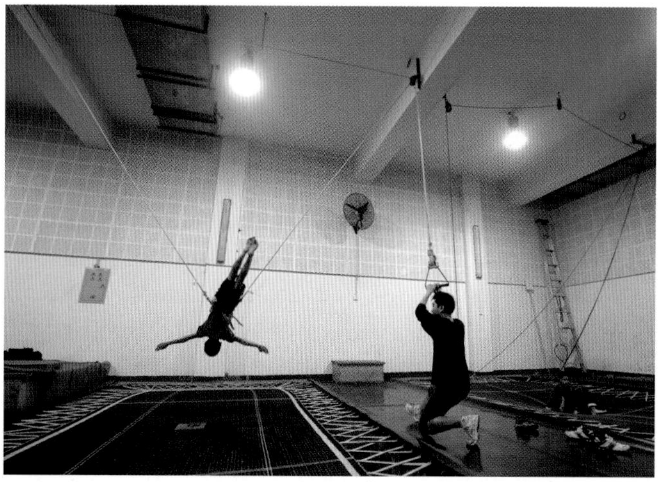
Figure 14.22 Mechanical guidance is often used when trampolining

The disadvantages of mechanical guidance are:

- It has limited use in group situations.
- It has limited use in fast/complex movements.
- The 'feel' of the movement is not experienced by the performer to the same extent as in an unaided movement.
- Kinaesthetic awareness can be limited.
- The performer may become reliant on the support.
- There is the risk of implied sexual misconduct.

### Activity 12

For each of the activities listed below suggest the most appropriate forms of guidance to use when introducing the skills to a group of novices. Justify your answers.

- High jump
- Back crawl in swimming
- Set plays in rugby
- Badminton smash shot
- Gymnast vault

### Exam-style question

1 Guidance is often used to enhance learning and understanding.

(a) Explain the term 'guidance'.

(b) Outline the advantages and disadvantage of using manual or mechanical guidance.

(5 marks)

## Types, structure and presentation of practice

In deciding how to use their allotted time to benefit learners effectively, teachers and coaches need to make decisions about when to practise, and how often. In making these decisions they should consider whether practice is better all at once (massed) or whether breaks are required (distributed). Within these blocks of practice they will consider whether the skill should be taught as a whole, in parts or in various combinations. The question of mental practice or rehearsal also needs to be considered.

As ever, there are no easy answers. Decisions regarding questions as to which type of practice will be most effective depend on the:

- individual's stage of learning;
- nature of the task;
- nature of the specific situation;
- time available.

## Feedback

The final part in the information-processing system is feedback. Strictly speaking, feedback is a processing term referring to information coming from within the system rather than information coming from the outside world. Feedback is now generally referred to as all the information that a performer receives as a result of movement (response-produced information).

When a performer is taking part in physical activity in any shape or form, information is fed back into the system either during or after the activity. This information can come from within the performer or from outside, relating to the adequacy of their performance. This information is used both to detect and to correct errors during the activity, and to make changes/improvements the next time the skill is performed.

As well as changing performance, feedback can also be used to reinforce learning and motivate the performer. It has been argued that without feedback, learning cannot occur. The nature of the feedback will alter depending on the performer's stage of learning, but it is vital that all information is accurate, limited to key points and relevant. Feedback in the early stages should be as frequent as possible – reducing as learning progresses in order to reduce the possibility of feedback dependency.

### Types and forms of feedback

#### Intrinsic feedback

Sometimes referred to as internal or inherent feedback, this type of feedback comes from within the performer, from the proprioceptors. When a golfer swings at the ball, they can feel the timing of the arm movement and the hip movement in conjunction with a perfect strike of the ball. This is also referred to as kinaesthetic feedback. The golfer can see and hear their club swing, and hear the ball being struck, which serves to back up the proprioceptive information being received. All this information is inherent to the task. The more experienced and skilled a performer is, the more effective their use of intrinsic feedback will be.

### Extrinsic feedback

Sometimes referred to as external or augmented feedback, this type of feedback is information received from outside the performer about the performance; it is given and used to enhance (augment) the already received intrinsic feedback. This is the type of feedback that is generally referred to in teaching and coaching. It can also be received from teammates within the context of a game. Performers usually receive this type of feedback by visual or auditory means; for instance, the coach or teacher tells or shows a performer the reasons why success or failure has occurred.

This form of information is used extensively during the cognitive and associative phases of learning. A less experienced performer will rely on guidance from the coach or teacher concerning their performance, as they have not yet developed their kinaesthetic awareness fully and cannot interpret feedback arising intrinsically.

Extrinsic feedback can be made up of a mixture of several different types and forms:

- continuous;
- terminal;
- knowledge of results;
- knowledge of performance;
- positive;
- negative.

### Continuous feedback

Continuous feedback is also referred to as ongoing or concurrent feedback. This type of feedback is received *during* the activity. It is most frequently received as proprioceptive or kinaesthetic information. For example, a tennis player can 'feel' the ball hitting the 'sweet spot' of the racket when playing strokes during a rally.

### Terminal feedback

This is feedback received by the performer *after* they have completed the skill or task. It can be given either immediately after the relevant performance or some time later.

### Positive feedback

This type of feedback occurs when the performance of a task is correct or successful. It can be used to reinforce learning, increasing the probability of the successful performance being repeated (e.g. a coach or teacher praising a beginner when they catch a ball successfully).

Although positive feedback is thought to facilitate perceived competence and help intrinsic motivation, it is important that a teacher does not give too much positive feedback, thereby distorting a performer's perceptions of their own performance and possibly affecting motivation.

### Negative feedback

This type of feedback occurs when the performance of a task is incorrect. For example, a basketball player will receive negative feedback in various forms if they miss a set shot: they see the ball has missed, friends comment, they realise they did not put enough power behind the ball, and the teacher or coach may indicate faults and suggest correction. All this should help to ensure that further shots are more successful.

## Knowledge of results and knowledge of performance

Knowledge of results (KR) is an essential feature of skill learning. Without knowing what the results of our actions have been, we will be unable to modify them in order to produce the precise movements needed for the correct performance of a skill. One of the more important roles of a teacher or coach is to provide this type of information. Knowledge of results is usually given verbally (e.g. a netball coach saying 'You missed the net by 10cm', or an athletics coach shouting out lap times during training). This type of feedback about goal or task achievement is thought to be very useful in the early phases of learning, when beginners like to have some measure of their successful performance. An eight-year-old child will see his/her performance in terms of 'I scored a goal today', or 'Our team won all the games', not in terms of the quality of his/her own performance.

Once KR has been given it is usually necessary for the teacher or coach to provide information about why or how the result came about. A hockey coach, when trying to develop passing, may give KR in the form of: 'Your pass was far too wide'. They may support this by adding: 'The reason it was so wide was because your left shoulder was not pointing towards your partner, your feet were not in the right position and your stick did not follow through in the direction the ball was meant to go'. This gives the performer additional (augmented) extrinsic information in order to help them know not only the result of the action (KR), but also why the result was incorrect and how to correct the performance. This type of feedback about the actual movement pattern is more like the feedback given by a teacher and is known as knowledge of performance (KP). Although most of the traditional research has been carried out with regard to KR, due to its ease of measurement, there has been a definite shift in emphasis towards researching KP, particularly with the increased availability of more modern computer and video technology allowing greater mechanical analysis of technique and performance.

Knowledge of results, as used in most psychology or coaching texts, is referred to as: 'Information provided to an individual after the completion of a response that is related to either the outcome of the response or the performance characteristics that produced that outcome' (R. Magill).

### Activity 13

For each of the activities listed below, give an example of knowledge of results and knowledge of performance which may be given to the performer:

- high jump;
- basketball shot;
- swimming race.

## The use of feedback

Feedback can be used to help with:

- the correction of errors;
- reinforcement;
- motivation.

There are numerous studies to support the importance of feedback (KR) in the learning process. In referring back to Fitts and Posner's phases of learning, feedback can be used to move the performer through the three phases of the learning process.

Once in the autonomous phase, the performer should be less reliant on KR and should, through their knowledge and understanding of the activity, be able to detect their own errors and, in conjunction with kinaesthetic feedback, be able to make corrections to their own performance.

Although skills can be learned without feedback, it is generally accepted that feedback makes the learning process more efficient by improving error correction and developing better performance. If we relate this to the discussion of motor programmes in the next chapter, we will see that if a performer receives additional information, the quality of his or her generalised patterns of movement (schemas which help initiate and control movement) can be effectively enhanced, particularly in the early phases of learning. When considering the use of feedback, the teacher or coach needs to be aware of the following:

- current skill levels of the performer (phase of learning);
- nature of the skill (complexity/organisation/classification) and its transferability.

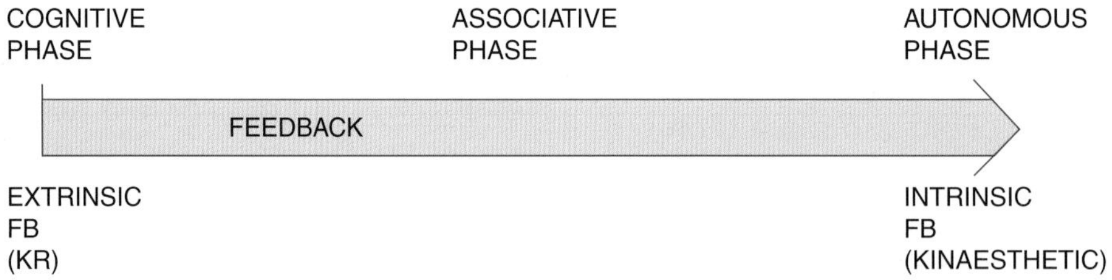


**Figure 14.23** How feedback moves the performer through the three-stage model

In relation to the above points, the coach or teacher has to decide on the following aspects of feedback:

- general or specific;
- amount (too much or too little);
- how to present it (visual/verbal);
- frequency (e.g. after every attempt, or a summary after several attempts – the performer must not become dependent on extrinsic feedback);
- time available for practice/processing.

Although the quantity, distribution and whether it is positive or negative are important considerations, the most crucial aspects of feedback are quality and appropriateness.

KR must not provide too much information, otherwise the performer will not know what to pay attention to or how to use the feedback to help future attempts. Attention must be directed to specific or major errors, particularly with beginners. If major errors are left out, this could lead to the performer assuming them to be correct, strengthening the incorrect S–R bond and making it much more difficult to deal with later. As well as telling the beginner what the problem is, a teacher or coach must provide information on how the performer can correct the error.

Feedback (KR) must be meaningful and relevant to the phase of learning. Beginners might need general information, whereas experienced performers may require more specific details. Sometimes, however, beginners may need much more specific information. For example, a more experienced badminton player would understand the comment, 'Your positioning is not right', and would probably rectify the fault immediately. The same statement made to a beginner would be of little value, as they would need much more specific feedback with regard to the position of the feet, the angle of the upper body, the preparation of the racket prior to the shot, and so on, in order for them to make the necessary corrections. It is important that the feedback given is useful to the performer and not just repetition of what is already obvious to them. Such repetition is called redundant feedback.

Researchers have found that time intervals after the performance have a bearing on how KR should be used. A teacher needs to be aware that once KR has been given, the performer has to have time to assimilate the information and put the KR into action. However, too long a delay could allow the performer to forget what has happened or to lose understanding of the relevance of the KR being given.

Feedback can also be used as reinforcement. Reinforcement, as you already know, increases the probability of certain behaviour being repeated. Using feedback to strengthen the bond between stimulus and response is useful.

Positive feedback has a great role to play in reinforcement. Both KR and KP can be useful in motivating a performer, maintaining interest and effort (direction and intensity). Seeing performance improve (e.g. an athlete improves their personal best or a tennis player increases the accuracy and percentage of successful first serves) should ensure that performers keep practising. It is very helpful if this is carried out in a formal way, with statistical evidence being logged by the teacher or coach. This information can be used both for the evaluation of current performance (error detection) and for future target setting. In this way, feedback can be used as an incentive. Using feedback in conjunction with goal setting has been recognised as being very effective in the learning process.

# Index